SOCIAL PSYCHOLOGY AND HEALTH

SECOND EDITION

Wolfgang Stroebe

OPEN UNIVERSITY PRESS
Buckingham · Philadelphia

To the members of ISAG
(Interdisziplinäre Sozialwissenschaftliche Arbeitsgemeinschaft)
In celebration of our twenty-fifth anniversary

Open University Press
Celtic Court
22 Ballmoor
Buckingham
MK18 1XW

email: enquiries@openup.co.uk
world wide web: www.openup.co.uk

and
325 Chestnut Street
Philadelphia, PA 19106, USA

First edition published 1995
Reprinted 1996, 1997

First published in this second edition 2000

A catalogue record of this book is available from the British Library

ISBN 0 335 19921 6 (pb)   0 335 19922 4 (hb)

Library of Congress Cataloging-in-Publication Data
Stroebe, Wolfgang.
    Social psychology and health / Wolfgang Stroebe. — 2nd ed.
      p. cm. — (Mapping social psychology series)
    Includes bibliographical references and index.
    ISBN 0–335–19922–4 (hb) — ISBN 0–335–19921–6 (pb)
    1. Clinical health psychology.   2. Social psychology.   I. Title.   II. Series.
  R726.7.S78   2000
    155.9—dc21   99–059166

Typeset by Graphicraft Limited, Hong Kong
Printed in Great Britain by Biddles Limited, Guildford and Kings Lynn

CONTENTS

PREFACE

This second edition of *Social Psychology and Health* has been so extensively revised that it essentially represents a new book. The parts which remained from the old text have been updated, a great deal of new text has been added, and more than a third of the original references have been replaced. The book has also grown in size, and the coverage of many of the areas has become more comprehensive. All this has been achieved within the old structure. Thus, hardly any of the chapter and section headings have been changed, and the number of chapters has remained the same.

There are at least three reasons for this extensive revision. First, health psychology is a very active research area. In the five years since the writing of the first edition, a substantial body of research has been published, much of which has had bearings on the topics covered in this book. Second, the book uses a great deal of epidemiological literature and this type of descriptive evidence does not age well. Third, and perhaps most importantly, my own perspective on health psychology has changed during the last few years. Since my move to the Netherlands, my research interests in health psychology have broadened from bereavement to obesity and sexual risk behaviour. This change in interest is reflected in some of the chapters of this book. What has not changed, however, is the basic scientific perspective which shaped this book. Although health psychology is an interdisciplinary endeavour, involving various areas ranging from medicine to sociology and economics, and although these perspectives are well represented, the main focus of this book is on social psychology and health. Therefore much of the health research presented here has been guided by social psychological theories and conducted by social psychologists.

It is important to recognize, however, that the relationship between social and health psychology has not been a one-way street. Health behaviour is notoriously difficult to change, and in conducting and evaluating interventions in the health area, shortcomings of social psychological theories and methods can sometimes be detected which would not show up in the more easy-going environment of the experimental laboratory. For example, the importance of skill training in behaviour change, which emerged from studies of health behaviour change, has been much less apparent in laboratory studies of attitude and behaviour change. There have also been theoretical developments in health psychology, such as the stage theories of change, which have not yet been assimilated by academic social psychology.

In the process of revising this book I lost my co-author. Such an event would normally not need to be discussed, but since this particular co-author also (still) happens to be my wife, a comment appears in order to prevent misunderstandings. I was (and still am) very sorry Margaret Stroebe decided to drop out of this project, but I had to accept her reasons, namely that other responsibilities would not have allowed her enough time to work on this book. She still managed to be a great support in this endeavour and to help me by providing a sounding board for many of my new ideas.

In writing a book one draws on the help and support of many others. The book profited from the insightful comments of a number of colleagues. I would like to express my gratitude to Klaus Jonas, Rinie Geenen and Mary Gergen for helpful suggestions. I am particularly indebted to Tony Manstead for his patience and for making many valuable suggestions for the improvement of the manuscript. I would also like to thank the members of the Interdisciplinary Workgroup on Social Sciences (ISAG). The biannual meetings of this workgroup during the last two decades, and particularly the many discussions with my friend Bruno Frey, have made me appreciate the value of economic analyses of social behaviour. Finally, I would like to thank Lizet Hoekert, Corrie Brouwer and Ilse Smulders for their assistance in the final preparation of this manuscript.

Wolfgang Stroebe

ONE

CHANGING CONCEPTIONS OF HEALTH AND ILLNESS

Good health and a long life are important aims of most persons, but surely no more than a moment's reflection is necessary to convince anyone that they are not the only aim. The economic approach implies that there is an 'optimal' expected length of life, where the value in utility of an additional year is less than the utility foregone by using time and other resources to obtain that year. Therefore, a person may be a heavy smoker or so committed to work as to omit all exercise, not necessarily because he is ignorant of the consequences or 'incapable' of using the information he possesses, but because the lifespan forfeited is not worth the cost to him of quitting smoking or working less intensively . . . According to the economic approach therefore, most (if not all!) deaths are to some extent 'suicides' in the sense that they could have been postponed if more resources had been invested in prolonging life.

(Becker 1976: 10/11)

THE MODERN INCREASE IN LIFE EXPECTANCY

Progress in medical science has been impressive. Knowledge of the body and understanding of disease processes have advanced continuously from the seventeenth century onwards, slowly at first but very rapidly since the turn of the century. This increase in medical knowledge appears to have resulted in a substantial increase in life expectancy. Today the life expectancy at birth in the USA is 76 years as compared to 48 years in 1900 (Matarazzo 1984; Fielding 1999). This increase in longevity has been due mainly to the virtual elimination of those infectious diseases as causes of death that were common at the turn of the twentieth century (e.g. pneumonia and influenza, tuberculosis, diphtheria, scarlet fever, measles, typhoid, poliomyelitis). Thus, whereas approximately 40 per cent of all deaths were accounted for by 11 major infections in 1900, only 6 per cent of all deaths were due to these infectious diseases in 1973 (McKinlay and McKinlay 1981). Between 1981 and 1995 the death rate due to infections has somewhat increased, mainly due to the appearance of a new infectious disease (AIDS). However, in 1996 the trend changed and infectious

Table 1.1 The 10 leading causes of death in the USA: 1900, 1940, 1980 and 1992

Cause of death	1900	1940	1980	1992
Pneumonia and influenza	1	5	6	6
Tuberculosis (all forms)	2	7		
Diarrhoea, enteritis and ulceration of the intestines	3			
Diseases of the heart	4	1	1	1
Intracranial lesions of vascular origin	5	3		
Nephritis (all forms)	6	4		
All accidents[a]	7	6	4	5
Cancer[b]	8	2	2	2
Senility	9			
Diphtheria	10			
Diabetes mellitus		8	7	7
Motor vehicle accidents		9		
Premature birth		10		
Cerebrovascular diseases			3	3
Chronic, obstructive pulmonary diseases			5	4
Cirrhosis of the liver			8	
Atherosclerosis			9	
Suicide			10	9
Human immunodeficiency virus infection				8
Homicide and legal intervention				10

[a] This category excludes motor vehicle accidents in the years 1900 and 1940, but includes them in 1980 and 1992.
[b] This category encompasses cancer and other malignant tumours in the years 1900 and 1940 and changes to malignant neoplasms of all types in 1980 and 1992.
Source: Matarazzo (1984); Gardner *et al.* (1996).

disease deaths began to decrease again (Armstrong *et al.* 1999). Table 1.1 illustrates the significant shift in causes of death during this century.

Because this decline in mortality from infectious diseases happened during a time when medical understanding of the causes of these diseases had vastly improved and when vaccines and other chemotherapeutic medical interventions became widely available, it was only plausible to attribute these changes to the efficacy of the new medical measures. However, this may be yet another example of a premature causal inference from purely correlational evidence. After all, during the same period conditions of life also improved considerably in most industrialized societies. For large populations in Western societies the problem of malnutrition has been solved and some of the most serious threats to health associated with water and food have been removed by improvements in water supply and sewage disposal.

As can be seen from Figure 1.1, which depicts the fall in standardized death rates for the nine common infectious diseases in relation to specific medical measures for the United States, the decline in mortality from these major infectious diseases took place *before* effective medical interventions became available. McKinlay and McKinlay (1981: 26) concluded

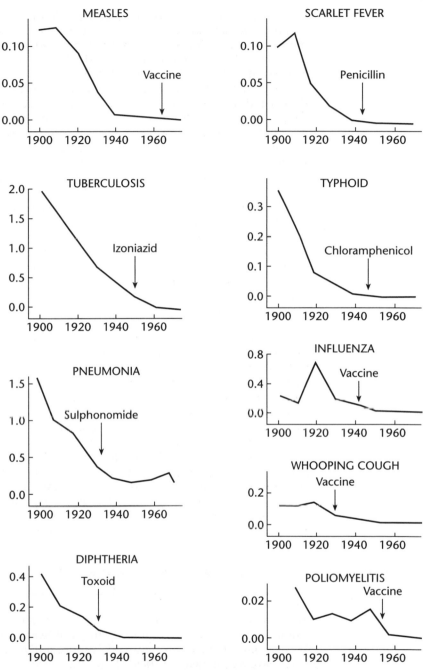

Figure 1.1 The fall in the standardized death rate (per 1000 population) for nine common infectious diseases in relation to specific medical measures in the USA, 1900–1973.
Source: McKinlay and McKinlay (1981).

from their analysis that 'medical measures (both chemotherapeutic and prophylactic) appear to have contributed little to the overall decline in mortality in the United States since about 1900 . . .' Similar conclusions were reached by McKeown (1979) on the basis of an even more extensive analysis of data from England and Wales.

Today, the major killers are cardiovascular diseases (i.e. heart disease and stroke) and cancers, with cardiovascular diseases accounting for approximately 40 per cent of deaths in the USA and other industrialized countries. Although deaths from cardiovascular diseases increased during the first half of this century, this pattern has recently begun to reverse. During the last four decades there has been a small but steady decline in deaths due to heart disease and stroke in the United States and several other industrialized countries.

Improvements in medical treatment undoubtedly contributed to this decline, but the significant changes in lifestyle that occurred in the USA during that period were also responsible. Goldman and Cook (1984) even estimated that more than half of the decline in heart disease mortality observed in the United States between 1968 and 1976 was related to changes in lifestyle, specifically the reduction in serum cholesterol levels and cigarette smoking.

Unfortunately, despite advances in medical treatment and significant lifestyle changes, deaths due to cancer have increased since 1950 in most industrialized countries. This increase in cancer deaths has been almost entirely due to an increase in lung cancer which is responsible for more than one fourth of all cancer deaths (Breslow 1990). However, from 1990 to 1995, there occurred for the first time a continuous and sustainable decline in cancer mortality in the USA of 0.6 per cent per year (Cole and Rodu 1996). Nearly 40 per cent of this decline in cancer mortality resulted from a reduction in lung carcinoma mortality and is thus likely to be due to the reduction of smoking in the USA.

To summarize, the significant increases in life expectancy at birth that occurred during this century in most industrialized countries seem to have been only partially attributable to improvements in medical treatment. There is substantial evidence that a purely medical explanation of these changes would be too narrow. Changes in sanitation, nutrition and lifestyles contributed importantly to the increase in life expectancy.

FROM DISEASE CONTROL TO HEALTH PROMOTION

The marked decline in mortality due to infectious disease during the twentieth century, the vast improvement in average living conditions in Western industrialized nations, and the substantial increase in life expectancy have stimulated considerable rethinking of the meaning of health and of the role of public health institutions in helping to achieve and maintain it (Breslow 1990). Whereas health had long been considered merely the absence of disease and infirmity, people were beginning to emphasize the positive aspects of health. This change in perspective was reflected in the influential definition of health offered by the World Health

Organization (WHO) in its constitution in 1948. The WHO defined health as 'a complete state of physical, mental, and social well-being and not merely the absence of disease or infirmity' (WHO 1948).

There are two important aspects of this definition of health which set it apart from previous definitions (Kaplan *et al.* 1993). First, by emphasizing well-being as the criterion for health, the WHO definition abandoned the traditional perspective of defining health in negative terms, namely as the absence of disease. Second, by recognizing that health status can vary in terms of a number of different dimensions, namely physical, mental and social well-being, the definition abandons the exclusive emphasis on physical health which had been typical of previous definitions (Kaplan *et al.* 1993).

The growing interest in interventions designed to prevent diseases and promote health has led to a change in focus of public health strategies towards a greater emphasis on health promotion. *Health promotion* can be defined as 'any planned combination of educational, political, regulatory, and organizational supports for action and conditions of living conducive to the health of individuals, groups, or communities' (Green and Kreuter 1991: 432). Countries adopting health promotion as policy have directed it mainly at primary prevention through modification of lifestyle factors that account for the largest numbers of deaths (e.g. smoking, drinking too much alcohol, eating a fatty diet, leading a sedentary life). Health promotion influences lifestyles through two strategies, namely health education and fiscal and legislative measures. Education involves the transfer of knowledge or skills. Thus, health education provides individuals, groups or communities with the knowledge about the health consequences of certain lifestyles and with the skills to enable them to change their behaviour. Fiscal or legislative measures such as increasing the tax on tobacco or introducing seat belt legislation are used to change the incentive structure that influences behaviour. Health promotion also uses strategies not directed at lifestyles such as environmental changes aimed at the protection of health (e.g. car safety measures).

THE IMPACT OF BEHAVIOUR ON HEALTH

No single set of data can better illustrate the fact that our health is influenced by the way we live than the findings of a prospective study on the health impact of some rather innocuous health behaviours, conducted by Belloc, Breslow and their colleagues (Belloc and Breslow 1972; Belloc 1973; Breslow and Enstrom 1980). In 1965, these researchers asked a representative probability sample of 6928 residents of Alameda county, California, whether they engaged in the following seven health practices:

1 Sleeping seven to eight hours daily.
2 Eating breakfast almost every day.
3 Never or rarely eating between meals.
4 Currently being at or near prescribed height-adjusted weight.
5 Never smoking cigarettes.

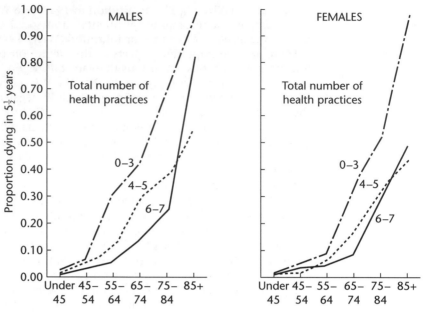

Figure 1.2 Age-specific mortality rates by number of health practices followed by sub-groups of males and females.
Source: Matarazzo (1984).

6 Moderate or no use of alcohol.
7 Regular physical activity.

At the time, it was found that good practices were associated with positive health status, those who followed all the good practices being in better health than those who failed to do so, and that this association was independent of age, sex, and economic status (Belloc and Breslow 1972).

Most striking, however, were the findings of two follow-up studies in which the relationship between these health habits and longevity was explored by using death records. At the first follow-up, conducted five and a half years later, 371 deaths had occurred (Belloc 1973). When the initial health practices in 1965 were then related to subsequent mortality, it was found that the more of these 'good' health practices a person engaged in, the greater was the probability that he or she would survive the next five and a half years (Figure 1.2).

These findings were confirmed at a second follow-up investigation conducted nine and a half years after the initial inquiry, when again an inverse relationship between health practices and age-adjusted mortality rates was observed (Breslow and Enstrom 1980). Men who followed all seven health practices had a mortality rate which was only 28 per cent of that of men who followed zero to three practices; the comparable rate for women who followed all practices was 43 per cent of those who followed zero to three practices. The authors also observed a great stability in the health practices of each individual over the nine and a half year period.

The importance of lifestyle factors for the maintenance of health and the prevention of disease has also been underlined by the outcome of analyses of the contribution of lifestyle factors and other modifiable causes to mortality in the United States. These analyses were conducted by the Centers for Disease Control and Prevention in 1977 and 1990 (McGinnis and Foege 1993). Since both analyses reached very similar conclusions I will focus here on the more recent report. McGinnis and Foege (1993) estimated that of the approximately 2,148,000 deaths that occurred in the USA in the year 1990, nearly 50 per cent were due to modifiable factors. More than 40 per cent of these premature deaths were due to lifestyle factors (e.g. smoking, eating the wrong diet, leading a sedentary lifestyle, consuming too much alcohol, sexual risk behaviour, illicit drug use, fire-arms, motor vehicle accidents). In addition, the list of modifiable causes includes preventable infectious diseases (excluding HIV) and death caused by toxic agents which may pose a threat to human health as occupational hazards, environmental pollutants, contaminants of food and water supplies, and components of commercial products. All these deaths were premature in the sense that they could have been postponed if individuals or communities had taken appropriate measures.

Findings such as these tend to support Becker's (1976) argument that most deaths are to some extent self-inflicted, at least in the sense that they could have been postponed, if people had engaged in 'good' health practices, like the ones listed by Belloc and Breslow (1972). The important implication of this research at the individual level is that the responsibility for health does not rest with the medical profession alone. Each of us can have a major impact on the state of our own health. At the institutional level, it emphasizes the potential effectiveness of preventive measures (i.e. primary prevention) that focus on persuading people to adopt good health habits and to change bad ones.

It is important to note, however, that life extension (i.e. mere quantity) is only one of the goals of health promotion, and perhaps not even the most important one. We may have to accept that there is a natural limit to our life expectancy and that we are unlikely to reach the age of 140, even with the healthiest of lifestyles (Fries et al. 1989). People are persuaded to engage in a healthy lifestyle not merely to lengthen their lives but to help them to stay fit longer and lead an active life right into old age without being plagued by pain, infirmity and chronic disease. Thus, the second major goal of health promotion is to increase the quality of life and to contribute to healthy and successful aging by delaying the onset of chronic disease and extending the active lifespan (Fries et al. 1989). Low probability of disease and disease-related disability and high cognitive and physical functional capacity in old age are two of the main components of successful aging (Rowe and Kahn 1987).

THE IMPACT OF STRESS ON HEALTH

The concept of stress has become so much part of common culture that it does not seem to need definition. Reports about health consequences of everyday stress pervade the advice columns of popular magazines and even teenagers complain to their teachers that they are under undue stress due to an overload of homework. It has become public knowledge that stress, like smoking or drinking too much alcohol, can have adverse effects on physical as well as mental health.

As we will see later in this book (Chapter 6), there is now ample evidence that psychosocial stress results in health impairment. To some extent these health consequences of stressful life events are mediated by the same changes in endocrine, immune and autonomic nervous systems which have been described in the classic work of Selye (e.g. 1976) on the health impact of physical stressors. However, the experience of psychosocial stress also causes negative changes in health behaviour that contribute to the stress–illness relationship (e.g. irregular eating habits, increases in smoking, alcohol consumption and drug intake). Furthermore, stress is often also a result of people's lifestyles. Thus, research on stress and illness is closely related to our interest in the impact of behaviour on health.

FROM THE BIOMEDICAL TO THE BIOPSYCHOSOCIAL MODEL OF DISEASE

That lifestyle factors and psychosocial stress are important determinants of health and illness is difficult to accept within the framework of the biomedical model which has been the dominant model of disease for several centuries (Engel 1977). This model assumes that for every disease, there exists a primary biological cause that is objectively identifiable. Let us exemplify this approach with statements from a typical medical textbook, *Introduction to Human Disease* by Kent and Hart (1987). According to these authors, diseases are caused 'by injury which may be either external or internal in origin . . . External causes of disease are divided into physical, chemical and microbiologic . . . Internal causes of disease fall into three large categories' (vascular, immunologic, metabolic) (1987: 8/9). Because behavioural factors are not considered to be potential causes of disease, they are also not assessed as part of the process of diagnosis.

By focusing only on biological causes of illness, the biomedical model disregards the fact that most illnesses are the result of an interaction of social, psychological and biological events. The logical inference of such a biological conception of disease is that physicians need not be concerned with psychosocial issues because they lie outside their responsibility and authority. Thus, the model has little to offer in guiding the kind of preventive efforts that are needed to reduce the incidence of chronic diseases by changing health beliefs, attitudes and behaviour.

In recognition of these problems, Engel (1977) proposed an expansion of the biomedical model which incorporates psychosocial factors into the scientific equation. The biopsychosocial model maintains that biological, psychological and social factors are all important determinants of health and illness. According to this approach, medical diagnosis should always consider the interaction of biological, psychological and social factors to assess health and make recommendations for treatment.

SOCIAL PSYCHOLOGY AND HEALTH

The growing recognition that lifestyle factors and psychosocial stress contribute substantially to morbidity and mortality from cardiovascular disease, cancer, injuries and other leading causes of death in industrialized countries was one of the factors which in the late 1970s led to the development of health psychology as a field which integrates psychological knowledge relevant to the maintenance of health, the prevention of illness, and the adjustment to illness. Social psychology had, and still has, an important contribution to make to this endeavour, because lifestyles are likely to be determined by health attitudes and health beliefs. Effective prevention has to achieve large-scale changes in lifestyles and such attempts will have to rely on mass communication and thus on an application of social psychological techniques of attitude and behaviour change.

The interest of social psychologists in the study of stress developed more recently, because many of the most stressful life events (e.g. divorce, bereavement) involve a break-up of social relationships. Furthermore, the health impact of stressful events not only depends on the nature of these events but also on the individuals' ability to cope with the crisis and on the extent to which they receive social support from relatives, friends and other members of their social network. Finally, the impact of stress on health, although to some extent due to the brain's influence on physiological processes such as the body's immune response, is also mediated by the adoption of health-impairing habits as coping strategies (e.g. smoking, alcohol abuse). Thus, social factors are not only important in determining the stressful nature of many life events but also as moderators of the stress–health relationship.

Social psychologists have also made important contributions to another major area of health psychology, namely the analysis and improvement of health care systems. This involved issues such as physician–patient relationships, compliance with medical procedures, anxiety as related to medical procedures, and burnout in the helping profession. Although a review of social psychological research on these topics would have been highly relevant in the context of this book, these issues will not be discussed. Due to space limitations any attempt at completely reviewing social psychological contributions to health psychology would have had to remain at a superficial level. Instead I decided to present an in-depth analysis of a number of selected areas. The reader interested in social psychological contributions to research into the health care system should consult the excellent overviews provided by Sarafino (1998) or Taylor (1995).

PLAN OF THE BOOK

Why do people engage in health-impairing behaviour and how can they be influenced? To answer these questions we need to know and understand the factors and processes that determine the adoption and maintenance of health behaviour. Chapter 2 presents the major models of behaviour from health and social psychology, to provide the theoretical framework for the analysis of determinants of health behaviour. Chapter 3 discusses strategies of behaviour change. I will argue that there are basically two stages to the modification of health behaviour. Individuals first have to be informed of the health hazards of certain behaviour patterns and persuaded to change. This can be achieved by public health interventions such as health education. Because people are often unable to change health-impairing behaviour patterns, a second stage may be necessary in which people are taught how to change and how to maintain this change. This second stage often relies on clinical intervention. Chapter 3 gives an overview of both the public health approach and the methods of clinical intervention.

The next two chapters discuss the major behavioural risk factors that have been linked to health. Chapter 4 focuses on health-impairing behaviour such as smoking, alcohol abuse and overeating. These behaviours are addictive in the sense that, once excessive, they are difficult to control. The self-protective behaviour covered in Chapter 5, such as eating a healthy diet, safeguarding oneself against accidents, and avoiding behaviour associated with the risk of AIDS, are in general somewhat more under the volitional control of the individual. In my discussion of these risk factors I will review both the empirical evidence that links these behaviours to negative health consequences and the effectiveness of public health strategies and/or therapy in modifying these behaviour patterns.

Chapter 6 discusses causes and consequences of psychosocial stress. Stressful life events have been related to an increased risk of morbidity and this health impact is not only mediated by the brain's influence on physiological processes but also by the adoption of health-impairing behaviours as coping strategies.

Chapter 7 reviews extra- and intrapersonal coping resources which help the individual cope with stressful life events. The review of extrapersonal coping resources focuses mainly on the beneficial effects of social support in moderating the impact of stress and discusses psychological mechanisms assumed to mediate this relationship. The discussion of intrapersonal coping resources focuses on hardiness and dispositional optimism. Finally, hostility is discussed as a personality moderator of stress which does not reflect a coping resource.

In summarizing my overall perspective in Chapter 8, I reflect on the contribution of social psychologists to the public health effort through theories and strategies that help to change health-impairing behaviour patterns and reduce psychological stress. I argue for integrated public health interventions that use both persuasion and changes in incentives to influence health-impairing behaviour patterns. I also argue for a reorientation of research on behavioural risk factors which focuses less on extension of total life expectancy and more on the extension of *active* life expectancy and successful aging. It is the reduction of morbidity rather than mortality which makes healthier lifestyles worthwhile for both the individual and society as a whole.

FURTHER READING

McKeown, T. (1979) *The Role of Medicine.* Oxford: Blackwell. A fascinating analysis of the role of medical measures in the decline of mortality over the last few centuries in England and Wales. It shows that for practically all infectious disease the major reduction in mortality occurred long before medical measures to cure them had been discovered.

TWO

DETERMINANTS OF HEALTH BEHAVIOUR: A SOCIAL PSYCHOLOGICAL ANALYSIS

Why do people engage in health-impairing behaviour such as smoking or eating a poor diet even if they know that they are damaging their health? Is there any way to influence them to change their behaviour? This chapter will present theoretical models from health and social psychology which will provide the framework for the analysis of the determinants of health behaviour. Knowledge of these determinants will help us to evaluate the potential effectiveness of the strategies of behaviour change that will be discussed in the following chapters.

There are several psychological models of behaviour which have either been developed specifically to predict health behaviour (health belief model, protection motivation theory) or as general models of behaviour (theory of reasoned action, theory of planned behaviour). Because these models all agree on the central role of attitudes and beliefs as determinants of behaviour, the first part of the chapter will define these central concepts and discuss the relationship between them. The second and third parts will then describe and compare these models of behaviour. Finally, the implications of these models for the planning of interventions aimed at changing health behaviour change will be discussed.

HEALTH BEHAVIOUR

The concept

Before discussing the determinants of behaviour, it might be useful briefly to consider the behaviour of interest in this book, namely health behaviour. Health behaviour is typically defined as behaviour undertaken by individuals to enhance or maintain their health (e.g. Kasl and Cobb 1970).

Sometimes researchers further distinguish between health-impairing behaviours like smoking or drinking too much alcohol which have a negative effect on health, and health-protective or health-enhancing behaviour such as exercising or eating a healthy diet which may have a positive effect (Matarazzo 1984). However, even health-enhancing behaviours are frequently undertaken for reasons unrelated to health. For example, many people who diet deprive themselves to improve their looks rather than their health. One could therefore also argue for an alternative definition in terms of objective rather than intended consequences of health behaviour. Thus, researchers have often used the term health behaviour to refer to behaviours which have been shown to have beneficial health consequences for those who practise them.

The structure of health behaviour

It would seem plausible that at least those health behaviours which are undertaken by individuals with the intention to maintain or improve their health should be strongly correlated. Thus, people who exercise should also use seat belts, drink no alcohol and be non-smokers. However, with few exceptions (i.e. people who smoke also over-indulge in alcohol), this does not seem to be the case. Research on the relationship between different health behaviours has found only weak correlations (e.g. Belloc and Breslow 1972; Mechanic 1979).

One reason for this apparent lack of a relationship could be the existence of different dimensions of health behaviour. As a result, different health behaviours would only show a strong relationship if they reflected the same dimension, but would be weakly related or even unrelated if they were situated on different dimensions. A factor analytic study of ratings of health behaviours conducted by Vickers et al. (1990) supported the assumption that the domain of health behaviour is structured in terms of different dimensions. These authors identified the following four dimensions of health behaviour:

- *wellness behaviour*, reflected by items such as 'I exercise to stay healthy', 'I limit my intake of food like coffee, sugar, fats, etc.' or 'I take vitamins';
- *accident control*, consisting of items such as 'I have a first aid kit at home', 'I fix broken things around my home immediately';
- *traffic risk taking*, reflected by items such as 'I don't speed while driving', or 'I carefully obey traffic rules to avoid accidents'; and
- *substance risk taking*, which consists of items such as 'I do not drink' or 'I do not smoke or use smokeless tobacco'.

Since smoking and drinking too much alcohol both fall into the category of substance risk taking, the finding that smoking and drinking are highly related, but much less related to other health behaviours, would be consistent with this dimensional framework.

ATTITUDES, BELIEFS AND BEHAVIOUR

The concept of attitude

Attitudes are considered major determinants of behaviour. Attitudes can be defined as the tendency to evaluate a particular attitude object with some degree of favour or disfavour (Eagly and Chaiken 1993). An attitude object can be any discriminable aspect of the physical or social environment, such as things (cars, drugs), people (doctors, the British), behaviour (jogging, drinking alcohol), and even abstract ideas (religion, health). Social psychologists typically divide the evaluative tendencies that reflect an attitude into three classes, namely cognitive reactions, affective reactions, and behaviour (e.g. Rosenberg and Hovland 1960; Ajzen 1988; Eagly and Chaiken 1993).

Evaluative responses of the cognitive type are thoughts or beliefs about the attitude object. For example, a positive attitude towards jogging might be associated with the belief that jogging helps one to keep one's weight down, increases fitness and decreases high blood pressure. Such beliefs are perceived linkages between the attitude object (i.e. jogging) and various attributes which are positively or negatively valued (i.e. low weight, high blood pressure).

Evaluative responses of the affective type consist of the emotions that people experience in relation to the attitude object. These evaluative responses also range from extremely positive to extremely negative reactions. For example, these days, many people feel revulsion when they think of fatty foods, whereas the idea of physical exercise makes them feel good.

Evaluative responses of the behavioural type consist of overt actions towards the attitude object which imply positive or negative evaluations. Thus, people go jogging regularly regardless of weather conditions and ask smokers not to smoke in their presence. Behavioural responses can also consist of behavioural intentions. Thus, the experience of not fitting into ski pants that were too big last season might lead one to form the intention to start a weight loss programme next week. Similarly, a smoker who learns that a colleague and fellow smoker has just died from lung cancer might form the intention to stop smoking.

The relationship between attitude and beliefs

It is plausible that people's attitudes should be related to their beliefs about these attitude objects. And indeed, most cognitive theories of attitude share the assumption that the attitude towards some attitude object is a function of the attributes associated with that object and the evaluation of these attributes (e.g. Rosenberg 1960; Fishbein and Ajzen 1975; Sutton 1987). Similarly, a person's attitude towards performing a given behaviour is assumed to be a function of the perceived consequences of that behaviour and the evaluation of these consequences.

The relationship between attitudes and beliefs can be expressed quantitatively in terms of expectancy–value models (e.g. Fishbein and Ajzen 1975).

According to these models an individual's attitude towards some action depends on the subjective values or utilities attached to the possible outcomes of that action, each weighted by the subjective probabilities that the action will lead to these outcomes. Thus, one's attitude towards personally engaging in physical exercise would be a function of the *perceived likelihood* (i.e. expectancy) with which physical exercise is associated with certain consequences such as low blood pressure or physical fitness and the *evaluation* (i.e. value, subjective utility) of these consequences. The way such beliefs combine to produce an attitude can be expressed by the following equation:

$$A = \Sigma b_i e_i$$

As can be seen, the subjective probability with which the attitude object is associated with a particular attribute (b) is multiplied by the subjective evaluation (e) of this attribute. The resulting products are summed.

The relationship between attitude and behaviour

It would also seem plausible to expect that people who have a positive attitude towards health have healthful lifestyles and refrain from health-impairing behaviours. However, the relationship between attitudes and behaviour has not proved to be quite so simple. In fact, social psychological research has sometimes failed to find substantial relationships between attitudes and behaviour that would seem relevant to these attitudes, particularly when very general attitudes were related to much more specific behaviour (for reviews, see Ajzen 1988; Eagly and Chaiken 1993). For example, a study of health attitudes and behaviour found that specific health behaviour, such as having regular dental check-ups or eating vitamin supplements, were largely unrelated to general attitudes towards health protection (Ajzen and Timko 1986).

The lack of correspondence that has frequently been observed in studies of the attitude–behaviour relationship does not imply, however, that we should abandon the idea that attitudes are predictors or determinants of behaviour. Since the early seventies social psychologists have studied the conditions under which measures of attitude predict behaviour. In their extensive analyses of attitude–behaviour research, Fishbein and Ajzen (1975) and Ajzen and Fishbein (1977) identified two conditions which were usually fulfilled by those studies that found attitude strongly related to behaviour: a relationship between attitude and behaviour was most likely to emerge if both attitude and behaviour had been assessed by measures which were (a) reliable and (b) compatible.

Reliability

Many of the classic studies of the attitude–behaviour literature which failed to observe a relationship between attitude and behaviour related attitudes to single instances of behaviour. As Ajzen and Fishbein (1977) and Epstein (1979) argued, single instances of behaviour are determined by a unique set of factors and are thus unreliable measures of behavioural tendencies, that is, the tendency to show a specific behaviour over time. For example, even a heavy smoker may refuse a cigarette offered on a particular occasion if he or she is suffering from a severe cold or does not like the particular brand of cigarettes. Only when one computes the average behavioural response over repeated occasions does the influence of factors that vary from one occasion to another tend to 'cancel out'. Thus, when one compares the number of cigarettes smoked on average by a heavy smoker with that smoked by a light smoker or a non-smoker, the cigarette consumption of the heavy smoker is likely to be higher. That aggregation across multiple instances of the same behaviour will increase the measure's temporal stability has been amply demonstrated (e.g. Epstein 1979).

However, this kind of aggregation does not solve the issue of attitude–behaviour consistency in the health area. Health psychologists typically enquire about the frequency with which a set of individuals engage in health-related behaviour during a particular period of time. For example, Belloc and Breslow (1972) asked their respondents whether they often, sometimes or never engaged in active sports, or how often they drank alcohol, and so on. Individuals are thus required to provide summary statements about their typical behaviour. If these statements are truthful, they are based on a person's recall of repeated instances of performing a given class of behaviour like 'engaging in active sports' or 'drinking alcohol' at different times and in different contexts. Therefore, such estimates reflect *aggregates* across multiple instances of the same behaviour and should be reasonably reliable measures of behavioural tendencies. And yet, they have often been found to show rather low correlations with global health attitudes (Ajzen and Timko 1986).

Compatibility

The use of reliable measures is a necessary but not a sufficient condition to achieve high correlations between measures of attitudes and behaviour. To assure a strong relation between measures of attitudes and behaviour, these measures need to be not only reliable but also compatible. Measures of attitude and behaviour are compatible if both are assessed at the same level of generality. Ajzen and Fishbein (1977) developed some criteria which help to evaluate the degree of compatibility between measures of attitude and behaviour. Every instance of behaviour involves four specific elements: (a) a specific action, (b) performed with respect to a given target, (c) in a given context, and (d) at a given point in time. The principle of compatibility specifies that measures of attitude and behaviour are compatible to the extent that their target, action, context and time elements are assessed at identical levels of generality or specificity (Ajzen 1988).

For example, a person's attitude towards a 'healthful lifestyle' only specifies the target, but leaves action, context, and time elements unspecified. A healthful lifestyle comprises numerous health practices that can be performed in many different contexts at many different times. A behavioural measure that would be compatible with this global attitude would have to aggregate a wide range of health behaviour across different contexts and times.

Consistent with this assumption, Ajzen and Timko (1986) reported that a measure of global attitudes towards health maintenance, which did not correlate significantly with the self-reported frequency with which respondents performed *specific* health protective behaviours, showed a substantial correlation with a behavioural index that aggregated the performance of a wide variety of different health protective behaviours. These behaviours related to different aspects of health and had been performed in a wide variety of contexts and times.

On the other hand, if we are interested in predicting *specific* behaviour, then an attitude measure would be compatible if it assessed the attitude towards performing the specific behaviour. Thus, Ajzen and Timko (1986) were able to predict specific health behaviour from equally specific attitudes towards these behaviours. For example, the reported frequency with which respondents had 'regular dental check-ups' correlated .46 with respondents' attitudes 'towards having regular dental checkups'.

In an elaboration of the psychological processes that underlie the principle of compatibility, Ajzen (1996) has suggested that to 'the extent that the beliefs salient at the time of attitude assessment are also salient when plans are formulated or executed, strong attitude–intention and attitude–behaviour correlations are expected' (p. 393). Thus, compatibility is assumed to affect these correlations between two types of measure because it determines the likelihood that the same beliefs are salient on each occasion. In contrast, if the contexts in which plans are made or executed stimulate beliefs which are vastly different from those salient when attitudes were assessed, attitudes will be poor predictors of intentions and action (Ajzen 1996; Ajzen and Sexton 1999).

The importance of compatibility between attitude and behaviour measures for establishing substantial attitude–behaviour relationships has been demonstrated in a recent meta-analysis. Meta-analyses are a set of techniques for statistically integrating the results of independent studies. These techniques make it possible to quantify study outcomes of a comprehensive sample of studies on a given topic in terms of a common metric (effect size). This enables one to compare outcomes across studies and to examine the overall outcomes of findings of all studies combined. Kraus (1995) identified eight studies that manipulated levels of compatibility between attitude and behaviour measures while holding other factors constant. The behaviours studied ranged from participation in a particular psychology experiment to blood donations and self-reported use of birth control pills. Kraus reported a mean correlation of r = .13 at the lowest level of compatibility as compared to r = .54 when compatibility was high.

The principle of compatibility has implications for strategies of attitude and behaviour change. As with prediction, compatibility should be observed in attempts to change behaviour. Thus, mass media campaigns designed to change some specific health behaviour should use arguments mainly aimed at changing beliefs relating to that *specific* behaviour rather than focusing on more general health concerns. For example, to persuade people to lower the cholesterol content of their diet, it would not be very effective merely to point out that coronary heart disease is the major killer and/or that high cholesterol levels are bad for one's heart. To influence diets one would have to argue that very specific changes in one's diet, such as eating less animal fats and less red meat, would have a positive impact on blood cholesterol levels and that the reduction in serum cholesterol should in turn reduce the risk of developing coronary heart disease.

A number of recent meta-analyses of studies of the attitude–behaviour relationship reported substantial relationships between attitude and behaviour, suggesting that most studies use measures of these constructs which are reliable and compatible. Based on a meta-analysis of 88 attitude–behaviour studies, Kraus (1995) reported a mean correlation of $r = .38$. An even more extensive meta-analysis based on 644 independent studies found a similar mean correlation of $r = .36$ (Six 1996). However, with $r = .23$ (based on 69 studies), the mean correlation for the domain of health behaviour was somewhat lower than the overall mean for all behavioural domains taken together.

MODELS OF BEHAVIOUR

The assumption that attitudes and beliefs are major determinants of behaviour is shared by four models of behaviour, from each of which predictions about health behaviour can be made. These models are the health belief model, protection motivation theory, theory of reasoned action and theory of planned behaviour. These theories belong to the family of expectancy–value models. As explained earlier, expectancy–value models make the assumption that decisions between different courses of action are based on two types of cognition: subjective probabilities that a given action will lead to a set of expected outcomes, and evaluation of action outcomes. Individuals will choose among various alternative courses of action that action which will be most likely to lead to positive consequences or avoid negative consequences. The models described in this section elaborate the basic model by specifying the *types* of beliefs and attitudes which should be used in predicting a particular class of behaviour and/or by incorporating *additional* variables such as subjective norms or perceived behavioural control to predict behaviour.

These models are rational reasoning models which assume that individuals consciously deliberate about the likely consequences of behavioural alternatives that are available to them before engaging in action. It would seem uneconomical if people who are regularly confronted with the same behavioural alternatives in a stable situational context were to devote a great deal of cognitive effort in making a choice. Thus, action generation and control is likely to vary on a continuum from conscious deliberation about likely outcomes of behavioural alternatives to automatic repetition of past acts. In the final section, it will be discussed how the notion of habitual behaviour can be integrated into cognitive models of behaviour.

The health belief model

The health belief model was originally developed by social psychologists in the US Public Health Service in an attempt to understand why people

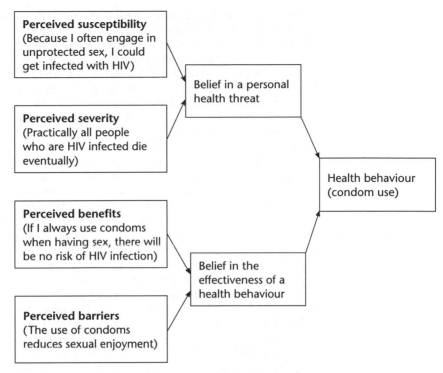

Figure 2.1   The health belief model applied to the reduction of sexual risk behaviour.
Source: Adapted from Stroebe and de Wit (1996).

failed to make use of disease prevention or screening tests for the early detection of diseases not associated with clear-cut symptoms, at least in the early stages. Later, the model was also applied to patients' responses to symptoms and compliance with or adherence to prescribed medical regimens. In the course of these applications, the model was considerably expanded (for reviews, see Wallston and Wallston 1981; Janz and Becker 1984; Harrison *et al.* 1992; Sheeran and Abraham 1996).

The model

The health belief model assumes that the likelihood that an individual engages in a given health behaviour will be a function of the extent to which a person believes that he or she is personally *susceptible* to the particular illness and of his or her perceptions of the *severity* of the consequences of getting the disease. Susceptibility and severity jointly determine the *perceived threat* of the disease (see Figure 2.1). For example, a sexually active student who frequently has unprotected sex with a variety of partners might fear that he or she runs the risk of contracting a sexually transmitted disease (perceived susceptibility). Obviously, getting such an infection could have severe consequences (perceived severity).

Given some threat of contracting a disease, the likelihood of engaging in a particular health behaviour will further depend on the extent to which the individual believes that the action yields *benefits* that outweigh the *barriers* associated with the action such as the costs, inconvenience or pain. For example, whether the student will decide to use condoms will depend on his or her estimate of whether the benefits to health associated with this action would really outweigh the costs in terms of the reduction of sexual enjoyment as a result of condom use or the embarrassment of negotiating with the partner.

Rosenstock (1974) further suggested that a *cue to action* might be necessary to trigger appropriate health behaviour. This could be an internal cue like a bodily symptom, or an external cue such as a mass media campaign, medical advice, or the death of a friend of similar age and lifestyle. For example, our sexually active student might continue to hesitate about using condoms until he or she develops some strange skin condition following a sexual encounter, or until there is a report in the papers that the spread of AIDS among heterosexuals is accelerating. Thus, one reason cues to action might be effective is by increasing the personal relevance of a health threat. A second reason why a cue to action might trigger behaviour is because it forms part of an implementation intention (Gollwitzer 1999). Implementation intentions are subordinate to goal intentions and specify when, where, and how a response leading to goal attainment should be enacted. By forming implementation intentions, people delegate the control of their behaviour over to anticipated situational cues, which when actually encountered, elicit these responses automatically. There is persuasive evidence that the formation of implementation intentions substantially increases the likelihood that individuals act in line with their intentions to engage health-promoting behaviours such as performing a breast self-examination (Orbell *et al.* 1997) or regularly take their pills (Sheeran and Orbell 1999).

The relation between the variables of the health belief model has never been formalized or even explicitly spelled out. However, in most studies an additive combination is assumed. The additive combination of the variables of the health belief model implies that the influence of each of the variables on health behaviour is not moderated by any of the other factors. For example, the assumption that the threat of a disease is a function of the *sum* of the perceived *susceptibility* of contracting a disease and the perceived *severity* of the disease implies that there is a moderate threat as long as one of these two variables is high, even if the other approaches zero. In contrast, intuition suggests that the perceived threat of an illness would be very low if either of the two factors had a value of zero. For example, there may be many deadly diseases in the world (high severity) which do not worry us, because there is not the slightest chance that we could contract them (low susceptibility). With other diseases, the chance of contracting them might be high, but the consequences might be so minor that we would not really take preventive action.

The type of relationship in which the impact of each of the factors on health behaviour is dependent on the level of the other factor would be better represented by a model using some kind of multiplicative combination of the components. However, even though a multiplicative combination of the components is intuitively more plausible than the additive combination, researchers in the health area have often failed to demonstrate the multiplicative combination between severity and probability of threat (e.g. Rogers and Mewborn 1976; for a review, see Jonas 1993). Jonas (1993) argued that the failure to support a multiplicative model may be due to the fact that people are unable to perform the kind of trade-offs between expectancies and valences (i.e. the values attached outcomes or consequences of behaviour) that are required by a multiplicative combination of the two variables. He presented empirical findings which support this assumption. As Weinstein (1988) suggested, one way out of this dilemma may be the postulation of a more complex decision rule that incorporates cut-off points. Thus, people may only attend to a problem once both the likelihood and the severity are above a certain level. Once both variables are above a certain level, the level of perceived threat may be an additive function of the two factors.

A further weakness of the health belief model is that a number of important determinants of health behaviour are not included. For example, the model does not consider potentially positive aspects of health-impairing behaviour patterns (e.g. the enjoyment of smoking) or that many health behaviours are popular for reasons totally unrelated to health (e.g. weight control and exercise behaviour is often motivated by the wish to look good rather than to be healthy). The model also fails to include self-efficacy or perceived behavioural control as factors influencing behaviour. There is a great deal of evidence that if people think they are unable to engage in a health-protective behaviour like keeping to a diet, they are unlikely to do so (for a review, see Schwarzer and Fuchs 1996). A further weakness of the model is its failure to consider social influence variables such as the subjective norm component of the models of reasoned action and planned behaviour to be discussed later (p. 27). Finally, the model assumes that the beliefs in a personal health threat and in the effectiveness of a health behaviour have a direct influence on behaviour that is not mediated by behavioural intention. This assumption is inconsistent with evidence indicating that the influence of beliefs on behaviour is mediated by behavioural intentions (e.g. Wurtele *et al.* 1982; Wurtele 1988).

According to the health belief model there can be many reasons why individuals do not change their health behaviour even if their actual vulnerability is high. For example, people show a pervasive tendency to underestimate their own health risks compared to those of others (Weinstein 1987). Thus, even if they accept that eating a fatty diet increases the risk of heart disease, they might feel protected by a particularly hardy constitution. But even if individuals perceive a threat realistically, they are unlikely to engage in health-protective measures if they doubt their effectiveness or if they feel that the effort is just too great to make it worthwhile. Thus, any media campaign aimed at modifying health behaviour should contain arguments which persuade them that serious health consequences are likely to occur, unless they change certain aspects of their lifestyle *and* that the adoption of specific health behaviour would considerably reduce this risk.

Empirical evaluation of the model

Janz and Becker (1984) reviewed 46 studies based on the health belief model, of which 18 used prospective and 28 retrospective designs. In order to assess support for the model, they constructed a 'significance ratio' for each dimension, which divided the number of positive, statistically significant findings for a given dimension of the model by the total number of studies reporting significance levels for this dimension. The results were as follows: barriers (89 per cent), susceptibility (81 per cent), benefits (78 per cent) and severity (65 per cent). The authors interpret these results as providing substantial support for the model.

However, the fact that the association between two variables is statistically significant is not very informative concerning the strength of the relationship. To evaluate the strength of an association we would need information about 'effect sizes' which would allow us to estimate the variance in health behaviour that is accounted for by the various components of the model either separately or jointly. This information has been provided by a meta-analytic review conducted by Harrison and colleagues (1992). Unfortunately, these authors were unusually restrictive in their selection of studies and based their analysis on only 16 studies (of which six had been included in the review of Janz and Becker 1984). Harrison and colleagues found overall that all four dimensions of the health belief model were significantly and positively related to health behaviours, but that less than 10 per cent of the variance in health behaviour could be accounted for by any one dimension. This would indicate a weak relationship compared to findings of meta-analyses of the models of reasoned action and planned behaviour which suggest that these models account for one third of the variance in behaviour (e.g. van den Putte 1991; Godin and Kok 1996; Six 1996; Armitage and Conner 1998). However, these results cannot easily be compared because Harrison and colleagues did not analyse the *joint* effect of the four dimensions of the model. The joint effect of all predictors taken together could be substantially greater than their independent effects.

Implications for the planning of interventions

According to this model, interventions are most likely to induce people to adopt some precautionary action if they can be persuaded that they are susceptible to some disease, that developing that disease will have severe consequences, that adopting the preventive action will make them less susceptible or reduce the severity of the illness, and that the perceived benefits of taking the precautionary action will outweigh the anticipated costs. The usefulness of this model can be illustrated with a study applying the health belief model to condom use among teenagers (Abraham *et al.* 1992). This study of more than 300 sexually active Scottish teenagers, which investigated the relation between the various components of the health belief model and intention to carry and use condoms, found perceived severity of HIV infection, perceived vulnerability to HIV infection and perceived effectiveness of condom use to be only weakly related to intention. In contrast, perceived barriers to condom use (e.g. beliefs concerning pleasure reduction, awkwardness of use, and partners' likely response to suggested use) were found to be substantially related to intentions to carry and use condoms. These findings suggest that instead of emphasizing young people's vulnerability to infection, the severity of infection and condom effectiveness, as had been done in most previous interventions, it might be more effective to focus on social acceptability barriers in future interventions.

Protection motivation theory

The original model

Although protection motivation theory has mainly been tested in the context of fear-arousing communications, the original version of the theory (e.g. Rogers and Mewborn 1976) constituted an attempt to specify the algebraic relationship between some of the components of the health belief model. According to the theory, protection motivation (that is the motivation to engage in some kind of health-protective behaviour) depends on three factors:

1 the perceived severity of the noxious event;
2 the perceived probability of the event's occurrence or perceived susceptibility; and
3 the efficacy of the recommended response in averting the noxious event.

The model does not include the costs of the recommended response as a variable.

According to this model, the response of a smoker exposed to a campaign that emphasizes the causal role of smoking in the development of lung cancer will depend on his or her answer to the following questions:

1 How bad is it to have lung cancer?
2 How likely is it that I will get lung cancer?
3 How much would stopping smoking reduce my risk of getting lung cancer?

The model assumes that the three factors combine multiplicatively to determine the intensity of protection motivation. More specifically, the intensity of protection motivation is assumed to be a monotonically increasing function of the algebraic product of these three variables.

An empirical test of the original model

Rogers and Mewborn (1976) tested the predictions of protection motivation theory in a series of three experiments, which used fear appeals on the topics of smoking, traffic safety and venereal diseases. In these experiments, fear-arousing communications manipulated each of the three crucial variables of the theory at two levels: high vs low noxiousness of the depicted event, high vs low probability of that event's occurrence and high vs low efficacy of the recommended coping response. The results differed across the three studies and did not provide clear support for the model.

In particular, in none of the three experiments was there any evidence of the three-way interaction (perceived susceptibility x perceived severity x perceived efficacy of coping) that would be expected on the basis of the multiplicative combination of the three factors of the model.

As Sutton (1982) pointed out, the failure of the study of Rogers and Mewborn (1976) to support the model could have been due to the fact that perceived efficacy and susceptibility are not independent of each other, as the model assumes. The recommended action is perceived as effective to the extent that it is thought to reduce the risk of occurrence of the noxious event. Therefore, perceived efficacy can never be greater than perceived susceptibility. This, he argued, leads to inconsistencies in some conditions of the experiment. For example, under conditions of *high effectiveness and low vulnerability*, respondents are told that taking certain protective actions would considerably reduce their risk of contracting a certain disease, even though they had been informed beforehand that there was little chance of their getting this disease anyway. This kind of inconsistency may account for the fact that experimental tests failed to find many of the interactive effects predicted by the model.

The revised model

In a revision of protection motivation theory, Rogers (1983; Rippetoe and Rogers 1987; for a review, see Boer and Seydel 1996) abandoned the notion that the various factors combine multiplicatively and also expanded the theory by including additional determinants of protection motivation. Probably the most important variable added was self-efficacy. The concept of self-efficacy refers to a person's belief that he or she is able to perform a particular action (Bandura 1986). Because people might not be motivated to stop smoking or drinking alcohol, despite a negative attitude towards these behaviours, if they think that they would be too weak or too addicted to do so, the inclusion of self-efficacy in a model of health protective behaviour should improve predictions. The revision also incorporated the health belief model's perceived barrier construct (labelled 'response costs') and added a related one, the rewards associated with 'maladaptive' responses (e.g. the enjoyment of continuing to drink or smoke, the time and energy saved by not having health check-ups).

The revised model assumes that the motivation to protect oneself from danger is a positive function of four beliefs:

1 the threat is severe;
2 one is personally vulnerable;
3 one has the ability to perform the coping response; and
4 the coping response is effective in reducing the threat.

The motivation to perform the adaptive response is negatively influenced by the costs of that response and by potential rewards associated with maladaptive responses.

More specifically, Rogers divided these six variables into two classes, which he named threat appraisal and coping appraisal (Figure 2.2). It is plausible that threat appraisal is based on a consideration of the factors of

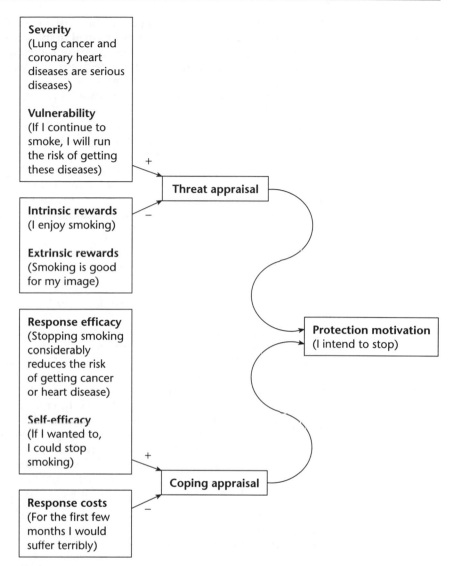

Figure 2.2 Protection motivation theory applied to the reduction of smoking.
Source: Adapted from Stroebe and de Wit (1996).

severity and susceptibility. After all, the threat experienced from continuing to smoke would be reflected by the severity of the likely health
consequences and of the probability of contracting them. It is less plausible, however, also to include the intrinsic and extrinsic rewards of the
maladaptive response (e.g. of continuing to smoke) under the concept of
threat appraisal. These rewards would probably have been better subsumed
under the category of response costs. After all, the adaptive response to
the threat from the consequences of health-impairing behaviour is to

stop and as a result to deprive oneself also of the rewarding qualities this behaviour may have had. The factors assumed to influence coping appraisal are the effectivity of the coping response, the individual's perception of his or her ability to execute the coping response (i.e. self-efficacy), and the costs of the recommended behaviour.

Rogers postulated an additive combination of factors within a given class but a multiplicative influence between classes. Thus, severity and vulnerability are assumed to combine additively to determine threat appraisal. However, coping appraisal and threat appraisal are expected to combine multiplicatively. Thus, increases in threat appraisal should increase protection motivation only when coping appraisal is moderate to high. When coping appraisal is low, due, for example, to low self-efficacy, then increased threat appraisal should not result in an increased intention to take protective action. Research assessing these assumptions has been reviewed by Rogers (1983).

Empirical tests of the revised model

Empirical comparisons of the revised protection motivation theory with the health belief model typically favour protection motivation. For example, Seydel et al. (1990) found a superiority of protection motivation theory due to the inclusion of self-efficacy. Wurtele and Maddux (1987) observed in a study on exercise behaviour that the predictors of the health belief model affected behaviour through behavioural intentions rather than directly as assumed by the health belief model. Research was less supportive of the predictions regarding the way in which different components of the model combine to influence protective intentions. Only partial support could be found for the assumption that variables within a given class are combined additively, but variables belonging to different classes should combine multiplicatively. Although some findings were consistent with the assumption of an interaction of variables belonging to different classes (e.g. Kleinot and Rogers 1982; Self and Rogers 1990), others were not (e.g. Maddux and Rogers 1983; Rippetoe and Rogers 1987; Mulilis and Lippa 1990).

Implications for interventions

These assumptions have important implications for the planning of interventions. For example, if self-efficacy for a given behaviour domain has been found to be relatively high in a target population (i.e. if most individuals feel competent to engage in a recommended health-protective action) the provision of information which increases vulnerability or severity should increase protection motivation and thus intention to act. Under these conditions individuals should be more likely to take action, the greater they perceive their individual risk. When self-efficacy is low, however, that is, when individuals feel that they are unable to engage in a given action (e.g. dieting to lose weight), increases in vulnerability should not result in increments in intentions. Under the latter conditions, rather than emphasizing risk, it might be more effective to provide individuals with information which increases their self-efficacy.

Conclusions

Both the health belief model and protection motivation theory have generated a great deal of research in the health area. During the last few decades, however, a number of more general models of behaviour have been developed which have also been applied to the health area. Obviously, it is not very economical to continue to entertain specific theories of health behaviour unless the predictive success of these models is greater than that of general models of behaviour. As we shall see later in our discussion of specific health behaviours (Chapters 4 and 5), the general models of behaviour to be presented in the following sections of this chapter have typically been more successful in predicting behaviour than the two theories of health behaviour which have just been described.

The theory of reasoned action

One of the more general social psychological models of behaviour, namely the theory of reasoned action (e.g. Fishbein and Ajzen 1975), has been tested extensively and has been successful in predicting a wide range of behaviour (for reviews, see Ajzen 1988; Eagly and Chaiken 1993).

The model

The theory of reasoned action predicts behavioural intention and assumes that behaviour is a function of the intention to perform that behaviour. A behavioural intention is determined by one's attitude towards performing the behaviour and by subjective norms. As outlined earlier (p. 14), a person's attitude towards stopping smoking will be a function of the perceived likelihood with which cessation is associated with certain consequences such as being healthier and fitter or reducing the risk of developing heart problems or lung cancer and the evaluation of these perceived consequences (Figure 2.3).

Subjective norms combine two components, namely normative beliefs and motivation to comply. Normative beliefs are our beliefs about how people who are important to us expect us to behave. For example, a woman might believe that her husband does not want her to indulge in dangerous sports or that he would like her to lose some weight. However, whether such normative beliefs influence intentions will also depend on one's willingness to comply with this norm. Thus, subjective norms are normative beliefs weighted by motivation to comply. The model quantifies these subjective norms by multiplying the subjective likelihood that a particular other (the referent) thinks the person should perform the behaviour by the person's motivation to comply with that referent's expectation. These products are analogous to the Expectancy x Value products computed for attitudes to the behaviour and are also summed over various salient referent persons. Because both attitudes and subjective norms reflect expectations regarding the consequences of a given behaviour weighted by the valence of these consequences, the model of reasoned action also belongs to the class of expectancy–value models.

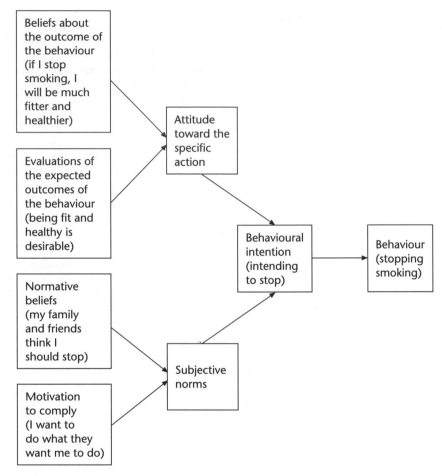

Figure 2.3 The theory of reasoned action applied to the decision to give up smoking.

Empirical evaluation of the model

Empirical tests of the model have mainly assessed its success in predicting behavioural intentions and actual behaviour for a wide range of behavioural domains. The model has been applied to blood donation, family planning, eating at fast food restaurants, smoking marijuana, mothers' infant feeding practices, dental hygiene behaviour and having an abortion (for a review, see Eagly and Chaiken 1993). In an extensive meta-analysis of research on the model based on 113 articles, van den Putte (1991) reported the following estimates of the various relations of the model based on 150 groups of respondents: The mean R for predicting intention from attitudes and subjective norms was .68, and the mean r for predicting behaviour from intention was .62. Thus, attitudes and subjective norms accounted for approximately 46 per cent of the variance in intentions and intentions for 38 per cent of the variance in behaviour. Van den Putte also found that the relation between intention and attitude was stronger than the relation between intention and subjective norms. More recent meta-analyses reported somewhat lower correlations between intentions and behaviour: based on 98 studies, Randall and Wolff (1994) computed an average correlation of $r = .45$. With a weighted mean correlation of $r = .40$ (N = 170 studies), Six (1996) found an even lower correlation between intention and behaviour.

Implications for interventions

According to the model, the effectiveness of strategies aimed at modifying health behaviour depends on the success in influencing the individuals' intention to engage in the specific behaviour. Since intentions are assumed to be the immediate determinants of behaviour, a change in a behavioural intention should result in a change in the correspondent behaviour. Intentions to engage in a specific behaviour are determined by attitudes towards that behaviour and relevant subjective norms which in turn are based on behavioural beliefs and normative beliefs respectively. These beliefs should be the target of the intervention.

Whether one should focus more on behavioural or normative beliefs in designing a campaign to influence a specific behaviour will depend on the relative importance of attitudes and norms in determining the behaviour in question. For example, subjective norms seem to be *less* important than attitudes for women's choice between breast and bottle feeding (Manstead *et al.* 1983), especially for women who are having a second (or later) child. On the other hand, women's decisions to have an abortion (Smetana and Adler 1980) or a couple's decision to have another child (Vinokur-Kaplan 1978), have been found to be *more* strongly affected by perceived social pressure than by personal attitudes. If behaviour is primarily under attitudinal control, attempts to change that behaviour by influencing normative beliefs will not be very successful. Similarly, if the members of some group perform a given behaviour because they believe that people who are important to them expect them to perform this behaviour, trying to change their attitudes towards that behaviour will have little impact on their intentions. Since the relative importance of the attitudinal and normative components is likely to vary between different populations, it is important in designing an intervention to conduct pilot tests with groups selected from the population to be targeted by the intervention.

Once one has determined whether a given behaviour (or intention) is primarily attitudinally or normatively controlled, one must identify salient outcomes of the behaviour and/or reference persons which are important for this particular behavioural domain. However, not all outcomes which are salient for a given behavioural domain are also strongly related to the relevant behaviour. For example, even though the negative health consequences of smoking are salient outcomes of this behaviour, the belief that smoking is unhealthy no longer discriminates between smokers and non-smokers (Leventhal and Cleary 1980). Thus, information about the negative health consequences of smoking is unlikely to persuade smokers to abandon their habit. Similarly, the perceived threat of contracting HIV infections has been found to have only a small association with heterosexual

condom use in an extensive meta-analyis of the determinants of heterosexual condom use (Sheeran *et al.* 1999). Interventions which focus on
the dangers of HIV and AIDS are therefore unlikely to be effective in
increasing condom use. To be effective, interventions have to focus on
those beliefs which most strongly discriminate between people who do
and do not intend to perform the behaviour in question.

According to the model, it should also be possible to change attitudes
towards some health-impairing behaviour by modifying the environment
so as to increase the costs of the behaviour (e.g. increases in the price
of tobacco, restriction of the sale of alcoholic beverages, introduction of
legal sanctions for non-use of seat belts). However, increasing the costs
of health-impairing behaviour will affect behaviour only if the person is
aware of these changes and if the costs are sufficiently high to outweigh
benefits. For example, the introduction of financial sanctions for failing
to use seat belts will influence the relevant behaviour only if the person
realizes that the law has been changed, thinks that there is a good chance
of getting caught if he or she does not comply and feels that the penalty
is large enough to outweigh the expected discomfort of wearing belts.

Omissions from the model

Despite being reasonably successful in predicting intention and behaviour, the model has been criticized by researchers who have argued that
intentions and actions are affected by a number of factors which are not
included in the model of reasoned action. The most interesting of these
additional determinants in the context of health behaviour is past behaviour. In a test of the theory of reasoned action that used self-reported
consumption of alcohol, marijuana and hard drugs as dependent measures, Bentler and Speckart (1979) found that reported past behaviour added
to the prediction of future behaviour even when intention was statistically controlled. This finding has been replicated in a number of further
studies for exercise (Bentler and Speckart 1981), condom use (de Wit *et al.*
1990; Schaalma *et al.* 1993) and seat belt use (Sutton and Hallett 1989). In
these later studies, multiple regression analyses showed that the prediction of behaviour was improved by the addition of past behaviour over
and above the prediction achieved on the basis of intention.

The problem of volitional control

The finding that measures of past behaviour add to the prediction of future
behaviour even when intentions are statistically controlled could represent the impact of any number of factors that influence behaviour but are
not taken into account by the theory of reasoned action. In interpreting
these findings, we have to remember that the theory of reasoned action
offers a theoretical account of the factors that determine intentions. Intentions only reflect the motivation to act. Execution of an action not only
depends on motivation but also on whether the behaviour is under volitional control of the individual. A behaviour is under volitional control if
the individual can decide at will whether or not to perform it. Thus, past

behaviour might reflect the influence of factors that are not under volitional control of the individual.

There are many factors which could lower the control individuals have over their actions. Some actions may have become so routinized and habitual that people perform them without thinking. For example, smokers might light a cigarette or pipe without intending to do so or without even realizing they are doing it. Because past behaviour would have also been influenced by their habit, using past behaviour to predict future behaviour would then improve predictions even when intentions are statistically controlled.

The control individuals have over their actions might also be lowered by the fact that these behaviours require skills, abilities, opportunities and the cooperation of others. As Eagly and Chaiken (1993) have pointed out, the great majority of studies that have supported the theory of reasoned action have involved relatively simple behaviours that do not require much in the way of resources and skills. Fishbein and Ajzen (1975) were not unaware of this issue, but they argued that people would take the need for resources or others' cooperation into account in forming their intentions. Changes in resources will then result in changes in intention. For example, if somebody who intended to play tennis with a friend on Monday evening learns that the friend has fallen ill, that person is likely to change his or her intention. Such unexpected changes in external conditions are one of the reasons why intentions predict behaviour better if the time lag between the assessment of intentions and behaviour is short.

Although this position is reasonable, the restriction of the model of reasoned action to behaviour that is under complete volitional control seriously limits the applicability of the model. Closer inspection reveals that very few behaviours are under the complete volitional control of the individual. Even the execution of such simple actions as brushing one's teeth depends on the availability of one's toothbrush and toothpaste.

The theory of planned behaviour

The model

This type of reasoning has led Ajzen to modify the theory of reasoned action and to develop the theory of planned behaviour (Ajzen 1988, 1991). The model of planned behaviour incorporates perceived behavioural control over the behaviour to be predicted as an additional predictor. Perceived controllability of a behaviour can be assessed directly by asking respondents to what extent performing a given behaviour was under their control, or by assessing the control beliefs assumed to determine perceived behavioural control. The concept is thus very similar to the construct of self-efficacy, which reflects people's judgements of their ability to execute certain courses of action required to attain intended levels of performance (Bandura 1986). The model of planned behaviour assumes that perceived behavioural control affects behaviour indirectly through intentions. Under certain conditions, it can also have a direct effect on behaviour that is not mediated by intentions (Figure 2.4).

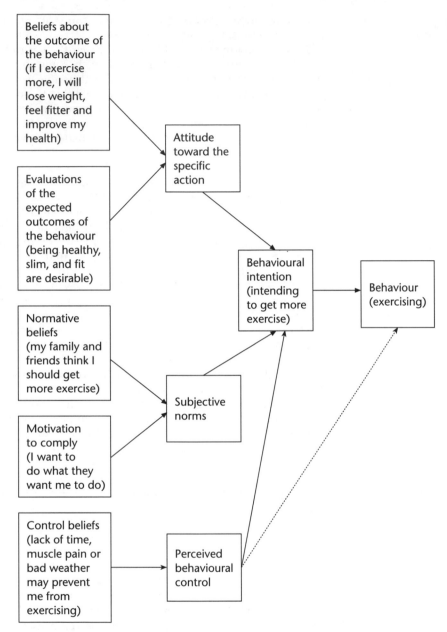

Figure 2.4 The theory of planned behaviour applied to the intention to engage in physical exercise.

The assumption that perceived behavioural control affects intentions is consistent with expectancy–value theories of motivation. People who lack the ability or the opportunity to achieve some goal will adjust their intentions accordingly, because intentions are partly determined by people's perception of the probability that a goal can be reached by them. For example, students who have learned from past performance that they lack the ability to achieve the kind of outstanding grades in their courses that they had hoped for are likely to adjust their intentions and aim for lower but more realistic grades.

The direct relationship between perceived behavioural control and behaviour which is not mediated by intentions (indicated by the broken line in Figure 2.4) is intuitively less plausible but can be illustrated by the following example. A businesswoman who likes to jog every evening may also know that on many evenings she has to entertain out-of-town customers and that their visits will prevent her from exercising. Thus, although she might indicate that she has every intention to jog daily, she would also have to admit that her time is not her own. Her *realistic* rating of the extent to which she has control over whether or not she jogs every evening will therefore be an additional predictor of her jogging that is not mediated by her intentions.

It is important to note that the direct link of perceived behavioural control to behaviour has a somewhat different theoretical status from the link that is mediated by intention. Whereas perceived behavioural control has a causal influence on intentions (e.g. the present author's knowledge of his lack of will-power has prevented him from ever forming the intention to jog), it is not the perceived but the *actual* lack of control which *causally* influences behaviour (via the direct route). Thus, it is not the businesswoman's expectation that out-of-town customers might have to be entertained which prevents her from jogging, but the actual visit of customers who have to be entertained.

The latter example can also be used to illustrate that perceived behavioural control should only improve the prediction of behaviour (which is exclusively based on intentions) if it realistically reflects actual levels of control. Suppose there is an unexpected slump in business and none of the expected out-of-town customers turn up. As a consequence the woman would have much more control over her jogging than she had anticipated earlier. It is plausible that under these conditions, perceived behavioural control as assessed earlier would not improve predictions of behaviour.

In line with this assumption Ajzen and Madden (1986) found in a study of students' intentions to get an A in a course (best grade), and their actual grades, that the direct link between perceived behavioural control and behaviour only emerged when perceived behavioural control was assessed toward the end of their semester *after* 'students had received considerable information concerning their performance in the course by means of feedback on class projects and examinations' (p. 466). A measure of behavioural control taken at the beginning of the semester did not improve the prediction of behaviour based on intention. Supposedly, students' estimates of their own control over grades had become more realistic in the course of the semester.

Determinants of perceived behavioural control

The factors that influence perceived behavioural control can either be internal or external to the individual (Ajzen 1988). Examples of internal factors are information, skills, abilities, and also urges and compulsions. Our control over health behaviour is often threatened by those internal factors that are collectively referred to as 'will-power'. Thus, despite the firm intention to visit a doctor or to lose weight, a person with medical or weight problems may know from past experience that he or she is unlikely to execute these intentions. Examples of external factors are opportunity and dependence on others (Ajzen 1988). For example, we know that we can only go cross-country skiing tomorrow if the snow does not melt and if our boss allows us to leave the office on time.

Terry and O'Leary (1995) and Armitage and Conner (1999) have suggested that control over internal and external factors should be assessed separately. Belief in the control of internal factors (i.e. motivation or ability) would be reflected by self-efficacy. Self-efficacy, defined as the confidence in one's own ability to carry out a behaviour, is a concept that was introduced by Bandura (e.g. 1986, 1997). The measure of perceived behavioural control, on the other hand, would reflect the control over the more external factors influencing behaviour. In a study of exercise behaviour, Terry and O'Leary (1995) demonstrated that self-efficacy only influenced the intention but had no direct effect on behaviour whereas perceived behavioural control was only related to behaviour but not to intention. However, Armitage and Conner (1999) failed to replicate these findings in their study of eating a low-fat diet, possibly because eating behaviour is much more under volitional control than is exercising.

A related distinction is that between efficacy expectancy and outcome expectancy. An *efficacy* expectancy is the expectation that, if one tried to perform a certain behaviour, one would be able to do it. For example, an obese individual might be fairly confident that he or she could substantially reduce daily calorie consumption. However, a reduction in calorie intake does not necessarily result in substantial weight loss. Thus, whereas the perceived likelihood that one is able to reduce one's calorie intake is an *efficacy* expectancy, the expectation that this reduction will actually result in substantial weight loss is an *outcome* expectancy. The concept of perceived behavioural control as originally introduced by Ajzen and Madden (1986) refers to both outcome expectancy and efficacy expectancy.

Empirical evaluation of the model

The model of planned behaviour has been applied to a variety of behaviours ranging from academic grades to shoplifting (for a review see Ajzen 1991). The first published test of the model was a study of weight loss (Schifter and Ajzen 1985). Female college students were asked at the beginning of the study to express their attitudes, subjective norms, perceived behavioural control and intentions with respect to losing weight during a six-week period. In addition, the extent to which participants had made detailed weight reduction plans was assessed, as were a number of general attitudes and personality factors. Consistent with the theory, the intention to lose weight was predicted quite accurately on the basis of attitudes, subjective norms and perceived behavioural control. However, perceived behavioural control and intentions were only moderately successful in predicting the amount of weight that participants actually lost during the six weeks (i.e. an outcome), with perceived behavioural control being the better predictor. As expected, there was also an interaction between perceived behavioural control and intention on weight reduction: a strong intention to lose weight increased weight reduction only for those participants who believed that they would be able to control their calorie intake, if they wanted to. Respondents who had made a detailed plan at the beginning of the period also tended to lose more weight.

Since then a great number of empirical studies testing the model of planned behaviour have been published. The results of these studies tend to support the central predictions of the model of planned behaviour that, unless a given behaviour in question is under complete volitional control of the individual, predictions of behaviour from the model of planned behaviour are superior to those based on the theory of reasoned action (e.g. Godin and Kok 1996; Armitage and Conner 1998). In a recent meta-analysis based on 142 independent tests of the theory of planned behaviour, Armitage and Conner (1998) reported an average multiple correlation of attitude, subjective norm and perceived behavioural control with intention of R = .63, accounting for 40 per cent of the variance. The average multiple correlation of perceived behavioural control and intention with behaviour was R = .54, accounting for 29 per cent of the variance in behaviour. Perceived behavioural control added an average of 6 per cent to the prediction of intention (controlling for attitude and norms) and two per cent to the prediction of behaviour, over and above intention.

A meta-analysis which focused only on applications of the theory of planned behaviour to the health domain reported similar findings. Based on 56 studies, Godin and Kok (1996) reported an average multiple correlation of R = .64 for the prediction of intentions. Attitudes towards the action and perceived behavioural control were most often significant contributors to the variation in intention. The prediction of behaviour yielded an average multiple correlation of R = .58. Thus, approximately one-third of the variation in the health behaviours studied can be explained by the combined effect of intention and perceived behavioural control. In half of the studies reviewed perceived behavioural control added significantly to the prediction of behaviour, although intention remained the most important predictor. As one would expect, the contribution of perceived behavioural control to the prediction of behaviour was greatest for addictive behaviours, a behavioural domain where volitional control can be assumed to be weak.

Implications for interventions

Because the model of planned behaviour is an extension of the model of reasoned actions, the two models share many implications for interventions. However, there are also important differences. For example, in contrast to the model of reasoned action, the model of planned behaviour recognizes behavioural control as a second predictor of behaviour. Thus, the first step in designing a successful intervention according to the model of planned behaviour is to assess empirically whether the behaviour is mainly determined by behavioural intentions or by perceived behavioural control. In the exceptional case where behaviour is mainly predicted by perceived behavioural control, one has to examine further the reasons for the lack of association between intention and behaviour. In the area of health behaviour, this is often due to the fact that there is little variance in intention. For example, most homosexual men intend to avoid engaging in unprotected anal sex with casual partners, but some do not succeed. Since those who do not succeed usually have low perceived behavioural control, the control variable becomes a better predictor of behaviour than intention. In this case, one might try to increase their control, for example through skill training.

In the more usual situation where behaviour is mainly determined by the relevant behavioural intention one then has to assess the extent to which the intention to engage in this behaviour is determined by attitudes, norms or perceived behavioural control. Once one knows which of the determinants of intention (i.e. attitude, subjective norm, perceived behavioural control) is most important, one should identify the salient beliefs which underlie this factor. Finally, one should focus one's persuasive communication on those of the elicited salient (attitudinal, normative, and/or control) beliefs which distinguish individuals who already perform the targeted behaviour from those who do not.

If interventions were always designed on the basis of this type of analysis, many costly failures could be avoided. This can be illustrated with the findings of a study of the effectiveness of a health education programme on AIDS developed by Dutch Educational Television (de Wit *et al.* 1990). Two groups of male and female students at secondary schools were assessed at two time-points, using a questionnaire which measured AIDS-relevant knowledge as well as attitudes towards condom use, perceived norms regarding condom use, perceived behavioural control over condom use, and intention to use condoms. In the interval between the two assessments, half the respondents were exposed to the health education programme on AIDS whereas the other half were not exposed to the information.

Students reported that they learned a great deal of new information through the programme. Consistent with these self-reports, the intervention group showed a significant increase in relevant knowledge. However, despite its impact on AIDS knowledge, the intervention did not influence intentions to use condoms. Intentions were solely determined by attitudes towards condom use, perceived norms and perceived effectiveness. This finding is in line with the results of other studies indicating that neither knowledge nor perceived susceptibility seem to be related to behavioural risk reduction regarding HIV infection (e.g. Richard and van der Pligt 1991; Abraham *et al.* 1992). The obvious implication from such findings is that future AIDS campaigns should give less emphasis to AIDS knowledge and focus more on attitudes towards condom use, subjective norms, and perceived effectiveness.

Beyond reasons and plans: the role of habits in planned behaviour

The models of behaviour discussed in the last section conceive of people as fairly rational decision makers who tend to deliberate about future actions to form a behavioural intention. Even though none of these models assumes that individuals have to weigh all the consequences of the behavioural alternatives at each behavioural opportunity, the fact that they all more or less imply that behaviour is mediated by intentions suggests that behaviour involves at least a minimum of cognitive deliberation.

Habits and behaviour

As argued earlier, much of the behaviour of interest to health psychology is enacted on a regular basis. It is therefore likely to have become habitual. Habits are 'learned sequences of acts that have become automatic responses to specific cues, and are functional in obtaining certain goals or end states' (Verplanken and Aarts 1999). Bargh and Barndollar (1996) have argued that not only is the execution of habitual acts automatic, but goals or intentions themselves can be activated by environmental stimuli. Thus, these authors suggest that the 'environment can directly activate a goal, and this goal can then become operative and guide cognitive and behavioural processes within that environment, all without any need or role for conscious decision-making' (Bargh and Barndollar 1996: 462). For example, when people have formed implementation intentions which specify the when, where and how of a goal-directed action, they have passed the control of their behaviour to the environment and switched from conscious, deliberative control of their goal-directed behaviour to being automatically controlled by the selected situational cues (Gollwitzer 1999).

What are the conditions under which behaviour becomes habitual? The two conditions emphasized by most authors are frequency of behaviour and stability of context (Bargh and Barndollar 1996; Ouelette and Wood 1998; Verplanken and Aarts 1999). Behaviour becomes habitual if it is performed frequently and regularly, and under environmental conditions which are stable. Behaviours are unlikely to become habitual if they are performed only once a year, or if they have to be performed under environmental conditions which are unstable. Once behaviour has become habitual, it should no longer be guided by conscious deliberations which are represented by the formation of intentions and the attitudes, subjective norms or perceived behavioural control on which intentions are based. Ouelette and Wood (1998) therefore hypothesized that such habitual behaviour should be directly related to future behaviour, unmediated by intentions. In contrast, when behaviour is not habitual and requires deliberative thoughts, the impact of past behaviour on future behaviour should be mediated by intentions.

Ouelette and Wood (1998) tested these assumptions in a meta-analysis of studies that included measures of past behaviour in tests of the models of reasoned action or planned behaviour. In line with predictions, measures of past behaviour that were only performed once or twice a year and in unstable contexts were much poorer predictors of future behaviour than intentions. In contrast, past behaviours which were performed regularly and in stable contexts were much stronger predictors of future behaviour than were measures of intentions.

These findings were confirmed in a study of choice of travel mode by Verplanken et al. (1998). The study was conducted in a small village and

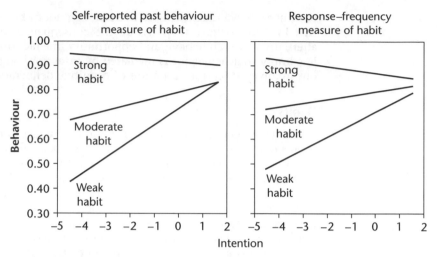

Figure 2.5 The relationship between intention and behaviour by habit strength.
Source: Verplanken *et al.* (1998).

the target behaviour was the choice of car for travelling outside the village rather than alternative travel options. Habits were measured in addition to the determinants of behaviour incorporated in the model of planned behaviour. The study is particularly interesting because in addition to assessing self-reported past behaviour (SPB) as a measure of habit strength, it also used a newly developed response–frequency measure (RF). To assess habits in the use of travel modes (e.g. car, bus, bicycle, airplane) with this measure, research participants were presented with a number of locations for trips and had to indicate how they would travel to these locations. Habit strength for a given mode of travel was reflected by the proportion of times this mode had been chosen. Thus, habitual car users would decide to go everywhere by car. Behaviour was assessed through a diary in which individuals had to list their travel destinations and modes of travel for a three-week period. In line with predictions, habit and intention interacted to influence behaviour (Figure 2.5). As we can see from Figure 2.5, which presents the simple regression slopes of intention on behaviour for participants with weak, moderate and strong habits, this effect emerged for both measures of habit strength. Intention was a significant predictor of behaviour when habit was weak. However, when habit was very strong, the predictive power of intention decreased. In other words, for individuals who habitually went almost everywhere by car, behavioural intention became a poor predictor of their choice of travel mode.

Habits and the prediction of behaviour

Does one have to conclude from these findings that rational reasoning models such as protection motivation theory or the model of planned behaviour should not be applied to behaviours that have become habitual?

In addressing this question one has to distinguish between two aspects of these models, namely process and prediction. Rational reasoning models of action are process as well as predictive models. They outline how behavioural responses are guided by conscious intentions which in turn reflect attitudes towards this behaviour, subjective norms and perceived behavioural control. From this perspective, attitudes, subjective norms and control perceptions are linked to behaviour through their effects on behavioural intentions (Eagly and Chaiken 1993; Ouelette and Wood 1998). This description of the action process is invalid for habitual actions which are cued directly by recurring features of the environment.

The automatic instigation and execution of habitual behaviour is in some aspects similar to the spontaneous processing or MODE model suggested by Fazio (1990; Fazio and Towles-Schwen 1999). According to this model, the attitude-to-behaviour sequence is initiated when attitudes are accessed from memory by the presentation of cues related to the attitude objects. The likelihood of such automatic activation of the attitude upon mere observation of the attitude object is a function of the accessibility of the attitude. The accessibility or ease of recall of an attitude will depend on the strength of the association that exists in memory between the attitude object and the individual's evaluation of the object. Only if the evaluation is strongly associated with the object is it likely that the evaluation will be activated spontaneously upon observation of the attitude object. If the association between object and evaluation is weak, the automatic attitude-to-behaviour sequence will not occur. Because there is some evidence that attitudes are highly accessible in domains of habitual behaviour (Verplanken and Aarts 1999), spontaneous processing may facilitate the instigation of habitual behaviour sequences even though the influence of spontaneous processing is not restricted to habitual behaviour sequences.

The fact that rational reasoning models of behaviour have become less valid as process models for response sequences which have become habitual and thus relatively automatic does not imply that these models are also invalid as a predictive model. After all, habitual behaviours were once controlled consciously. Therefore, we must have once held attitudes, norms, and control beliefs which were in line with the behaviour. Furthermore, when asked about our attitudes, subjective norms and intentions with regard to habitual behaviour, we are likely to base our inferences partly on our perception of this behaviour (Bem 1965). For example, if asked whether they are intending to have a shower the following morning, individuals who shower regularly are likely to answer in the affirmative, even though this behaviour is automatic and no longer regulated by conscious intentions. One would therefore expect intentions to be good predictors even of habitual behaviour, unless individuals are just in the process of trying to break their habits. It is puzzling that this assumption has not been supported by the findings of Verplanken and colleagues (1998) described earlier.

Under conditions where habits conflict with intentions, intentions and attitudes become poor predictors of behaviour. Under these conditions control beliefs will be the most valid predictors of behaviour, because they reflect the individual's assessment of the extent to which he or she has control over a given behaviour. Thus, in a study of alcoholics who attended psychotherapy to give up alcohol, Jonas (1995) found perceived behavioural control to be the best predictor of therapy success.

The breaking of habits: implications for interventions

The fact that habitual behaviours are instigated and executed more or less automatically, without the individual consciously intending or choosing this behaviour, has implications for interventions aimed at changing the behaviour. First, there is some evidence to suggest that the existence of strong habits makes individuals less interested in attending to information relevant to the habitual behaviour (Verplanken and Aarts 1999). But even if a persuasive communication succeeds in inducing individuals to form the intention to change a habitual behaviour, they are likely to experience difficulties in acting on this decision. These difficulties might merely be due to the fact that the individual has to remember consciously to control the behaviour sequences which have previously been enacted automatically. Even though the joke of the bus driver who stops at every bus stop when she takes her family shopping in the family car is probably exaggerated, most of us will have experienced situations where we walked to the old address of friends even though we knew they had moved, or dialled an old telephone number even though we were well aware of the new number.

In these cases we merely have to remember to replace a habitual sequence of behaviour by an alternative sequence. Breaking habits is likely to be even more difficult if there is no alternative sequence to replace the old one. For example, individuals who want to stop smoking, to reduce their alcohol consumption, or to eat less have to interrupt a given sequence of behaviour without being able to replace it by an alternative set of responses. According to Mandler (1975), the interruption of an integrated response sequence produces a state of arousal that, in the absence of certain alternative responses (completion or substitution), develops into an emotional expression which could often be anxiety. Furthermore, in the case of appetitive behaviours, attempts at consciously interrupting the habitual sequence of events might give rise to urges and cravings (Tiffany 1990). Dieters might be unable to ban the thought of food, just as smokers cannot avoid thinking about cigarettes. Furthermore, in cases of addictive behaviour such as smoking or drinking too much alcohol, nicotine or alcohol deprivation is likely to result in physiological reactions which impair normal functioning. Thus, for interventions to be successful, we not only have to persuade individuals to stop smoking, or to reduce their consumption of alcohol, we also have to teach them to break the link that associates their behaviour with the environmental and internal stimulus conditions which trigger and support it.

SUMMARY AND CONCLUSIONS

The first part of this chapter discussed the conditions under which attitudes are related to behaviour and stressed the need for measures of attitude and behaviour which are both reliable and compatible. The second part of the chapter discussed models of behaviour from health and social psychology. The health belief model and protection motivation theory identified five determinants of health behaviour. According to these theories, individuals are likely to engage in health protective behaviour if they perceive a *health threat* which appears *serious*, and if they feel able to *perform some action* that is likely to *alleviate* the health threat and that is *not too effortful or costly*. The theory of reasoned action assumes that the performance or non-performance of a given behaviour depends on one's intention to perform the behaviour. Behavioural intentions are in turn determined by one's attitude towards performing the behaviour and by subjective norms. Thus, the beliefs that losing weight would lead to a number of consequences which are positively valued (attitude) and that friends, family members and/or one's partner would prefer one to lose weight (subjective norms) are likely to result in the intention to lose weight.

All these models are theories of motivation that describe the factors influencing the formation of behavioural intentions. However, even though intentions are important determinants of behaviour, actual performance depends also on other factors, such as ability, skills, information, opportunity and factors which are collectively referred to as 'will-power' (i.e. the ability to maintain one's motivation during the execution of an intention). The concept of perceived behavioural control is used as a summary index of all internal and external factors that might thwart our intentions. According to the model of planned behaviour, our intention to lose weight will be a function of perceived behavioural control over weight loss as well as of our attitude towards losing weight and our beliefs about the shape important others want us to have. Perceived lack of control with regard to weight loss could be due to perceived low self-efficacy (e.g. I will never be able to control myself), low outcome expectancy (e.g. even if I eat less, I will never lose any weight) and external influences (e.g. how can I lose when I have to attend several business lunches every week?).

These expectancy–value models are rational reasoning models of action which assume that behaviours are guided by conscious intentions. This is unlikely to apply to well-practised behaviours in stable environments which are likely to be cued directly by recurring features of the environment. However, the fact that the models of reasoned action and planned behaviour become invalid as process models does not imply that they also lose their power to be predictive of behaviour.

It is uneconomical to entertain specific theories of health behaviour such as the health belief model or protection motivation theory, unless the predictive success of these specific models is greater than that of general models such as the theory of planned behaviour. It is also unlikely that these specific models will do better in predicting behaviour than the theory of planned behaviour, because all the components of the specific model can be integrated into the more general theory of planned behaviour. Thus, an individual's attitude towards continuing to smoke will be the sum of the products of the positive (e.g. weight control, pleasure) and negative consequences of smoking, each weighted by its valence. Individual perceptions of susceptibility to lung cancer as well as the severity of lung cancer would therefore enter into this attitude. The attitude toward stopping, on the other hand, would reflect the perceived costs of stopping as well as beliefs about the efficacy of smoking cessation in preventing lung cancer. The concept of perceived behavioural control, as one of three determinants of intention in the theory of planned behaviour, incorporates perceived self-efficacy as well as outcome expectancies. Finally, the model also considers subjective norms which have no place in the health belief model but might be important determinants of health behaviour such as smoking or weight loss.

FURTHER READING

Ajzen, I. (1988) *Attitudes, Personality and Behavior*. Milton Keynes: Open University Press. A very readable account of the conditions under which attitudes predict behaviour. Discusses the principles of aggregation and compatibility as well as the theories of reasoned action and planned behaviour.

Conner, M. and Norman, P. (eds) (1996) *Predicting Health Behaviour*. Buckingham: Open University Press. Contains excellent and detailed descriptions of the different models of health behaviour and comprehensive reviews of health psychological research conducted to test these models. Particularly relevant are the chapters on the health belief model (Sheeran and Abraham), protection motivation theory (Boer and Seydel) and the theory of planned behaviour (Conner and Sparks).

Eagly, A.H. and Chaiken, S. (1993) *The Psychology of Attitudes*. Fort Worth, TX: Harcourt Brace Jovanovich. Still the most comprehensive and authoritative review of the social psychology of attitudes. Chapters 1 (the nature of attitudes) and 4 (the impact of attitudes on behaviours) are most relevant to the material discussed in this chapter.

Verplanken, B. and Aarts, H. (1999) Habit, attitude, planned behaviour: is habit an empty construct or an interesting case of goal directed automaticity?, in W. Stroebe and M. Hewstone (eds) *European Review of Social Psychology*, Vol. 10. Chichester: Wiley. An excellent discussion of the role of habits as determinants of behaviour. The chapter also discusses how the habit concept could be integrated into models such as the theory of planned behaviour.

THREE

BEYOND PERSUASION: THE MODIFICATION OF HEALTH BEHAVIOUR

If we accept estimates like those from the Centers for Disease Control (1980) and McGinnis and Foege (1993) that more than 40 per cent of the mortality from the ten leading causes of death in the USA is due to modifiable lifestyle factors, health promotion offers challenging opportunities to social psychologists. During the last decade, there has been great progress in social psychological understanding of processes of persuasion, attitude and behaviour change (for reviews see Eagly and Chaiken 1993; Chaiken *et al.* 1996b; Petty *et al.* 1997), and health promotion would constitute a worthwhile field of application of this knowledge. Social psychologists should help to design mass media campaigns to inform people of the health hazards involved in smoking, drinking too much alcohol, eating a fatty diet, failing to exercise and other behaviours that are detrimental to their health, and to persuade them to change their lifestyles.

Unfortunately, persuasion is often not enough to achieve lasting changes in health behaviour. For example, even though the first report in which the US Surgeon General pointed out the health hazards of smoking had a considerable impact on smoking behaviour, particularly among males, many of the people who still smoke would like to give it up but do not succeed in doing so. Survey data show that about one-third of all current smokers make an attempt to stop at least once per year and that only one-fifth of these succeed in any single attempt (Centers for Disease Control 1994). Although there is probably no harm in reminding these smokers of the damage they are continuing to do to their health, what most of them need is help not only in quitting but also in staying off cigarettes.

THE NATURE OF CHANGE

Before we approach the main topic of this chapter, namely strategies of attitude and behaviour change, we have to clarify whether to conceive of change as movement along a continuum or a progression through qualitatively different stages. The models discussed so far view the process of health behaviour change as movement along a continuum. To predict behaviour, these theories combine the assumed determinants of behaviour in an algebraic equation assuming that the numerical value of the equation locates the individual on a single continuum that indicates the probability of action. Any intervention that increases the value of the prediction equation is presumed to enhance the prospects for behaviour change (Weinstein and Sandman 1992).

The example of smoking presented earlier is more in line with stage theories of change. These theories propose that health behaviour change involves progression through discernible stages from ignorance of a health threat to completed preventive action. The different stages are assumed to represent qualitatively different patterns of behaviour, beliefs and experience, and factors which produce transitions between stages vary, depending on the specific stage transitions being considered. Consistent with this view, our example of smoking implied that there are at least two qualitatively different stages in the modification of health behaviour. The first involves the *formation of an intention* to change. Individuals have to be informed of the health hazards of certain behaviours and to be persuaded to change. However, even if people accept a health recommendation and form the firm intention to change, they are likely to experience difficulty in *acting* on these intentions over any length of time. Thus, a second stage involves teaching people how to change and how to maintain this change. Whereas the first stage of this process can be most effectively achieved through persuasion or other social psychological procedures of social influence, with behaviour such as substance abuse or excessive eating clinical intervention may sometimes be needed at the second stage.

This simple stage model allows one also to illustrate the important characteristics of stage models, namely that people at different points in the process of changing their behaviour are confronted with different problems, that they use different strategies to deal with these problems, and that different types of interventions are therefore needed to influence them. Stage models offer a systematic analysis of the different problems which confront individuals as they move from being unaware of a health problem to taking action and maintaining it. Two stage theories will be presented, namely the precaution adoption process model of Weinstein (1988; Weinstein and Sandman 1992) and the transtheoretical model of behaviour change (e.g. Prochaska *et al.* 1992).

Precaution adoption process model

The precaution adoption process model of Weinstein (1988; Weinstein and Sandman 1992) was originally developed as a dynamic version of the health belief model and of protection motivation theory. I will present here the most recent version of the model (Weinstein and Sandman 1992).

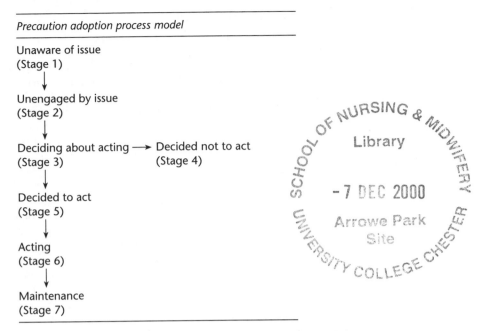

Precaution adoption process model

Unaware of issue
(Stage 1)

↓

Unengaged by issue
(Stage 2)

↓

Deciding about acting ——► Decided not to act
(Stage 3)   (Stage 4)

↓

Decided to act
(Stage 5)

↓

Acting
(Stage 6)

↓

Maintenance
(Stage 7)

Figure 3.1   Stages of the precaution adoption process model.

The model

The starting point for this model is the individual who is unaware of a given health risk, either out of personal ignorance or because the risk is as yet generally unknown (Stage 1). Examples for the latter are the risk of HIV infection before 1980, but also the dangers involved in smoking before anti-smoking campaigns started in 1964. When people first learn about some issue, they are no longer unaware of the risk, but they may not really be concerned by this knowledge either (Stage 2). However, further communication from friends or the mass media may convince them that the risk is really a serious one and that they are personally at risk. This would move them to Stage 3 of the precaution adoption process, the stage at which decisions are being considered. This decision-making process can result in the decision either not to take action or to take action. If the individual decides not to take action, the precaution adoption process ends, or at least it ends for this particular point in time. This outcome represents a separate stage (Stage 4), although not a stage along the route to action. If people have decided to adopt a precaution (Stage 5), the following step is to initiate action (Stage 6). Stimulated by the transtheoretical model of behaviour change, Weinstein and colleagues added a 'maintenance' stage (Stage 7) to indicate repetitions that may be required after a preventive action has first been performed. Whereas with lifestyle change such as adopting physical exercise or stopping smoking, maintaining the new behaviour is essential, there are other precautions, such as buying a burglar alarm or having asbestos removed from one's home, where actions need not be continued.

Evaluation of the model

One strength of the model is that it offers a systematic analysis of the factors which influence people as they move from stage to stage. For example, reading about some previously unknown risk factor should be important in moving people through the first two stages, but information which makes personal vulnerability salient (e.g. a health scare) and outlines some effective remedy should be most important in determining whether someone will adopt the precautionary action (move from Stage 3 to 5). Finally, the presence of situational obstacles and constraints should be most important when intentions have to be translated into action (Stages 5 and 6).

However, the precaution adoption process model has not stimulated a great deal of published research (Weinstein and Sandman 1992; Blalock *et al.* 1996). In one of the few applications to health issues, Blalock and colleagues (1996) studied stages in the adoption of health behaviours that protect individuals against the risk of developing osteoporosis, a disorder characterized by decreased bone mass and increased susceptibility to fracture from which women are most at risk. Two behaviours are recommended to reduce the risk of developing osteoporosis, namely calcium consumption and weight-bearing exercise. Participants in this cross-sectional study were 620 women between the ages of 35 and 45 years. They were sent a questionnaire assessing their precaution adoption stage with regard to both calcium consumption and exercise, and measuring the variables assumed by the model as predictors for the various stages. Examples of these predictor variables were health motivation, barriers against exercising or eating calcium-rich food, self-efficacy and osteoporosis knowledge.

Findings indicated that most of these predictor variables significantly discriminated between respondents in the relevant stages. For example, in line with theoretical expectations, the level of individual self-efficacy with regard to exercising was highest for individuals in Stages 6 and 7 who were currently exercising, lower in Stages 4 and 5 who were contemplating action, and lowest in Stages 1 to 3. Similar patterns were observed for most predictors and both kinds of health precautions.

Although findings like this are consistent with the stage model suggested by Weinstein and his colleagues, they are not actually inconsistent with the assumptions underlying continuum models such as the models of planned behaviour and reasoned action (Ajzen 1988). For example, since self-efficacy is one of the determinants of the intention to act and of actual behaviour in the model of planned behaviour, this model would also predict that individuals who hold very weak intentions should differ significantly in their self-efficacy regarding this particular behaviour from those who hold strong intentions or those who are actually engaged in this particular behaviour (Weinstein *et al.* 1998).

The transtheoretical model of behaviour change

The model

At present, the transtheoretical model is undoubtedly the most popular stage theory of health behaviour change. It distinguishes five stages of change through which individuals are assumed to move when they change

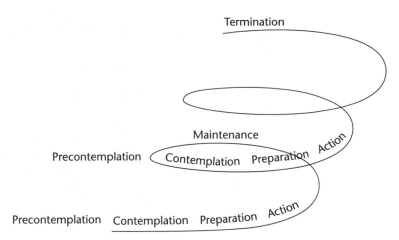

Figure 3.2 A spiral pattern of the stages of change of the transtheoretical model.
Source: Prochaska *et al.* (1992).

a given problem behaviour. Prochaska and his colleagues (e.g. 1992) originally considered change as a linear progression through these stages. Because relapse is the rule rather than the exception, they changed the original conception to assume a spiral pattern. During relapse individuals regress to some earlier stage such as contemplation or even precontemplation. However, it is still assumed that these stages form a simplex pattern in which adjacent stages are more highly correlated with each other than any other stage. The following description of these stages will be based on Prochaska and colleagues (1992).

Precontemplation is the stage at which there is no intention to change behaviour in the foreseeable future. Individuals at this stage are typically not even aware that they have a problem, even though their family or friends might feel that there is a need for them to change. They can be identified by their negative answer to a question about whether they are intending to change the problem behaviour within the next six months. In terms of the precaution adoption process model of Weinstein and Sandman (1992), the precontemplation stage includes both people who have never thought about the desirability of changing and those who have thought about it, but arrived at the conclusion that they do not need or wish to change. For example, there will be few smokers who have never thought about stopping. Some smokers may have even stopped for some time and then decided that the benefits of not smoking were not worth their deprivation. It seems plausible that such people may need different types of arguments and will be more difficult to influence than individuals who never thought about a given health risk.

Contemplation is the stage in which people are aware that a problem exists and are considering doing something about it without having reached a definite decision. There is no commitment to act. A smoker who is at this stage may feel some unease about the potential health damage due to smoking or the impact smoking may have on his family, but he or she will not yet have made the decision to stop. Individuals at this stage weigh the 'pros' and 'cons' of changing their behaviour. Individuals can remain in this stage for long periods of time. Contemplators will indicate that they are seriously considering changing the health-impairing behaviour in the next six months.

Preparation is a stage at which individuals have not only formed a firm intention to change, but have also begun to make small behavioural changes. An example would be a smoker who has formed the intention to stop and has already begun to reduce his or her cigarette consumption, or to delay smoking the first cigarette of the day. Although they have made some reductions in their problem behaviour, they have not yet reached the criterion for effective action such as stopping smoking, or abstaining from drinking alcohol. They usually score high on measures of both contemplation and action.

Action is the stage at which individuals change their behaviour and/ or their environment in order to overcome their problem. Operationally, individuals are classified in the action stage if they have successfully altered their addictive behaviour for a period ranging from one day to six months. Successfully altering addictive behaviour means reaching a particular criterion such as abstinence.

Maintenance is the stage at which individuals expend great effort to prevent relapse and to consolidate the gains made during action. In the case of addictive behaviour, this stage begins at six months following the initial action and continues for an indeterminate period. For some behaviours maintenance can be considered to last for a lifetime.

The transtheoretical model specifies different types of cognitions that are assumed to change and different strategies of change which individuals are assumed to employ when moving through different stages. With regard to types of cognitions, the transtheoretical model borrowed concepts from Janis and Mann (1977) and Bandura (1986). Based on the theoretical ideas of Janis and Mann, it was assumed that individual perceptions of the 'pros' and 'cons' of engaging in a given problem behaviour (decisional balance) would change as individuals moved through the stages (e.g. Velicer *et al.* 1985; Prochaska *et al.* 1994). Following Bandura (1986) it was further assumed that the level of the individual's self-efficacy would be important in the change process. Self-efficacy represents the individuals' level of confidence that they are able to change a given problem behaviour and to maintain this change. The model does not state precisely how these variables relate to stages of change beyond describing them as 'intertwined and interacting variables in the modification of mental and health behaviours'.

The strategies of change reflect the behavioural or cognitive techniques employed by individuals to modify a particular problem behaviour. A list of ten change processes has been developed inductively from a scrutiny of recommended change techniques in systems of psychotherapy (Prochaska *et al.* 1992). The ten strategies of change can be divided into two broad categories. Experiential or cognitive processes include activities related to thinking and experiencing emotion about changing a health-impairing behaviour (consciousness raising, self-evaluation, dramatic relief, environmental re-evaluation, and social liberation). Behavioural processes are categories of behaviour which are assumed to be helpful for changing this behaviour (counterconditioning, stimulus control, reinforcement management, self-liberation and helping relationships). Whether individuals really use these strategies in modifying problem behaviour, and whether the sets of techniques and methods assumed on the basis of the conceptual analysis to reflect a given change process really form a coherent scale, was then investigated empirically in a number of different samples (e.g. Prochaska and DiClemente 1983; Prochaska *et al.* 1988).

Evaluation of the model

There are three lines of evidence used to support the transtheoretical model (Budd and Rollnick 1996). The first line claims support for the hypothesis that individuals move through *each* of the various stages. With the development of questionnaires measuring individual stages of change, it has become possible to assess this assumption. Thus McConnaughy and colleagues (McConnaughy *et al.* 1983, 1989) claim to have demonstrated that scores of adjacent stages of change were more highly correlated than were scores for stages that were non-adjacent. However, this conclusion has recently been challenged by Sutton (1996) who argued that the correlation between non-adjacent stages was often *nearly* as high as that for adjacent stages. Further evidence inconsistent with the assumption that there is an 'orderly' progression through each of the stages has been reported by Budd and Rollnick (1996). Using a newly constructed Readiness to Change Questionnaire on a sample of men with drinking problems, the authors found that adding a direct path in their structural equation model between precontemplation and action fitted their data better than the structure assumed by the stage model. This finding is inconsistent with the assumption that individuals can only move to action via the contemplation stage.

The second line of argument offered in support of the transtheoretical model claims that in different stages individuals employ different strategies of change. In a review of this research, Prochaska and colleagues (1992) reported that individuals in the contemplation stage were most open to consciousness-raising techniques, and also tended to re-evaluate the effects of their addictive behaviour on their environment, especially on the people with whom they were closest. Successful action and maintenance, on the other hand, entailed effective use of behavioural processes such as counterconditioning, stimulus control and reinforcement management, but also support and understanding from helping relationships (Prochaska and DiClemente 1983; Prochaska *et al.* 1991).

Although data from cross-sectional studies tend to support this assumption (e.g. Prochaska *et al.* 1991), a recent longitudinal study of smoking cessation failed to find support for this type of progression (Herzog 1999). This study used data collected as part of a larger study of worksite cancer prevention from 600 smokers who completed a baseline and two annual follow-up surveys. Cross-sectional results replicated previous findings with virtually all the processes of change increasing in a linear fashion from precontemplation to preparation. However, when strategies of change at baseline were used to predict stage movement prospectively no support was found for the transtheoretical model. None of the strategies of change measured at baseline was significantly related to progressive change out of the precontemplation or contemplation stages at the follow-up measurements one and two years later.

Decisional balance has also been related to stages of change (Velicer *et al.* 1985). In a cross-sectional study of the relationship between stages of change and decisional balance across 12 problem behaviours Prochaska and colleagues (1994) reported clear commonalities. Thus, for all 12 problem behaviours the 'cons' of changing the behaviour were higher than the 'pros' for respondents in the precontemplation stage, whereas the reverse was true for respondents in the action stage. Similarly, in a prospective study of a sample of smokers, decisional balance scores allowed the prediction of movements from contemplation to other stages (Velicer *et al.* 1985). Contemplators who saw the advantages of stopping smoking outweighing the disadvantages were most likely to move to action and were found to be more likely to have given up smoking six months later, whereas contemplators with the reverse balance were more likely to have moved back to precontemplation status. However, these findings were not replicated by Herzog and colleagues (1999).

Because the pro and con statements reflect beliefs about the perceived advantages and disadvantages of changing the problem behaviour, the difference between the number of pro and con statements endorsed by individuals forms a crude measure of their attitude. Thus the relationship observed between stages and change and decisional balance may merely indicate a positive relationship between individuals' attitudes towards changing a given problem behaviour and their intention to do so. In line with this assumption, Kraft *et al.* (1997) reported from a study of a sample of smokers that intention to try to stop smoking increased linearly with an increase in cons and decreased linearly with an increase in pros. Furthermore, although the measure of stages was significantly related to the measure of pro and cons when entered individually, this effect disappeared when intention was entered first into the regression analysis.

In conclusion, the transtheoretical model of behaviour change focuses on a number of interesting variables which, except for self-efficacy, have previously been neglected in research on health behaviour. The weakness of the model is that it does not allow the derivation of theoretically based predictions about the relationship between the different variables. So far as there is any knowledge about the relationship between stages and processes of change, it has been derived empirically and is of a correlational nature. Furthermore, research guided by this model has not yet resulted in consistent support of the model.

Implications of stage model for interventions

The major implication for interventions to be derived from stage models of change is that the nature of the interventions has to be matched to the stage of change of the target individuals. For example, information about the health consequences associated with a given health-impairing behaviour is most likely to be effective for individuals who are in a precontemplation or contemplation stage. Once a decision to act has been taken, action- or maintenance-oriented information, for example information which enhances the self-efficacy of the individual with regard to changing the behaviour, is likely to be more effective.

There is limited systematic evidence with regard to these hypotheses. In one of the few published studies, Dijkstra *et al.* (1996) tested some of these predictions in a longitudinal field experiment with a sample of just over 1000 smokers who were given information matched to their stage of change. In a pre-test, these smokers had to assign themselves to one of four stages of change on the basis of descriptions of these stages. The authors added a stage to the original stage model, by dividing precontemplators into 'immotives' who were not considering changing within the next five years, and 'precontemplators' who were considering stopping in less than five years. Smokers in each of the four stages of change were then randomly assigned to one of four information conditions:

- information about the health consequences of smoking;
- self-efficacy enhancing information about how to stop smoking;
- both types of information combined; and
- a control condition with no information.

The post-test questionnaire sent 12 weeks after these communications assessed intentions to stop, changes in stage, attempts to stop for 24 hours, and refraining for more than seven days from smoking.

The authors predicted that the immotives should be most affected by information about health consequences, precontemplators and contemplators by the combined information condition, and preparers by the self-efficacy information without information about health consequences. Three outcome measures were assessed, namely forward transition from one stage to the next, intention to stop, and actual cessation for at least seven days. Impact was assessed for each of the different stages by comparing the effect of the matched messages against the 'No information' control condition and by inferring the relative effectiveness from whether or not a given difference reached significance. The authors claim that their findings were fairly consistent with their predictions. Immotives were the only group benefiting from the health consequences information only. Precontemplators benefited most from self-efficacy enhancing information only, contemplators from the combination of both kinds of information, and preparers most from self-efficacy-enhancing information. However, only for the preparers could these effects be observed for all three dependent measures. For the other groups, the impact of matched messages was restricted to stage transitions.

In a later publication of these data, Dijkstra *et al.* (1998b) reported a more appropriate analysis in which they compared smokers who received communications that matched the stage they had reached with smokers who received a communication that did not match their stage of change. For immotives and precontemplators the matched communications were no more effective than the mismatched ones. However, for the contemplators and preparers combined, the matched communications proved to be marginally more effective with regard to stage transitions than the messages which were mismatched.

Matching the arguments in a communication to the stage of change of the target individual is only one way in which information can be tailored to individual characteristics. Once the information about individual characteristics has been collected through interviews or questionnaires, the communication can be personalized in many ways and made to appear, and actually to be, more relevant to the individual. Since the tailoring can be done by computer, this procedure can be used as a public health strategy (Dijkstra and de Vries 1999). The effectiveness of this type of tailoring will be discussed in the review of research on the change of specific health behaviours (p. 97).

Conclusions

Stage models describe the different tasks assumed to confront individuals at different stages of behaviour change and the types of intervention which would induce these individuals to move to the next stage. They thus offer an interesting heuristic framework for the design of interventions and for the tailoring of interventions to particular target populations, and they also help us to understand why some mismatched interventions fail to have any impact (e.g. giving information on health consequences to individuals in the action stage or giving self-help manuals to precontemplators). However, the kind of tailoring of communications suggested by these models often requires an individualized matching of communications based on personal information. It would therefore be important to know whether giving the mismatched information *in addition* to the matched information (i.e. the combined information) has substantial negative effects. If adding the mismatched to the matched communication does not *reduce* the impact of the matched information, matching of components to individual characteristics of the target population may not be essential.

Although the evidence presented in this section indicates that for purposes of research it is often important to divide the continuum of change into several different stages, discussion in the remainder of this chapter will be structured in terms of the simple distinction into two stages introduced earlier, namely the formation of intentions and their realization. This distinction is not being proposed here as a stage theory, but is used as a heuristic device to structure the discussion of change. Whereas the processes that motivate change and aim at the formation of an intention to change a given health behaviour can be subsumed under the public health model which relies on strategies of health promotion, clinical interventions may be needed to help individuals to change health-impairing behaviours such as excessive eating, smoking, or alcohol abuse. Thus, sometimes it may be necessary to employ therapy to teach individuals the skills they need to act on their intentions.

THE PUBLIC HEALTH MODEL

The term 'public health model' is used here to refer to interventions that rely on health promotion and are designed to change the behaviour of large groups, such as the members of an industrial organization, or the citizens of a state or country (Leventhal and Cleary 1980). The objective of this type of health promotion is primary prevention, that is, to induce people to adopt good health habits and to change bad ones. There are basically two ways to effect this change, namely through *persuasion* and through *modification of relevant incentives*.

Persuasion is used in health promotion to influence individual health beliefs and behaviour. People are exposed to more or less complex messages that reflect a position advocated by a source and arguments designed to support that position. The source may be a medical expert or a public health institute and the message may point out that a specific unhealthy practice such as overeating or leading a sedentary life is likely to result in a number of very unpleasant health consequences.

Modification of relevant incentives is often employed as a health promotion strategy to increase the effort or costs of engaging in certain unhealthy practices or to decrease the costs of healthful practices. Thus governments may use fiscal and legal measures to alter the contingencies affecting individuals as they drink, smoke or engage in other health-damaging behaviour. Often persuasion and incentive modification strategies are combined. Thus a health promotion campaign aimed at preventing alcoholism might involve mass media messages pointing out the dangers of alcoholism, worksite health promotion programmes, and changes in incentives such as an increase in the tax on alcohol or a legal restriction on the sale of alcoholic beverages.

A third health promotion strategy relies on passive protection through the regulation of product designs or the engineering of the physical environment to make it safer. However, this strategy is of less interest in the context of a book on social psychology and health and will therefore only be mentioned briefly. The main focus of our discussion in this section on the public health model will be on persuasion and modification of incentives.

Persuasion

Persuasion can be defined as the effects of exposure to relatively complex messages from other persons on the attitudes and beliefs of the recipients. Research has studied the impact of characteristics of the communicator, the message or the recipient on influencing attitude change. Before highlighting empirical research on persuasion in laboratory and field settings, a brief theoretical analysis of persuasion will be presented. This should improve understanding of the processes or variables which mediate the impact of communications on beliefs and attitudes.

Theories of persuasion

Although theories of persuasion typically incorporate motivational and affective principles, most of the more recent theories have been based on a cognitive analysis of persuasion processes. In the decades following

World War II persuasion research has been dominated by an information-processing paradigm that emphasized reception and learning of the arguments contained in persuasive messages (e.g. Hovland *et al*. 1959; McGuire 1985). This perspective stimulated a great deal of interest in the relationship between recipients' retention of the message content and the extent to which they were influenced by a message (see Eagly and Chaiken 1993). However, the findings that emerged from this type of research seemed to be inconsistent with the notion that attitude change was a function of the reception and learning of the arguments contained in the persuasive message (although see Eagly and Chaiken 1993: 264).

This confronted researchers with a puzzling problem. If it was not the actual content of the arguments which resulted in persuasion, how then do persuasive communications influence beliefs and change attitudes? One answer to this question was provided by the *cognitive response theory* developed by Greenwald (1968) and refined by Petty, Cacioppo and others (see Petty *et al*. 1981b). The cognitive response approach stresses the mediating role of the thoughts or 'cognitive responses' which recipients generate as they reflect upon persuasive communications. According to this model, listening to a communication is like a mental discussion in which the listener responds to the arguments presented in the communication. Cognitive responses reflect the content of this internal communication. The model assumes that these cognitive responses mediate the effect of persuasive messages on attitude change. Since cognitive responding is assumed to vary both in magnitude and favourableness, persuasion should be a function of the *extent* of cognitive responding that occurs as well as its *favourableness*.

The extent to which individuals engage in argument-relevant thinking is determined by their processing motivation and ability. The more motivated and able individuals are to think about the arguments contained in a communication, the more they will engage in argument-relevant thinking. Whether increases in processing ability or motivation increase or decrease the persuasive impact of a communication will depend on the favourableness of individual responses to the communication. The favourableness of cognitive responses depends mainly on the quality of the arguments contained in a communication. A persuasive communication which contains many strong arguments will stimulate predominantly positive thoughts whereas a communication containing weak arguments will elicit unfavourable cognitive responses. With strong arguments stimulating favourable thoughts, increases in processing motivation and/or ability should result in an increased persuasion. With weak arguments eliciting unfavourable thoughts, increased motivation or ability to engage in argument-relevant thinking will decrease the persuasive impact of the communication.

These predictions have been tested in numerous experiments (see Eagly and Chaiken 1993). The impact of processing motivation on persuasion has typically been studied by manipulating the personal relevance of the topic of the communication. Consistent with prediction, increasing the personal relevance of a communication resulted in decreased persuasion for communications containing mainly weak arguments, but increased persuasion for messages which consisted of strong arguments (Chaiken 1980; Petty *et al*. 1981a).

The impact of processing ability or capacity has often been studied through the use of distraction. Distracting individuals while they are listening to a message should decrease their ability to process the message. Petty *et al.* (1976) manipulated distraction by having respondents record visual stimuli while listening to a message. The degree of distraction was varied by the frequency with which the stimuli flashed on a screen. The favourableness of respondents' cognitive responses was manipulated by using either very strong or very weak arguments. In line with expectations from cognitive response theory, distraction increased persuasion for weak messages and decreased persuasion for strong messages. Furthermore, an analysis of the thoughts which respondents reported having had during the communication indicated that distraction inhibited the number of counter-arguments to the message which contained weak arguments and reduced the number of favourable thoughts for the version consisting of strong arguments. Capacity may also be low because the individual possesses little knowledge about the topic in question (Wood *et al.* 1985) or is under time pressure (Ratneshwar and Chaiken 1991).

The cognitive response model shares with the earlier information processing theories the assumption that individuals who listen to a communication systematically evaluate the arguments contained in the communication to arrive at a decision about the validity of any conclusions or recommendations given. However, individuals sometimes may not be motivated or able to evaluate an argument and still want to form an opinion on the validity of a recommended action.

The *dual-process models* of persuasion which have recently dominated persuasion research, namely the elaboration likelihood model (e.g. Petty and Cacioppo 1986) and the heuristic–systematic model (e.g. Chaiken 1980; Chaiken *et al.* 1996), suggest that the kind of systematic processing implied by the cognitive response model is only one of two different modes of information processing that mediate persuasion. If individuals are either unwilling or unable to engage in this extensive and effortful process of assessing arguments, they might base their decision to accept or reject the message on some peripheral aspect such as the credibility of the source, the length of the message or other non-content cues. This has been called heuristic processing (Chaiken 1980; Eagly and Chaiken 1993).

In heuristic processing people often use simple schemas or decision rules to assess the validity of an argument. For example, people may have learned from previous experience that health recommendations from physicians tend to be more valid than those from lay persons. They may therefore apply the rule that 'doctors can be trusted with regard to health issues' in response to indications that the communicator is a medical doctor, and agree with the health message. Because the individual agrees with the message without extensive thinking about the content of the arguments, dual-process theories assume that attitudes formed or changed on the basis of heuristic processing will be less stable, less resistant to counter-arguments, and less predictive of subsequent behaviour than those based on systematic processing. In support of these assumptions a number of studies show that attitude change accompanied by high levels of issue-relevant cognitive activity are more persistent than changes that are accompanied by little issue-relevant thought (e.g. Haugvedt and Petty 1992).

A central prediction of dual-process models is that heuristic cues have a greater impact on attitudes than argument quality when motivation or ability to engage in issue-relevant thinking is low, whereas argument quality has a greater impact when motivation or ability to process is high. Experiments manipulating variables which were assumed to affect processing motivation or ability, such as personal relevance, time pressure, message comprehensibility or prior knowledge have also yielded results supportive of the theory. As one would expect, the influence of peripheral cues on attitudes is low when processing ability and motivation is high, but increases substantially when recipients lack the motivation or ability to process the message extensively (e.g. Petty *et al.* 1981a; Wood and Kallgren 1988).

This pattern of finding has typically been explained by assuming that systematic and heuristic processing are mutually exclusive processing modes, with systematic processing being employed when processing motivation and ability are high, and heuristic processing being used when motivation and ability are low (Chaiken 1980; Petty and Cacioppo 1986). However, disregarding peripheral cues because processing motivation is high seems wasteful, given that these cues may contain valid and easily accessible information. Chaiken and her colleagues (e.g. 1996a) have recently developed an alternative conception which implies that heuristic processing is the default option which is always employed in assessing the validity of a persuasive argumentation. Like earlier theoreticians, they argued that individuals need to be economical with their limited processing capacity. Individuals will therefore invest only as much effort into processing a given set of arguments as is warranted by the importance of the issue at hand. Chaiken and her colleagues introduced the notion of a 'sufficiency principle' which reflects a trade-off between minimizing effort and reaching an adequate level of confidence in one's judgement. If an issue is of no great importance (e.g. low personal relevance), individuals will require not a great deal of confidence. They will invest little effort and rely solely on heuristic processing, even though heuristic processing is not very effective in creating subjective confidence in the validity of an attitude. With increasing importance of a particular issue the level of subjective confidence desired by the individual will also increase. Therefore individuals will increasingly rely on systematic processing. Even though systematic processing requires greater processing capacity, it is generally more effective in increasing subjective confidence because it provides the individual with more judgement-relevant information than does heuristic processing. Conclusions based on systematic processing typically override the judgemental impact of heuristic processing and, as a result, the impact of heuristic cues is attenuated.

There are two conditions, however, under which individuals will rely on heuristic processing even when highly motivated to process a persuasive message systematically, namely, if their processing capacity is limited or if the information is ambiguous. The impact of processing motivation on systematic processing is limited by processing capacity. Even if individuals are highly motivated to engage in systematic processing of persuasive arguments, they may have to rely on heuristic processing due to low processing capacity. Second, individuals may rely on heuristic cues in their assessment of the validity of a position even after extensive systematic processing, if the persuasive arguments are so ambiguous that systematic processing does not result in clear-cut conclusions (Chaiken and Maheswaran 1994).

Implicit in our discussion so far has been the assumption that individual information processing is motivated by the desire to hold attitudes and beliefs that are objectively valid. Chaiken and her colleagues (e.g. 1996a) have modified the heuristic–systematic model to incorporate motives other than the need to be accurate. Of particular interest for health psychology is defence motivation, which reflects the desire to hold attitudes and beliefs that are consistent with existing central attitudes and values, for example the belief that one is healthy and safe. Defence motivation leads to a directional bias in accepting a given attitudinal position. Both systematic and heuristic processing might be employed in a biased way. Within the systematic mode, selective processing involves the biased evaluation of evidence and arguments. Material that is congruent with existing self-relevant beliefs, such as research supporting one's position on some issue important to one's self-definition, will be more easily accepted than incongruent material. Individuals are likely to read incongruent evidence more carefully and spend more time disproving it than they will with arguments that are congruent with the position they wish to defend. Within the heuristic mode, biased processing might be achieved by questioning the reliability or validity of a heuristic if it leads to conclusions that challenge the validity of a preferred position. For example, even if a patient usually follows the heuristic that 'doctors can be trusted with regard to health issues', when receiving a particular threatening diagnosis, the patient may introduce an additional heuristic, namely that one should always consult several experts before making important decisions.

To summarize, during recent years dual-process models have undergone a theoretical evolution which dramatically changed the assumptions underlying these models. Thus, the assumption that the two modes of information processing are alternatives, with one (heuristic processing) being employed when individuals are unmotivated or unable to engage in issue-relevant thinking and the other (systematic processing) when motivation and ability are high, has been replaced by the assumption that the two modes co-occur. Heuristic processing is assumed to serve as a default option. When individuals are motivated to use systematic processing because an issue is important, systematic processing typically overrides the impact of heuristic processing, unless individuals are unable to process systematically (due to capacity limitations or lack of knowledge) or the evidence is so ambiguous that they have to base their conclusions on heuristic cues. Second, the assumption that individuals always strive for accurate judgements has been replaced by the assumption that communications can arouse different processing motives (e.g. defence motivation rather than accuracy motivation).

The impact of persuasion

The major difficulty in persuading people to engage in healthful behaviour patterns is that they involve immediate effort or renunciation of gratification in the here and now in order to achieve greater rewards or to avoid worse punishment in the remote future. As religious leaders discovered centuries ago, when facing similar (or even worse) problems, fear appeals can be an effective way of achieving compliance. Today, fear or threat appeals are the mainstay of most mass media health promotion campaigns. These appeals frequently combine information that is fear-arousing with information that provokes a sense of personal vulnerability to the illness threat, because in order to arouse fear, a health risk must not only have serious consequences but the individual must also feel personally at risk. For example, even though HIV infection has very serious consequences, these consequences will not be fear-arousing to those heterosexuals who consider AIDS to be a disease which only affects homosexuals and drug users. Fear appeals are usually followed by some recommendation that, if accepted, would reduce or avoid the danger. The effectiveness of fear appeals has been studied extensively (for reviews, see Sutton 1982; Boster and Mongeau 1984). Because much of persuasion-based health promotion employs fear appeals, the following section on laboratory research on persuasion will discuss the effectiveness of this kind of persuasive appeal.

Persuasion in the laboratory: the case of fear appeals

In a typical early study of the impact of fear appeals smokers would be exposed to factual information about the danger of smoking in a low-threat condition. In a high-threat condition, they would in addition be exposed to a film which would make the nature of lung cancer more vivid by including a section on a lung cancer operation, showing the initial incision, the forcing apart of the ribs, and the removal of the black and diseased lung. Under both conditions, a recommendation would be given that these consequences could be avoided if respondents gave up smoking.

Early theoretical paradigms

Early research on fear arousal has been guided theoretically by the assumption that fear is a drive or motivator of attitude change (for a review of early studies, see Leventhal 1970). The risk information arouses fear which is reduced by the rehearsal of the communicator's recommendations. When a response reduces fear, it is reinforced and becomes part of one's permanent response repertory. The drive model therefore suggests that greater fear should result in greater persuasion, but only if the recommended action appears effective in avoiding the danger. If this is not the case, fear may be reduced by other means such as denying or ignoring the danger or derogating the communicator.

Because part of the empirical evidence was inconsistent with the drive model of fear-arousing communications, Leventhal (1970) developed the parallel response model. This introduced threat appraisal as the important mediator between environmental threat and action and abandoned the notion that emotional arousal is a necessary antecedent of the adaptation to danger. According to this model an environmental threat is cognitively evaluated by the individual and this appraisal can give rise to two parallel or independent processes, namely danger control and fear control. Danger control involves decisions to act as well as instrumental actions the individual performs after having weighed the information about the external threat against information about own coping resources. Information deriving from the emotional reaction to the threat about the need to act or the inability to act provides the cues for fear control. Actions which are in the service of fear control such as avoidance actions (including defences) as well as attempts to control the emotional response (e.g. drinking alcohol, smoking) frequently have no effect on the actual danger.

The important contribution of this model, which, as we shall see later, is structurally similar to stress-coping theory (Chapter 6), is the central role given to cognitive appraisal processes and the differentiation of emotional from cognitive responses to fear-arousing communications. Its weakness is that it does not specify the processes of cognitive evaluation which precede the action tendencies. This task was completed by later models which focused exclusively on cognitive processes. According to the health belief model (e.g. Rosenstock 1974) and to protection motivation theory (e.g. Rogers and Mewborn 1976; Rogers 1983), individuals accept a recommendation if they perceive it as *effective* (effectiveness) in averting *negative* consequences (severity) which would otherwise be *likely to happen to them* (vulnerability). In terms of these models, fear influences attitudes and behaviour not directly, but only indirectly through the appraisal of the severity of the threat. These models suggest that even the most vulnerable individuals would not adopt protective actions which they perceive as ineffective in averting the negative consequences. In addition to response efficacy, the revised version of protection motivation theory also emphasized self-efficacy, that is the person's confidence in his or her ability to enact the protective response. The effect of low self-efficacy should be similar to that of low response efficacy.

The empirical evidence is only partly supportive of the early theoretical interpretations of fear appeals. Consistent with predictions, the vast majority of experiments on the impact of fear or threat appeals have found that higher levels of threat lead to greater persuasion than lower levels (Sutton 1982; Boster and Mongeau 1984). This effect holds for behavioural intentions as well as actual behaviour, but tends to be stronger for intentions. The willingness of recipients to accept a recommendation has also been found to be affected by their perception of the effectiveness of the recommended action in averting a threat. However, although the main effects of perceived effectiveness on intentions to adopt the action have been found in a number of studies (e.g. Chu 1966; Rogers 1985), there is no evidence of any interactions.

Particularly damaging to the health belief and protection motivation theories have been the findings of studies which assessed the predicted effect of vulnerability on individuals' willingness to adopt a protective action. According to the predictions derived from these models, the greater their own vulnerability, the more willing individuals should be to protect themselves against a severe threat. In contrast, empirical studies assessing the impact of vulnerability have typically reported the opposite findings. The earliest study was conducted by Berkowitz and Cottingham (1960) who used fear appeals to motivate drivers to use seat belts. Respondents were subdivided in terms of the amount of driving they did, assuming that individuals who drive a great deal should also perceive themselves as more at risk. In contrast to what one would predict from the above models, the high-fear communication produced increasingly favourable attitudes towards seat belts only among non-drivers. Regular drivers were about equally favourable to the use of seat belts in the high- and low-fear conditions. Similarly, Niles (1964, reported in Leventhal 1970) exposed smokers, who were divided into two groups according to their self-rated vulnerability to lung cancer, to high- and low-fear communications. She found that high-fear communications increased acceptance of recommendations to stop smoking and take X-rays, but only for respondents who scored low on self-rated vulnerability. Respondents who scored high showed essentially no difference between high- and low-fear communications.

The problem with these correlational studies is that outcomes may be determined by other factors which are correlated with vulnerability. Thus, it is quite plausible that individuals who feel vulnerable to lung cancer but continue smoking do so because they have been unable to stop. Similarly, individuals who drive a great deal but do not use seat belts may have little confidence in their ability to buckle up regularly.

A dual-process theory of fear appeals

Interpretations of the impact of fear appeals in terms of dual-process theories focus on information processing as well as persuasive outcomes. As Gleicher and Petty (1992) and Liberman and Chaiken (1992) have argued, fear arousal can have two different effects, either acting as a motivator to induce recipients to engage in intensive (and accurate) message processing, or inducing defence motivation. Because defence motivation will be aroused when self-definitional beliefs are being threatened, one crucial variable in determining the effects of a fear appeal will be the perceived relevance of the threat. However, even if a threat is relevant and severe, it should arouse defence motivation only if individuals feel unable to master or reduce the threat, that is if they feel *vulnerable*. One would therefore predict that the perception of vulnerability to a severe (health) threat induces both fear *and* the motivation to reduce or eliminate the threat. The threat can be reduced or eliminated either by taking action (if an action alternative is available) or through biased thought processes (i.e. defensive processing). The motivation to engage in defensive processing will be the higher, the less the individual feels able to eliminate a severe threat by taking an effective action.

In predicting the impact of defence motivation on information processing and persuasion, it is important to note that the persuasive appeals used in fear communications consist of two parts:

- a *fear appeal* which emphasizes the severity of the threat and individual vulnerability; and
- an *action recommendation* which provides information on how to avoid the health threat.

Individuals exposed to a fear-arousing communication have to engage in two types of appraisal, namely appraisal of the threat and appraisal of coping strategies available for reducing or eliminating the threat. Defence motivation should bias the appraisal of the threat by *decreasing* willingness to accept the fear appeal. Individuals are likely to scrutinize carefully the information aimed at inducing their vulnerability to a severe threat, searching for inconsistencies and logical errors, and generally attempting to downgrade the threat. However, once individuals have accepted that they are at risk, and experience fear, they should be more willing to accept the action recommendation on how to cope with the threat. They should therefore be *less* motivated to scrutinize the arguments contained in the recommendation.

In the absence of vulnerability, increased severity of a threat should induce accuracy motivation. The motivation of individuals to engage in argument-relevant thinking should increase with increasing severity of a threat. After all, it is worthwhile thinking about some serious threat, even if it is not of immediate relevance. As a consequence, increasing the severity of the threat in the absence of vulnerability should motivate them to check the accuracy of the claims contained in both the threatening message and the recommended action. Increasing the severity of the threat under these conditions should therefore increase their attitude towards an action recommendation that is soundly argued and effective, but decrease their attitude towards an action recommendation which is poorly argued or obviously ineffective.

The theories of reasoned action and planned behaviour would suggest a third important distinction, namely that between outcome measures which rely on attitudes, and those that assess behavioural intentions or behaviour. In deriving predictions with regard to the action recommendation, one has to differentiate between the impact of fear appeals on attitudes towards the recommended action and on the intention to accept the recommendation (or actual behaviour). Information about the severity of a threat should increase intentions to act only if individuals feel vulnerable to the health risk. After all, why should one invest time and effort in taking protective action against a threat, if one does not feel vulnerable?

Given these predictions, and given that the manipulations used in most studies confounded vulnerability and severity, it is not surprising that even the more recent research which not only assessed outcomes but also levels of processing resulted in a complex pattern of findings (Jepson and Chaiken 1990; Baron *et al.* 1992, 1994; Gleicher and Petty 1992; Liberman and Chaiken 1992; Kuppens *et al.* 1996). However, if one sorts studies into those that focused on processing of fear appeals vs those that focused on the action recommendation, a somewhat more orderly pattern emerges.

The earliest evidence for selective processing of fear appeals was presented by Janis and Terwilliger (1962) who asked subjects to 'think aloud' as they read an anti-smoking communication which aroused either high or low fear. Content analysis of these responses indicated that subjects produced more unfavourable and fewer favourable thoughts when reading the high- rather than the low-fear message. The high-fear message also induced somewhat less persuasion although this difference was only marginal.

Further evidence for selective processing of the fear message has been presented by Liberman and Chaiken (1992) who exposed women who either did or did not drink coffee to messages which either supported or

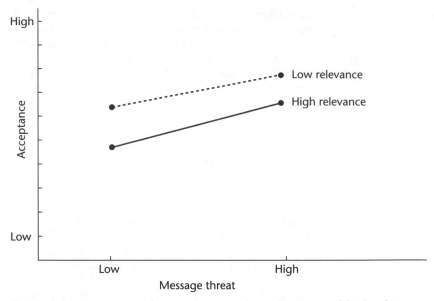

Figure 3.3 Acceptance of message among low-relevance and high-relevance subjects reading low-threat or high-threat messages.
Source: Adapted from Liberman and Chaiken (1992).

disconfirmed a purported link between coffee drinking and fibrocystic disease. Thus, the high-threat version of the message was threatening to coffee drinkers because it made them feel *vulnerable* to a serious health threat. In contrast, the low-threat version claimed that this link had been disconfirmed. These manipulations resulted in two main effects on beliefs in the negative health consequences of caffeine consumption (Figure 3.3). First, participants were more confident in the link between caffeine and fibrocystic disease after having received a high- rather than low-threat message. Second, and more interestingly, relevance significantly reduced this belief. Thus, individuals who drank a great deal of coffee and thus felt vulnerable to the threat were less likely to believe in the link than those who did not drink a great deal of coffee. The fact that individuals who felt vulnerable to threat were less likely to believe in the caffeine–disease link, tends to suggest defensive processing. However, there was no threat by vulnerability interaction suggesting that even the low-threat message was threatening enough to arouse defence motivation. There was also evidence for the predicted differences in processing. Compared to individuals who did not drink a great deal of coffee, vulnerable subjects were more likely to find weaknesses in the pro-link message and less likely to find weaknesses in the anti-link report.

Support for the predicted differences in processing action recommendations comes from a study by Jepson and Chaiken (1990). Subjects who were chronically fearful about cancer detected fewer logical errors that were planted in a message about cancer check-ups for adults, and also listed fewer issue-relevant thoughts than subjects who were not fearful. More-over, consistent with the dual-process assumptions that reduced systematic processing of poor arguments increases persuasion, fearful subjects also indicated more agreement with the message.

Gleicher and Petty (1992) also found that moderately to highly fearful subjects were more inclined to accept a recommendation aimed at redu-cing the threat without carefully scrutinizing the message than were low-fear subjects. However, it remained unexplained why they found these effects not only for a recommendation which was relevant to the threat but also for one which was irrelevant. The findings of a study of Baron and colleagues (1994) also do not really contribute to the clarification of this issue. Although they found that high-fear patients about to receive a dental filling processed the action recommendation more carefully than low-fear patients, their findings are not really relevant to our theoretical predictions, because the action recommendation (on water fluoridation) was not really designed to avert the present danger.

Conclusions and implications

It is difficult to draw conclusions from these studies with regard to design-ing health promotion interventions. Even though there was evidence of defensive processing, the overwhelming majority of studies on fear appeals has found that higher levels of threat resulted in greater persuasion than did lower levels. However, the effectiveness of high-fear messages appeared to be somewhat reduced for respondents who feel highly vulnerable to the threat. There is some evidence, however, that unless individuals feel vulnerable to a threat, they are unlikely to form the intention to act on the recommendation given (Kuppens et al. 1996). Thus, if a man believes that only homosexual men run the risk of HIV infection during inter-course but he is himself heterosexual, then he might readily accept the recommendation that homosexual men should always use condoms dur-ing intercourse and his readiness to accept this recommendation should be the greater, the greater the risk that is described. However, these beliefs will have no impact on his own sexual risk behaviour. Thus, unless the communication also stresses the risk to heterosexual men and thus makes him feel vulnerable, it will affect his attitudes but have no impact on his intentions.

There may also be limitations to the effectiveness of fear appeals which are not revealed by experimental studies that often use *novel* threats to influence behaviour which is completely under the *voluntary control* of the research participants. Fear appeals are most likely to be effective for individuals who are in a precontemplation stage because they are un-familiar with a given health risk. For example, when the dangers involved in unprotected anal intercourse among men became known in the early 1980s, this information appeared to result in a tremendous reduction of individuals engaging in this activity. However, there was a hard core of men who continued to engage in this high-risk activity and, as the inter-vention studies to be reviewed later illustrate, simply reiterating the dan-gers of HIV infection does not achieve risk reduction with these individuals. The extent to which they engage in risk behaviour is also unrelated to self-perceived vulnerability (Gerrard et al. 1996). They know the risk but

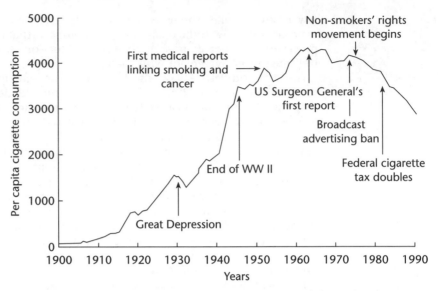

Figure 3.4   Per capita cigarette consumption among adults and major smoking and health events in the USA, 1900–1984.
Source: Novotny *et al.* (1992).

continue because they are unable or unwilling to use condoms. To induce behaviour change in these individuals, one has to persuade them that condoms do not necessarily reduce sexual pleasure and/or one has to teach them the technical and social skills involved in condom use.

Persuasion in the field

Although laboratory studies can tell us a great deal about how to develop persuasive appeals that have maximum impact on individuals who are exposed to them, they provide only limited information about the effectiveness of persuasion in a mass media context. In real life, audiences can actively or passively avoid exposure to health messages. There can be little doubt, however, that an extensive national campaign can produce meaningful behavioural changes in attitudes and behaviour. The data on changes in per capita cigarette consumption in the USA during the latter half of this century certainly suggest that the anti-smoking campaign, which began with the first *Report of the Surgeon General on Smoking and Health* in 1964 (USDHEW 1964), had great impact (Figure 3.4). Yet, even with such apparently clear-cut data, it is difficult to decide how much of the decline in smoking behaviour should be attributed to the media campaign, and how much to other causes. For example, as a result of the changing attitude towards smoking, there were large increases in local excise taxes on cigarettes between 1964 and 1978. Between 1965 and 1994 the average price of a pack of cigarettes increased from 27.9 cents to 169.3 cents (Sorensen *et al.* 1998). The increased cost of cigarettes is likely to have contributed to the decrease in cigarette consumption. Therefore, to assess the impact of the media campaign on smoking behaviour, one would need a control group which is comparable in every respect to the USA population but which was not exposed to the campaign. Without such a comparison, we will never be certain whether smoking behaviour would have changed even without the anti-smoking campaign.

The evidence from controlled studies suggests that mass media communications often result only in modest attitude change and even more modest behaviour change (for reviews, see McGuire 1985; Sorensen *et al.* 1998). For example, mass media campaigns persuading individuals to wear seat belts have not been terribly effective, resulting in a mere 4.4 per cent increase in seat belt use according to one meta-analysis (Johnston *et al.* 1994). Similarly, a mass media campaign to encourage family planning had no detectable effect on relevant indicators such as the sale of contraceptives, the number of unwanted pregnancies and the birth rate (Udry *et al.* 1972). Finally, the impact of the large community-based intervention trials conducted during the 1980s were rather disappointing (for a review, see Sorensen *et al.* 1998).

Limits to persuasion

Why is it so difficult to motivate people at least to *try* changing their poor health habits? The present discussion of the reasons why persuasive appeals used in health promotion campaigns often have rather modest effects on attitudes or intentions will focus on two issues:

1 The choice of the domains of health behaviour targeted by public health interventions.
2 The content of the persuasive communications used in those interventions.

The choice of health behaviour targeted by public health interventions

Jeffery (1989) has attributed the failure of many public health campaigns to persuade people to adopt healthful lifestyles to a discrepancy between individual and population perspectives of health risk. He argued that people are not persuaded to change because engaging in the kind of health-impairing behaviour patterns targeted by health promotion campaigns may not be all that risky. There is a discrepancy between individual and population perspectives of health risks. Public health policies are guided by the *population attributable risk*, that is, the number of excess cases of disease in a population that can be attributed to a given risk factor. Individual decision making, on the other hand, is determined by individual rather than population gain. Highest personal gain, however, is achieved when absolute risk to the individual and relative risk are both high. The problem with many health-impairing behaviour patterns is that the *relative risk*, that is the ratio of chance of the disease for individuals who engage in a risky behaviour and those who do not, is rather low. For example, a sedentary lifestyle is related to heart disease, but the relative risk is modest. And yet, because heart disease is the most common cause of death in most countries and because a sedentary lifestyle is very common, the excess burden in the population attributable to this risk factor is high. But even if the relative risk for a behavioural risk factor is high, the *absolute risk*, that is the probability of becoming ill or dying within a given period of time, may still be so low as to make it not seem worthwhile for the individual to change. For example, even though a smoker runs a much higher risk of developing lung cancer than a non-smoker, the 10-year absolute risk of lung cancer for a 35-year-old man who is a heavy smoker is only about 0.3 per cent, and the risk of heart disease is only 0.9 per cent (Jeffery 1989). And yet, these small numbers have a tremendous significance from a population perspective. In a group of one million heavy smokers aged 35, nearly 10,000 will die (prematurely) before age 45 because of the smoking habit. From the perspective of the individual, however, the odds are heavily in favour of individual survival with or without behaviour change.

But do people really know this? The few studies which have assessed individuals' perceptions of behavioural risks suggest that people vastly overestimate these risks. For example, when a national sample of Americans was asked to estimate how many of 100 smokers 'would die of lung cancer because they smoke', the average response was 42.6 (Viscusi 1990) which is far above the actual risk. It is doubtful, however, whether individuals would apply these risk estimates also to themselves. There is considerable evidence that individuals are much more optimistic about their own chances than they are about those of others, and this tendency has become known as the false optimism bias (Weinstein 1987). Thus, van der Velde and colleagues (1994), who asked a small random sample of citizens of Amsterdam to estimate both 'their chances of becoming infected with the AIDS virus within the next two years because of their sexual behaviour' and that of 'a man/woman of your age', reported that own risk was given at 5 per cent, other risk at 19 per cent. It is worth noting that, although these citizens estimated their own risk as much lower than that of their fellow men and women, their estimate was still above the (likely) 'true risk'.

A second question is whether individuals really use information about prevalence or base rates in making decisions about changes in their lifestyle. Information campaigns typically emphasize relative risks (i.e. the increase in risk due to a given health-impairing behaviour) and rarely mention base rates (i.e. absolute risk). They may be justified in doing this. There is ample evidence from other areas of judgement (e.g. attribution theory; Borgida and Brekke 1981) that people underuse prior probabilities derived from base rates. It would actually seem reasonable for people to take precautionary measures against risk factors which double or triple the risk of some terrible consequence occurring to them, even if the absolute risk of such and incidence were rather low. Thus, even though the evidence is not yet conclusive, we would expect that as long as the relative risk due to some behavioural risk factor was high, people may be persuaded to adopt precautionary measures even if the absolute health risk was rather modest.

The content of the persuasive communications used in public health interventions

Another reason for the modest impact of many public health interventions is that they use communications which have been developed on the basis of common sense and without the benefit of social psychological theorizing. More specifically, many of the community interventions use a 'one-size-fits-all' intervention (Sorensen *et al.* 1998), even though attitude theories suggest that most important determinants of attitude change vary across different segments of the population. Because we have discussed the implications of these theories for interventions earlier, we will focus here on a few examples to illustrate this point.

The most specific guidelines for the design of a successful intervention can be derived from the models of reasoned action and planned behaviour (Fishbein *et al.* 1994). According to these theories, persuasive arguments will only be effective if they influence the attitudes, norms and control perceptions which are relevant for the behaviour in question. Thus, to design an intervention, one will have to establish empirically the relative importance of attitudes, subjective norms and perceived behavioural control as determinants of the intention to engage in the targeted health behaviour. It makes little sense to try to change individuals' attitude towards a given health-impairing behaviour, when the reason they engage in this behaviour is that they feel unable to stop (i.e. perceived behavioural control) or that they think that their partner expects them to engage in this behaviour (subjective norms). Once one has determined which of the components of the model of planned behaviour exerts influence on the behaviour to be influenced, one has to conduct empirical studies to 'elicit' from members of the target population the salient beliefs which underlie these determinants. Because most of these factors vary across different sub-groups of the population, one will have to design different communications for these different groups.

For example, not everybody is interested in health issues and thus motivated to change as a result of health information. Adolescents are often not very concerned about their health. They are likely to feel that health warnings are not (yet) relevant to them and will therefore not be motivated to attend to health communications (Thompson 1978). Rather than trying to convince them of the importance of health issues, their lack of interest in health should be taken into account in the design of communications. Arguments should focus on those beliefs which are related to the targeted health behaviour in that particular age group. For example, Abraham and colleagues (1992) concluded from a study of young Scottish teenagers that, since young people's intentions to use condoms were mainly affected by perceived barriers to condom use, educational programmes should focus on acceptability barriers rather than emphasizing young people's vulnerability to infection, the severity of infections, and condom effectiveness.

Health communications are also less effective for individuals of lower socio-economic status. An analysis of 20 years of Belgian studies of the impact of health communications suggested that these programmes were most effective for individuals of high socio-economic status (Kittel *et al.* 1993). Similarly, in a study of the association of sexual risk behaviour and exposure to HIV health promotion folders, Janssen *et al.* (1998a) found that risk perception with regard to unprotected sex increased with exposure to health promotion materials only for gay men who were well educated. Among the uneducated there was even a negative relationship: higher exposure rates were related to lower perceived risk of unprotected intercourse.

One potential explanation for such differences is that most of these health communications have been designed by the well educated for the well educated. Thus, the less educated audiences might have been less able to understand the argumentation or, even if they understood them, might have found them less convincing. There is a great deal of evidence which is consistent with these assumptions:

1 There is a strong relationship between socio-economic status (SES) and ill health. High-SES individuals are also healthier and this gap has been widening over the years (for reviews, see Kenkel 1991; Adler *et al.* 1994; Williams and Collins 1995).
2 Socio-economic status is negatively related to knowledge about health risks (e.g. Kenkel 1991; Janssen *et al.* 1998b).
3 The lower individuals' socio-economic status, the more they are likely to live unhealthily by smoking, eating a poor diet, drinking too much alcohol and being physically inactive (e.g. Kenkel 1991; Adler *et al.* 1994; Williams and Collins 1995).
4 The more people know about adverse health consequences, the less they are likely to engage in health-impairing behaviour patterns (e.g. Kenkel 1991).
5 Finally, for smoking there is even evidence that the relationship with level of education only emerged after the health consequences of smoking became widely established (Farrell and Fuchs 1982).

However, there is evidence to suggest that the differential impact of health education and promotion on individuals of different socio-economic levels is not exclusively mediated by health knowledge. Thus, the impact of level of education on health behaviour is only partially reduced when health knowledge is controlled for (Kenkel 1991). Similarly, the impact of educational level on health is also only partly reduced if health behaviour is controlled for. This is consistent with earlier findings that health knowledge is neither the only, nor even the most important, factor mediating the relationship between socio-economic status and health outcome.

Beyond persuasion: changing the incentive structure

In view of the uncertain effects of health promotion via mass media persuasion, it is hardly surprising that governments often decide to influence behaviour by changing the rewards and costs associated with alternative courses of action rather than relying on persuasion. Thus, government policies can be introduced that alter the set of contingencies affecting individuals as they engage in health-damaging behaviour (Moore and Gerstein 1981). For example, governments can increase the costs of smoking or drinking by increasing the tax on tobacco and alcohol products, they can institute stricter age limits, or they can reduce availability by limiting sales.

Legal age restrictions

In most countries a large segment of the population (as defined by a minimal drinking or driving age) is not permitted to buy alcohol or drive a car. Although the value of such age limitations in reducing drinking problems or accident rates among the young has been doubted, the evidence from studies of changes in age limitations suggests that age limits do exercise a restraining effect. For example, evaluations of the impact of changes in minimal drinking age on alcohol problems and alcohol-related problems in the relevant age groups have indicated that raising the drinking age reduces both alcohol consumption and motor vehicle accidents (e.g. Ashley and Rankin 1988).

Price and taxation

One of the basic assumptions of economic theory states that, everything else being equal, the demand for a good should decrease if the price of that good is increased. The relation between changing prices and changing consumption can be expressed by price elasticities. Price elasticity reflects the way in which consumption responds to changes in price. It is defined as the percentage change in the quantity of a good demanded divided by the percentage change in the price associated with the change in demand. Thus, an elasticity of −0.7 means that a 10 per cent increase (decrease) in price would reduce (increase) the quantity of the good demanded by seven per cent. A commodity is said to have high price elasticity if the demand reacts to changes in price, that is, if demand goes up when prices go down, or goes down when prices go up. Similarly, income elasticity reflects the way the demand for a commodity reacts to changes in income.

There is ample evidence to demonstrate that the demand for alcoholic beverages, like the demand for most other commodities, responds to changes in price and income. In a review of econometric studies that estimated the values of price and income elasticities of alcoholic beverages for Australia, Canada, Finland, Ireland, Sweden, Great Britain and the United States, Bruun and colleagues (1975) concluded that, with everything else remaining equal, a rise in alcohol prices generally led to a drop in the consumption of alcohol, whereas an increase in the income of consumers generally led to a rise in alcohol consumption. There is similar evidence for smoking, although less research seems to have been conducted on this issue (for reviews, see Warner, 1981, 1986; Walsh and Gordon 1986).

Summary and conclusions

If one compares the effectiveness of public health strategies that use persuasion with those that change the contingencies associated with a given behaviour (e.g. price), the latter strategy often seems more effective. However, there are limitations to the use of monetary incentives or legal sanctions to influence health behaviour which do not apply to persuasion. First, these strategies cannot be applied to all health behaviours. Whereas it is widely accepted that governments should control the price of tobacco products and alcohol, a law forcing people to jog daily would be unacceptable and difficult to enforce. Second, the use of monetary incentives or legal sanctions to control behaviour might weaken internal control mechanisms that may have existed beforehand. Research on the effects of extrinsic incentives on intrinsic motivation and performance has demonstrated that performance of an intrinsically enjoyable task will decrease once people have been given some reward for performing that task (e.g. Lepper and Greene 1978). For example, if health insurance companies decided to offer lower rates to people who engage in regular physical exercise, such financial incentives might undermine the intrinsic motivation of people who exercise because they enjoy doing it.

Mass media communications can alert people to health risks that they might not otherwise learn about. Thus, public health education through the mass media has already resulted in a major change in health attitudes, which in turn may have increased popular acceptance of legal actions curbing health-impairing behaviour. For example, Warner (1981) attributed the large growth in state and local excise taxes for cigarettes between 1964 to 1972 to the anti-smoking campaign. The anti-smoking campaign in the USA is also an illustration of the fact that persuasion and incentive-related strategies do not preclude each other and are probably most effective when used in combination. Thus, the anti-smoking campaign resulted in a non-smoking ethos which was probably responsible for the legislative successes of the non-smokers' rights movements during the 1970s and 1980s.

SETTINGS FOR HEALTH PROMOTION

Following the review of public health approaches to health promotion, this section will give a few examples of the settings in which the strategies discussed in the preceding sections have been applied. We will begin this discussion with a somewhat unusual setting for a *public* health measure, namely the physician's office.

The physician's office

Although prevention has not been a strong component of traditional medical practice, medical school curricula are increasingly emphasizing the value of diagnosing health-impairing habits in healthy people and of advising them to change (Taylor 1995). As health experts who usually have a relationship of trust with their patients, physicians are particularly credible agents for inducing changes in health behaviour. Health advice is therefore more likely to be followed if it is issued by one's personal physician rather than some anonymous mass media source. Thus, physicians can become influential in health promotion by merely advising patients to change health-impairing behaviour. For example, there is evidence from 39 controlled trials of smoking interventions in medical practices that advice given to patients to stop smoking resulted in a moderate though significant reduction in the number of people who smoked (Kottke *et al.* 1988).

Physicians are likely to be even more effective in their traditional role of making health recommendations if they act on the basis of medical tests and examinations. For example, the advice to eat a low-cholesterol diet is more likely to be followed by a patient who has just received feedback that his serum cholesterol values are high, than without such feedback. To increase adherence in these situations it is important, however, that the information is made understandable to the patient and that specific recommendations are given. Instead of merely telling patients that they should lower their cholesterol intake, specific goals should be set (Locke and Latham 1990). Furthermore, the physician (or a dietitian working with the physician) should give specific information on the cholesterol content of various foods to help patients reach these goals. Finally, doctors and patients should agree on a date for new tests to be conducted to allow feedback on the success of these measures.

Schools

The school system is an ideal place for health promotion because, potentially, one can reach the total population and reach them early enough to prevent health-impairing habits from developing. For example, schools have been particularly active in instituting anti-smoking programmes (for reviews see Best *et al.* 1988; Rooney and Murray 1996). These programmes vary from lectures by school principals or physicians to fear-arousing films, teacher participation (e.g. introducing material on smoking into science and hygiene classes) and student participation (e.g. anti-smoking essays, group discussion). Evaluations of these programmes suggest that only moderate reductions in the number of students who start smoking have so far been achieved (Rooney and Murray 1996).

Worksite

The worksite is an advantageous setting for conducting health promotion activities because a very large number of people can be reached on a regular basis. This allows the use of strategies that combine the public health approach with some of the clinical approaches to be discussed later. There is also a potential for manipulation of the social and physical environments in order to create positive incentives for healthy behaviour. Furthermore, the possibility of reduced health care costs and absenteeism make such interventions attractive for organizations (Cataldo and Coates 1986; Terborg 1988). The advantages of instituting such worksite health promotion programmes seem to have been recognized by many industrial organizations. Thus, a national survey of worksite health promotion programmes based on a random sample of worksites with 50 or more employees conducted in the USA found that 65.5 per cent of these worksites reported at least one health promotion activity (Fielding and Piserchia 1989).

Taylor (1995) discussed three ways in which companies have dealt with poor health habits of their employees. The first is through on-the-job programmes that help employees to practise better health behaviour. Thus, the most commonly offered health promotion activities consist of advice on exercise, stress management, smoking cessation, weight loss, nutrition and hypertension detection and control (Fielding 1986; Terborg 1988). A second way in which industry has promoted good health habits is by structuring the working environment in ways that help employees to engage in healthy activities. For example, companies might provide on-site health clubs, or restaurants that provide a balanced diet, low in fat, sugar and cholesterol. Very few industries use a third approach, namely offering monetary incentives for health behaviour (Terborg 1988). Although there is great enthusiasm about the efficacy of these programmes, results of recent large trials conducted to evaluate the effectiveness of such worksite health promotion programmes have been mixed (e.g. Salina et al. 1994; Byers et al. 1995; Glasgow et al. 1995, 1997; Sorensen et al. 1996; Maes et al. 1998). There is evidence, however, that more intensive interventions can be effective (e.g. Salina et al. 1994; Byers et al. 1995).

Community

This type of intervention incorporates a variety of different approaches, ranging from door-to-door or mass media information campaigns telling people about the availability of a breast cancer screening programme to a diet modification programme that recruits participants through community institutions. Evaluation of community-based interventions using quasi-experimental control group designs which compare intervention communities to matched control communities suggest that these interventions can be effective although results are rather variable (Sorensen et al. 1998).

Two early community studies targeting cardiovascular disease prevention were the North Karelia Project and the Stanford Three Community Study. The North Karelia Project, a large-scale community intervention conducted in northern Finland, resulted in a substantial reduction in coronary risk factors (Puska et al. 1985). An intensive educational campaign was implemented using the news services, physicians, and public health nurses who staffed community health centres. An assessment of the effectiveness of these programmes based on self-report data showed that, compared to a neighbouring province used as a control group and not exposed to the campaign, there was a considerable improvement in several dietary habits in North Karelia (especially concerning fat intake). There was also a net reduction in smoking in North Karelia, as well as small but significant net reductions in serum cholesterol levels and blood pressure. Most importantly, however, there was a 24 per cent decline in cardiovascular deaths in North Karelia, compared with a 12 per cent decline nationwide in Finland. Although the generalizability of these results is limited by the fact that the project was instituted in response to concerns among the North Karelia population about the extremely high heart disease rate in the area, findings such as these suggest that community-based interventions can be effective in changing health-impairing behaviour patterns.

The Stanford Three Community Study exposed several communities to a massive media campaign concerning smoking, diet and exercise through television, radio, newspapers, posters and printed materials sent by mail

(Farquhar *et al.* 1977; Meyer *et al.* 1980). In one of the communities, the media campaign was even supplemented by face-to-face counselling for a small subset of high-risk individuals. A control community was not exposed to the campaign. The media campaign increased people's knowledge about cardiac risk and resulted in modest improvements in dietary preferences and other cardiac risk factors.

In the late 1970s three large community-based intervention trials were started, the Stanford Five-City Project, the Minnesota Heart Health Project and the Pawtucket Heart Health Project. These trials, which varied in length from five to seven years, were aimed at reducing coronary risk factors, including high blood pressure, elevated serum cholesterol levels, cigarette smoking and obesity. In two of the projects (Five-City, Minnesota) impact was assessed both by repeated measures taken in a cohort and independent cross-sectional surveys conducted periodically over the period of the intervention. In Pawtucket only cross-sectional surveys were employed. The overall results of these studies have been somewhat disappointing. Analyses of the differences for the cohort between measurements at baseline and at the end of the six-year intervention in the Five-City Project, which was the most successful of these trials, showed that the treatment cities produced significantly greater improvement in cardiovascular disease knowledge as well as greater reductions in blood pressure and smoking than the control cities (Farquhar *et al.* 1990). These findings could not be replicated with the cross-sectional samples. In the Minnesota Heart Health Project, the only treatment effect that could be detected was a small reduction in smoking among women (Luepker *et al.* 1994). There was also some indication of treatment effect on physical activity. But this effect could only be demonstrated for a one-item measure and not when a more extensive and reliable physical activity questionnaire was used. The intervention did not have any significant effects on blood cholesterol levels, blood pressure or weight. Finally in Pawtucket, only a slowing down of secular weight increases could be observed. Whereas the average weight (related to height) increased in the control city, it remained relatively stable in Pawtucket (Carleton *et al.* 1995). The community intervention had no detectable impact on smoking, blood cholesterol or blood pressure. In none of these studies has there been any impact on incidence or prevalence of coronary heart disease or mortality.

There has been much speculation about the reasons for the rather modest impact of these interventions. One plausible reason is that these studies were conducted during a time when major efforts were made by governmental institutions all over the United States to change health-impairing lifestyle patterns in the US population. These efforts included information campaigns as well as changes in taxation and legislation. That these efforts were successful is demonstrated by the pervasive health improvements which were observed in the non-intervention, control cities in all three studies. Since the community interventions in these studies also appeared to rely heavily on education about health risks, the added effect of these treatments was probably too weak to be demonstrated reliably. Thus the failure of these interventions to have pervasive effects on coronary risk factors and coronary health in these communities may yet be another demonstration that information about the negative consequences of health-impairing behaviour patterns is ineffective with populations who are already well informed about these consequences but do not know how to change. These interventions might have been more effective if they had provided the citizens of these communities with more information about how to go about changing their health-impairing behaviour.

Summary and conclusions

Drawing on different settings for health promotion allows one to reach different sections of the population. Therefore there are good reasons for pursuing each of the venues of health habit change. Community interventions and school programmes can be used to educate the population about unhealthy lifestyles and to motivate people either not to adopt health-impairing behaviours or to change such behaviours if they have already been adopted. Physicians can also play an important part in this endeavour. Schools are potentially able to play an important role in persuading individuals not to adopt certain unhealthy behaviours such as smoking, drug use and excessive drinking. Industrial organizations, on the other hand, can become important sources of motivation for individuals to change health-impairing habits. Because large industrial organizations can often also afford to employ professional counsellors in their health promotion classes, they can effectively combine the public health and clinical therapy approach. Finally, it should be remembered that the efficacy of health interventions is a function *both* of their *impact* in producing individual behaviour change and their *reach*, defined as the number of individuals who are affected in the population (Sorensen *et al.* 1998). Whereas the individual impact of public health interventions is likely to be smaller than that of clinical treatments, their efficacy could be larger because of their more extensive reach.

THE THERAPY MODEL: CHANGING AND MAINTAINING CHANGE

Even if people have formed the strong intention to change some problematic health behaviour, they are unlikely to succeed at their first attempt. Most people who seek therapy for problematic health behaviour will first have attempted to achieve the desired change on their own. Thus 90 per cent of an estimated 37 million people who stopped smoking in the two decades following the US Surgeon General's first report linking smoking to cancer have done so unaided (American Cancer Society 1986). After all, therapy is expensive and most people believe that they are quite capable of giving up smoking or losing weight on their own, at least until they try to do so.

Unlike the public health model, most therapy programmes involve a one-to-one relationship where 'patients' and therapists are in dyadic interaction, although group treatments and self-therapy programmes are also used (Leventhal and Cleary 1980). Because people who come to therapy programmes have already decided to change and are motivated to act on their decision, the function of therapy programmes is not to *persuade* people to change but to help them to *achieve* and *maintain* the desired change.

Cognitive–behavioural treatment procedures

Most therapy directed at changing problematic health behaviour has relied on behavioural techniques, although cognitive components have been included in more recent behavioural treatment programmes. Behavioural treatment procedures can be distinguished from other therapeutic orientations in that they involve one or a number of specific techniques that use learning-based principles to change behaviour. More recently, therapeutic methods designed to impact specifically on cognitive variables have become standard components of every contemporary approach to behavioural treatment (Ingram and Scott 1990).

The major behavioural or cognitive techniques that have been used in therapies aimed at changing health-impairing behaviour patterns are classical or Pavlovian conditioning (e.g. aversion therapies), operant procedures (e.g. contingency management, contingency contracting), self-management procedures, skill training, and cognitive restructuring. Earlier therapies often relied on only one of these techniques (narrow band approach). Present-day behavioural clinicians generally use a multitude of different techniques within one treatment programme. The obvious drawback of such a multi-component treatment is that it is difficult to know in use of a successful therapy which aspect or aspects of the treatment package were really effective.

This section will outline the theoretical principles underlying these therapeutic procedures. A more detailed description of specific therapies (e.g. for alcoholism, obesity, smoking), as well as an evaluation of their effectiveness, will be given in Chapter 4.

Classical conditioning

Classical conditioning was first described in 1927 by the Russian physiologist Pavlov who, in research on the digestive system of dogs, observed that many of these animals already began to salivate when they heard the footsteps of the assistant who normally fed them. Pavlov reasoned that the normal response to food (salivating) had become linked to the assistant's footsteps. Thus, by regularly preceding the stimulus that normally elicits salivation (i.e. the food), the assistant's footsteps had gained the power to elicit this response. Expressed more technically, salivation had become conditioned to the sound of the steps.

The first study which demonstrated that classical conditioning can be used to condition aversive reactions in humans was an experiment by Watson and Raynor (1920) in which they used a loud noise to instil fear of laboratory rats in a little boy. The noise was a very loud bang that was known to make the child cry and to display all signs of fear. Watson and Raynor demonstrated that the fear reaction which had initially been elicited by the noise became now linked to (i.e. conditioned to) the rat. Thus, through classical conditioning, the child's fear of the loud noise developed into a fear of a laboratory rat. Following this principle, Watson and Raynor (1920) developed the model for aversion therapy.

Early attempts at aversion therapy relied on electric shock (e.g. McGuire and Vallance 1964). However, although shocks are quite effective with laboratory animals, they did not seem to work well with humans. Modern behaviour therapies therefore employ aversive reactions that are *relevant* to the response that needs to be changed. Thus, aversion therapy with alcoholics has used vomiting-inducing drugs. The alcoholic is given alcohol just a few minutes before nausea and vomiting occurs (e.g. Lemers and Voegtlin 1950). Similarly, smokers might be induced to smoke continually, inhaling every six to eight seconds until they cannot stand it any longer (Lichtenstein and Danaher 1975). Sometimes aversion therapy uses imaginary rather than real stimuli to arouse aversion (e.g. Elkins 1980). In this procedure, both the target behaviour and the aversive stimulus are presented through imagination. For example, the subject has first to imagine himself preparing to smoke and then experiencing nausea and vomiting.

Operant conditioning

Operant procedures modify behaviour by manipulating the consequences of such behaviour. They involve the contingent presentation (or withdrawal) of rewards and punishments in order to increase desirable or decrease undesirable behaviour. Behavioural theorists assume that health behaviours, like any other behaviour, have been learned through processes of operant conditioning. For example, a widely accepted theory of alcohol abuse, the Tension Reduction Hypothesis, assumes that alcohol is consumed because it reduces tension. By lowering tension, and thus reducing an aversive drive state, alcohol consumption has reinforcing properties. Cigarette smoking may have similar tension-reducing functions.

Like the early forms of aversive conditioning, operant procedures initially used electric shocks to change behaviour. Because these procedures did not prove to have lasting effects, present-day operant procedures frequently employ some form of contingency management. For example, smokers or alcoholics may agree with their therapist on some set of rewards or punishments that will be enacted, contingent on their behaviour.

Self-management procedures

Classical and operant conditioning procedures are based on the assumption that the forces shaping a person's life lie primarily in the external environment. In contrast, self-management procedures are based on the assumption that individuals can organize their environment in ways which make certain behaviours more likely (e.g. Miller and Munoz 1976). For example, individuals can reward themselves for reaching certain behavioural goals (e.g. for losing a certain amount of weight) or punish themselves for transgressing a predetermined rule (i.e. not to drink before the evening).

Goal setting may be the most effective component of self-management. The application of self-reinforcement always involves some goal that has to be reached for the reinforcement to be applied. That this is an important determinant of the effectiveness of such procedures is suggested by research on goal setting in the context of task performance in industry. This work has consistently demonstrated that setting specific and challenging goals and providing relevant feedback leads to substantial increases in performance (for a review, see Locke and Latham 1990). Specific goals are likely to result in specific behavioural intentions. The greater effectiveness of specific over more global goals would therefore also be consistent with predictions derived from the models of reasoned action or planned behaviour. Because self-reinforcements are usually made dependent on reaching very specific goals, and because individuals provide themselves with relevant feedback through self-monitoring, these procedures are comparable to those used in goal-setting research.

Skill training

Skill training procedures have been used both as a primary treatment strategy in narrow-band approaches and as one of a number of approaches in multi-component treatment programmes (Riley et al. 1987). The main assumption underlying skill training techniques is that people engage in health-impairing behaviour because they lack certain skills. For example, people might become alcoholics because they lack the appropriate strategy to cope with stress (Riley et al. 1987). Relapsed addicts frequently report that stress and negative emotional states often immediately preceded their return to drug use (e.g. Baer and Lichtenstein 1988; Bliss et al. 1989). By providing individuals with the skills for coping with such stressful situations, there will be an alternative response to cope with the problem. This should reduce the need to turn to cigarettes or alcohol in order to be able to cope.

Cognitive restructuring

These techniques help patients to identify and correct the self-defeating thoughts which are frequently associated with emotional upset and relapse experiences. For example, Mahoney and Mahoney (1976) described the irrational and maladaptive cognitions that dieters often experience. These include thoughts about the impossibility of weight loss, the adoption of unrealistic goals which are soon disappointed, and self-disparaging statements. Using the methods of Beck (1976) and Meichenbaum (1977), patients are taught to discredit these arguments.

Relapse and relapse prevention

One distressing aspect of changing problematic health behaviour either through therapy or unaided is that people are often unable to maintain their changed habits. Thus relapse rates for addictions range from 50 to 90 per cent with approximately two-thirds of the relapses occurring within

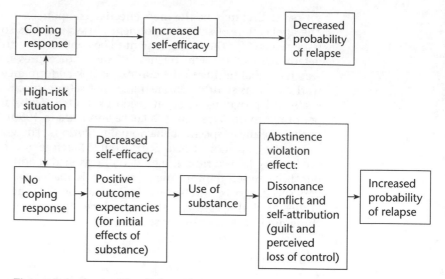

Figure 3.5 A cognitive–behavioural model of the relapse process.
Source: Adapted from Marlatt (1985).

the first 90 days (Marlatt 1985; Brownell *et al.* 1986). Similarly, in the field
of weight control, few of the dieters who succeed in losing substantial
amounts of weight are able to maintain their losses for any significant
period of time (Sternberg 1985).

Despite the high probability that clients who undergo therapy to change
some health-impairing habit will experience a relapse soon after the end
of their therapy, this possibility used not to be discussed (or even acknow-
ledged) during therapy. Thus, when it happened, clients were unprepared
to cope with relapse. During the last decade, this attitude has changed and
specific relapse prevention approaches have been developed (e.g. Marlatt
1985; Brownell *et al.* 1986). These models emphasize the similarities in
the precipitating conditions and consequences of relapse experiences across
different domains of health behaviour.

The most comprehensive theory of the relapse process has been developed
by Marlatt and colleagues (Marlatt and Gordon 1980; Marlatt 1985). Their
cognitive behavioural model of relapse (Figure 3.5) integrates elements
from social psychological theories such as social learning, attribution and
dissonance theory to account for the relapse process.

Central to the model is the concept of *perceived behavioural control* or
self-efficacy (Bandura 1986). It is assumed that individuals who manage to
maintain abstinence or to comply with some other rule regarding the target
behaviour (e.g. controlled drinking, smoking reduction, dieting) experience
a sense of control. This sense of control, which will become stronger the
longer the period of abstinence maintenance or successful rule following, will be threatened when individuals encounter a high-risk situation.
High-risk situations are situations which increase the risk of relapse.

Cummings *et al.* (1980) analysed more than 300 initial relapse episodes obtained from clients with a variety of problem behaviours such as

problem drinking, smoking, heroin addiction, compulsive gambling, and overeating. On the basis of these reports, three primary high-risk situations that were associated with almost three-quarters of all the relapses could be identified. Relapses happened most often in the presence of *negative emotional states* (35 per cent of all relapses) such as depression, anxiety, or stress. For example, depression resulting from the failure to pass an exam would significantly increase the likelihood of relapse. *Interpersonal conflicts* (16 per cent of the relapses) also appear to be a frequent antecedent of relapse. Thus, people who have gone through the break-up of a relationship or had a conflict with a family member or their boss might take a drink or smoke a cigarette in an attempt to calm themselves. *Social pressure* (20 per cent of the relapses) is another frequent cause of relapse, involving either direct social influence from people who exert pressure on the individual to engage in the taboo behaviour or indirect pressure via modelling (e.g. being in the presence of others who engage in the same target behaviour).

The study of Cummings and colleagues (1980) suffers from a methodological weakness which characterizes practically all studies of relapse episodes, namely a reliance on long-term retrospective recall. It is therefore encouraging that their basic findings could be confirmed by the first study to collect real-time data on temptation and lapse. Shiffman and colleagues (1996) asked a sample of over 100 ex-smokers who stopped smoking to record temptations (which did not result in lapses) and lapses in an electronic diary at the time they actually occurred. Shiffman and colleagues confirmed that negative affect played a significant role in smoking lapses. The evidence further suggested that acute interpersonal stressors were an important cause of the distress that resulted in relapse.

Smoking environments and smoking cues also played an important role in promoting relapse among abstinent smokers. Seeing other people smoke was a significant correlate of temptations and relapses. These effects were stronger when the people smoking were part of the abstinent smoker's immediate social group, which suggests that the effect was mediated by social modelling rather than the mere effect of being exposed to smoking cues. When smoking was discouraged, lapses were less likely to occur. Finally, alcohol consumption was associated with lapses but not temptations, which suggests that the effect of drinking did not operate by increasing temptations but by reducing resistance.

In contrast to Cummings and colleagues (1980), who found that 'urges and temptations' were associated with only 6 per cent of the relapse situations, Shiffman and colleagues (1996) found that lapses were strongly associated with the intense urge to smoke. This difference probably reflects the fact that physiological factors are more important for relapses in attempts to abstain from smoking or alcohol consumption than in attempts to stop compulsive gambling. Different but influential physiological factors may be involved in obesity. Even though food does not seem to be addictive in the way that cigarettes and alcohol are, the physiological pressure to regain lost weight may be extremely powerful (Brownell *et al.* 1986). Genetic factors that are implicated in alcoholism and obesity may also operate via physiological urges (e.g. Goodwin *et al.* 1973; Stunkard *et al.* 1986).

If individuals manage to cope effectively with the high-risk situation, the probability of relapse will decrease significantly. One reason for this emphasized by Marlatt and Gordon (1980) is that individuals who cope successfully will have validated their sense of control. They will therefore expect to cope with future high-risk situations. This expectancy is closely associated with the notions of self-efficacy (Bandura 1986) and perceived behavioural control (Ajzen 1988). High self-efficacy or high perceived behavioural control are positively related to behavioural intentions. Individuals are more motivated to engage in a behaviour if they perceive their ability to perform that behaviour successfully as high rather than low.

In contrast, failure to cope with the high-risk situation should decrease the sense of control or self-efficacy. The risk of failure should be particularly high if the situation also involves the temptation to engage in the prohibited behaviour as a means of coping with the stress. For example, if an individual is very anxious about the outcome of some examination and also feels that smoking a cigarette or having a drink would calm him or her down, the risk of relapse is very high. Thus, the sense of being unable to cope effectively in a high-risk situation combined with the positive outcome expectancies for the effects of the old habitual coping behaviour greatly increases the probability of an initial relapse.

Most people who attempt to change a health-impairing habit such as smoking or drinking perceive 'stopping' in a 'once and for all' manner. Thus, the transgression of an absolute rule will result in what Marlatt and Gordon (1980) termed the *abstinence violation effect* (i.e. the inference that the failure to remain abstinent is an indication of one's complete lack of will-power and self-control). However, because similar effects can be observed in dieters who have violated their diet norm, one should perhaps use the more general concept of a *'goal violation effect'* (Polivy and Herman 1987).

One major reason for the abstinence or goal violation effect is *self-attribution*. The concept of attribution refers to the processes by which individuals arrive at causal explanations for their own or other people's actions (Heider 1958). These explanations can vary on a continuum that ranges from attributions to internal causes to attributions to external causes. Examples of internal causes would be personality, ability or motivation. Examples of external causes would be task difficulty, or social pressure. Individuals who relapse are likely to make internal attributions. They tend to blame the relapse on personal weakness or failure and to interpret it as evidence of their lack of will-power and their inability to resist temptation. This self-attribution will further decrease the individual's sense of self-efficacy and control.

A second reason for the abstinence or goal violation effect is *dissonance*. The flagrant violation of a dietary goal or abstinence rule would also be inconsistent with the individual's self-concept (as a dieter or abstainer) and therefore arouse dissonance. Dissonance is an aversive internal state, as unpleasant as, for example, anxiety. Thus, whenever dissonance is aroused, individuals are motivated to reduce it (Festinger 1957). In the case of violations of abstention rules, dissonance can either be reduced by changing one's self-image or by changing one's attitude towards abstention. Thus, ex-smokers who relapse could reduce their dissonance either by deciding that they have no will-power or by persuading themselves that smoking is not so bad after all. Obviously, both mechanisms of dissonance reduction would increase the risk of future relapse.

A recent study of smokers participating in a smoking cessation programme supported these predictions (Gibbons *et al.* 1997). Gibbons and colleagues reported a decline in risk perception and in commitment to quitting after smoking resumption among those ex-smokers who relapsed. This effect was much stronger among relapsers who had moderate to high self-esteem than among those with low self-esteem. Thus, the recognition of having demonstrated weakness and lack of will-power by relapsing appears to be dissonant only with the self-concepts of high self-esteem individuals.

According to this analysis, the first step to take in the prevention of relapse is to teach clients to recognize high-risk situations that are likely to trigger a relapse (Marlatt 1985). The second step involves teaching them the coping skills that are necessary to master the high-risk situation. Such relapse prevention techniques have now been tested with a variety of health behaviours including alcohol abstinence (e.g. Chaney *et al.* 1978), smoking (e.g. Shiffman *et al.* 1985), and weight control (Sternberg 1985). A recent meta-analysis of 26 published and unpublished studies which employed relapse prevention techniques concluded that relapse prevention was generally effective, particularly for alcohol problems (Irvin *et al.* 1999).

SUMMARY AND CONCLUSIONS

This chapter presented and discussed two types of approaches to the modification of health behaviour, the public health model and the therapy model. The public health model involves health promotion programmes that are designed to change the behaviour of large groups (e.g. members of industrial organizations, students of a school, citizens of a community or even the population of a country). Three major strategies are used to achieve this objective: persuasive appeals, economic incentives and legal measures.

Mass media health appeals are quite effective in increasing people's knowledge of certain health hazards but they are often less effective in changing their behaviour. As we have tried to point out, the impact of many of these communications on attitudes and behaviour could have been increased if their design had been based on social psychological theory and methodology. However, it would be misleading to assess the impact of public health interventions solely on the evidence of their efficacy in producing individual behaviour change. The impact of an intervention is a function of both efficacy and reach. Reach has been defined as the penetration of the intervention within the population (Sorensen *et al.* 1998). Thus, even when the impact on individual behaviour is relatively small, the overall impact of public health interventions on the population can still be substantial. Furthermore, the effects of continuous public health campaigns are likely to accumulate.

Thus, as the anti-smoking campaign of the 1960s and 1970s illustrated, public health approaches can achieve significant behaviour change if extensive media campaigns are combined with economic and legal measures.

Thus, the mass media campaign that was initiated by the report of the US Surgeon General (USDHEW 1964) is likely to have played a causal role in the global change of attitudes toward smoking. This general change in climate was probably responsible for the increases in local and state taxation during the late 1960s and for the legislative successes of the non-smokers' rights movements during the 1970s.

However, the example of smoking can also serve to illustrate the weaknesses of the public health approach. It has been very successful in conveying information about the health risk of smoking – nearly everyone in the United States now believes that cigarette smoking is hazardous. It has been less successful in changing behaviour. Nearly one-third of the US population continues to smoke, despite the considerable reduction in the prevalence of smoking during recent decades.

The fact that many of the people who smoke today would like to stop suggests that a sizeable proportion of those individuals have been unable to stop on their own and would profit from clinical therapy. Thus, even though educational campaigns can be effective in motivating individuals to change, good intentions are often not enough in the case of health-impairing behaviour such as substance abuse or excessive eating. By teaching people strategies that help them to maintain the motivation and to execute their intention to change, clinical therapy can make an important contribution to changing these sorts of behaviours.

Thus, public health strategies and clinical therapy are complementary rather than contradictory approaches. To decide to undergo therapy, individuals must first be aware of having a problem and be willing to do something about it. Although in the case of problems such as alcoholism or obesity public health education may be less instrumental in creating problem awareness, with other problems health education has certainly played an important role in creating awareness.

FURTHER READING

Eagly, A.H. and Chaiken, S. (1993) *The Psychology of Attitudes*. Fort Worth, TX: Harcourt Brace Jovanovich. Still the most comprehensive and authoritative review of the social psychology of attitudes. Chapters 6 and 7 discuss the process theories of attitude formation and change.

Fishbein, M., Middlestadt, S.E. and Hitchcock, P. (1994) Using information to change sexually transmitted disease-related behaviors: an analysis based on the theory of reasoned action, in R.J. DiClemente and J.L. Peterson (eds) *Preventing AIDS: Theories and Methods of Behavioral Interventions*, pp. 61–93. New York, NY: Plenum. This chapter presents a detailed analysis and discussion of the use of the models of reasoned action and planned behaviour in designing interventions to change attitudes and behaviour.

Jeffery, R.W. (1989) Risk behaviors and health: contrasting individual and population perspectives. *American Psychologist*, 44: 1194–202. Argues that the discrepancy between individual and population perspective of health risk is responsible for the failure of many public health campaigns to influence health behaviour.

Liberman, A. and Chaiken, S. (1992) Defensive processing of personally relevant health messages. *Personality and Social Psychology Bulletin*, 18: 669–79. An experimental test of hypotheses about the impact of fear appeals on persuasion derived from dual process theories.

Marlatt, G.A. and Gordon, J.R. (eds) (1985) *Relapse Prevention*. New York, NY: Guilford. The book provides a comprehensive approach to relapse prevention.

Prochaska, J.O., DiClemente, C.C. and Norcross, J.C. (1992) In search of how people change: applications to addictive behaviours. *American Psychologist*, 47: 1102–14. The article presents and discusses the ideas underlying the transtheoretical model. A very good introduction.

Sutton, S. (1996) Can 'stages of change' provide guidance in the treatment of addictions? A critical examination of Prochaska and DiClemente's model, in G. Edwards and C. Dare (eds) *Psychotherapy, Psychological Treatments and Addictions*. Cambridge: Cambridge University Press. This chapter critically analyses the key assumptions underlying the transtheoretical and other stage models.

FOUR

BEHAVIOUR AND HEALTH: EXCESSIVE APPETITES

The two previous chapters examined determinants of health behaviour and the effectiveness of strategies of change. The present chapter and the next one will discuss the major behavioural risk factors that have been linked to health. The discussion of behaviour and health will be divided into two sections. Chapter 4 covers health-impairing behaviour related to excessive appetites, such as smoking, drinking too much alcohol and overeating. These are appetitive behaviours that, once they have become excessive, are exceedingly difficult to control. People who want to change often enter counselling or therapy programmes to help them to act according to their intentions.

In contrast, the self-protective behaviours such as eating a healthy diet, exercising, safeguarding oneself against the risk of injury from accidents (e.g. wearing a seat belt), and avoiding behaviour associated with contracting AIDS (needle sharing, unprotected sex) that are discussed in Chapter 5 are generally somewhat more under the voluntary control of the individual.

The structure of our discussion of behavioural risk factors is similar in both chapters. Each section will begin with a critical review of the empirical evidence that links these behaviours to negative health consequences. After a discussion of theories of the development and maintenance of these behaviours, the effectiveness of strategies of attitude and behaviour change in modifying the risk of health impairment will be discussed.

SMOKING

The health consequences of smoking

Since the US Surgeon General, in his first report on smoking (USDHEW 1964), identified cigarette smoking as the single most important source of preventable mortality and morbidity, smoking rates among adults in the United States have dropped from 42.5 per cent in 1965 to 25.5 per cent in 1990 (Klesges *et al.* 1996). However, not all societal groups have shared equally in this trend. In particular, young people, women, minority groups, and individuals of low socio-economic status have failed to contribute to the decline in rates of smoking (Adler *et al.* 1994; Klesges *et al.* 1996). As a result, the smoking rate of women is approaching that of men and the inverse relationship between cigarette smoking and socio-economic status has become more marked over the years (Kenkel 1991).

Moreover, even though smoking rates have declined in the United States and most Western industrialized countries, they have increased in many non-Western countries, particularly China. Since 1980, the number of cigarettes sold in the world has increased by 950 billion. In 1995 5422 billion cigarettes were smoked worldwide, more than 100 billion cigarettes a week, a pack a week for every man, woman and child in the world. China gets through a quarter of all cigarettes smoked, but Latin America and the former communist countries also account for large parts of worldwide consumption (*Independent*, 7 March 1996).

Mortality

The negative health effects of smoking are appalling. It has been estimated that close to 400,000 people die each year of smoking in the United States alone. This is more than the total number of American lives lost in World War I, Korea, and Vietnam combined (Fielding 1985). To claim an equivalent share of lives, the airline industry would have to experience three jumbo jet crashes every day of the year (Walsh and Gordon 1986). Of the deaths each year due to coronary heart disease (the leading cause of death in most industrialized countries), 30 to 40 per cent can be attributed to cigarette smoking (Fielding 1985). Overall, the mortality from heart disease in the USA is 70 per cent greater for smokers than non-smokers (USDHHS 1985). Similar excess rates have been reported for Canada, the United Kingdom, Scandinavia, and Japan (Pooling Project Research Group 1978).

The second leading cause of death in the United States and other affluent industrial nations is cancer. Smoking is responsible for approximately 30 per cent of all deaths from cancer. Lung cancer, which was nearly unknown in the USA at the start of the twentieth century, now accounts for 25 per cent of cancer mortality and 5 per cent of all deaths (Fielding 1985). Between 80 and 85 per cent of deaths from lung cancer have been attributed to smoking (USDHHS 1982). Current smoking rates among women have also resulted in a dramatic rise in lung cancer deaths among women. Lung cancer has now replaced breast cancer as the leading cause of cancer deaths among women (Klesges *et al.* 1996). However, contrary to popular beliefs, coronary heart disease and not lung cancer is the major cause of smoking-related deaths. Lung cancer is only responsible for one-seventh of the excess mortality attributed to smoking. Finally, smoking also doubles the risk of dying from stroke, the third leading cause of death in the United States (USDHHS 1990).

Morbidity

Morbidity is also considerably higher among smokers than among non-smokers. Current smokers report more chronic bronchitis, emphysema, chronic sinusitis, peptic ulcers and arteriosclerotic heart disease than do persons who have never smoked (Schwartz 1987). Data from the National Health Interview Survey conducted in the USA in 1974 suggest that there are more than 81 million excess work days lost and more than 145 million excess days of bed disability per year because of smoking (Schwartz 1987). By substantially increasing the risk of disability in the elderly, smoking also reduces the chance of enjoying an active and healthy old age (Ferrucci *et al.* 1999).

The risk of morbidity and mortality for pipe and cigar smokers who do not inhale deeply is somewhat smaller than that for cigarette smokers but still considerably higher than that for non-smokers (Fielding 1985). It is less clear whether smokers of filter cigarettes run a lower risk of morbidity and mortality than smokers of non-filter cigarettes (Fielding 1985).

Although there can be no doubt that smoking is unhealthy, estimates of smoking-related morbidity and mortality are likely to exaggerate the direct impact of smoking on health. Such estimates are usually based on the difference between the age-adjusted morbidity and mortality rates of smokers and non-smokers. To attribute these differences to smoking would only be justified if smokers did not differ from non-smokers except with respect to their smoking. This is clearly not the case. People who smoke live unhealthily in other respects as well and this could contribute to their elevated mortality risk. A national survey of behavioural risk factors conducted in the USA indicated that, compared to non-smokers, smokers had higher age-adjusted rates of 'acute drinking' (five or more alcoholic drinks per occasion at least once a month) and 'chronic drinking' (averaging two or more alcoholic drinks per day), more episodes of driving while intoxicated, and lower use of seat belts (Remington *et al.* 1985). Current smokers also differ from former and never smokers in their dietary intake and physical activity. For example, a study of 3250 working adults found that current smokers consumed more calories per day from high-fat and high-calorie foods, including dairy products, meat, eggs, french fries and fats, and reported less frequent leisure time physical activity than former and never smokers (French *et al.* 1996). All these behaviours may independently or synergistically contribute to higher chronic disease risk in smokers.

The health benefits of stopping

Smoking cessation has major immediate health benefits for men and women of all ages (USDHHS 1990). Former smokers live longer than continuing smokers. Only one year after stopping smoking, the risk of coronary heart disease is reduced by half. After 15 years it is the same as that of people who never smoked. The risk of lung cancer also declines steadily in people who quit smoking and after 10 years is less than half of that of continuing smokers.

Smoking and weight

Smoking has one effect that may be considered positive, particularly by women: it appears to lower body weight. Middle-aged smokers weigh less than non-smokers, and smokers who quit smoking tend to gain weight, women more so than men (for a review, see French and Jeffery 1995). However, there is no evidence that *young* people who start smoking reduce their body weight and no weight differences have been observed in a large sample of young men and women (Klesges *et al.* 1998). This suggests that the weight control benefits of smoking take years to accrue and are probably due to a slight attenuation of the commonly observed weight increase as people age. In contrast to the weight control benefits of smoking, the costs of stopping appear to be immediate. Smokers who stop smoking gain between 2.3 kg (USDHHS 1990) and 6 kg (Klesges *et al.* 1997) within one year, the higher gains being observed in those who manage to stop completely. Although this weight gain is unlikely to reduce the health benefits gained from stopping smoking, it can act as a deterrent for cosmetic reasons. There is persuasive evidence that weight gain following smoking cessation is mainly due to the removal of the stimulating effect of nicotine on metabolic rate: weight gain can be suppressed through nicotine replacement, there appears to be a linear relationship between nicotine dose during replacement and the extent to which weight gain is suppressed, and weight gain occurs once nicotine replacement is stopped (e.g. Doherty *et al.* 1996). However, there is also evidence to suggest that people eat more after they stop smoking (USDHHS 1990).

Passive smoking

In addition to the impact on their own health, smokers also endanger the health of others. Epidemiological data suggest that cigarette use during pregnancy may be related to spontaneous abortion, premature birth, low birthweight, and death of the infant during the first day of life (McGinnis *et al.* 1987; Kaplan 1988). In the past two decades, there has also been increasing awareness of the health hazards due to exposure to *environmental tobacco smoke* (USDHHS 1986; Brownson *et al.* 1997). There is evidence from studies assessing mortality from lung cancer among non-smokers exposed to smoking spouses that these 'involuntary' or 'passive' smokers have a substantial elevation in their risk of lung cancer and of heart disease (Brownson *et al.* 1997). Evidence is also beginning to emerge that passive smoking at work is associated with increased coronary heart disease and that the health risk increases linearly with increasing exposure (He *et al.* 1994). The evidence of the health impact of environmental smoking has led to the introduction of much more stringent restrictions in the places where tobacco can be smoked in the United States (USDHHS 1986); the same is increasingly happening in many European countries.

The economic costs of smoking

While the cost of smoking in terms of human lives is beyond question, the argument that smoking also imposes a financial burden on society (as advanced by several US state governments in court cases against the tobacco industry in 1996) can be challenged. Although smokers impose considerable costs through hospitalization, medical costs, and higher absenteeism rates, they also produce extra tax income via tobacco taxes. Furthermore, with their early death they subsidize the collectively financed retirement plans of non-smokers, and contribute less to the high health costs of an aging population (Manning *et al.* 1989; Barendregt *et al.* 1997). Economic analyses have repeatedly indicated that these financial benefits outweigh the costs imposed by smoking (Barendregt *et al.* 1997; Manning *et al.* 1989). It is poetic justice that the tobacco industry could not use these arguments in their defence against the accusation of economic damage because at the time they had still to admit that smoking posed a serious threat to health.

Conclusion

The case of smoking provides an intriguing example of how individual and population perspectives intersect. There can be no doubt that smoking endangers the lives of smokers and of those who are involuntarily exposed to tobacco smoke. These facts are well known. According to a 1989 Gallup survey, nearly 70 per cent of smokers aged 18 to 49 said that they would like to stop (USDHHS 1990). Furthermore, at least in the United States, governments have introduced stringent laws to protect non-smokers from the damaging effects of environmental tobacco smoke. However, with smokers being vilified in many countries, it is only fair to mention that at least financially they do not appear to impose a burden on society.

Determinants of smoking

In attempting to explain why people smoke, one has to distinguish between becoming a smoker and maintaining the habit. Social pressure from peers or older siblings is probably the prime factor in experimenting with smoking (Leventhal and Cleary 1980; Spielberger 1986). For example, a recent prospective study of the initiation of smoking which followed two cohorts of teenagers for several years from 9th grade (14–15 years old) found that the number of friends who smoked at the beginning of the study was strongly associated with experimenting with cigarettes during the study (Killen *et al.* 1997). This initial experimentation is a crucial step. Some data suggest that 85 to 90 per cent of those who smoke four cigarettes become regular smokers (Salber *et al.* 1963). This is one of the reasons why the prevention of smoking should begin in school and target young people before they have experimented with it (Best *et al.* 1988).

Reasons for smoking

The reasons smokers give for why they maintain the habit, once initiated, have been extensively analysed (Ikard *et al.* 1969; Leventhal and Avis 1976; Spielberger 1986). Factor analyses of self-report data collected from samples of smokers have led to very similar factor structures (Shiffman 1993b). For example, a study conducted by Leventhal and Avis (1976) resulted in the following factors: pleasure–taste (e.g. 'I like the taste of tobacco'); addiction (e.g. 'I get a real gnawing hunger for a cigarette when I haven't smoked for a while'); habit (e.g. 'I smoke cigarettes automatically without even being aware of it'); anxiety (e.g. 'When I am nervous in social situations, I smoke'); stimulation (e.g. 'Smoking makes me feel more awake'); social rewards (e.g. 'I smoke to be sociable'); and fiddle (e.g. 'Handling a cigarette is part of the enjoyment of smoking').

Leventhal and Avis (1976) and Ikard and Tomkins (1973) examined the validity of these reports by dividing respondents on the basis of their responses to such questionnaires into high and low scorers on a particular dimension. When the actual smoking behaviour of these respondents was examined under experimentally manipulated conditions, respondents' behaviour validated their reported reasons for smoking. For example, when smokers were given cigarettes adulterated with vinegar, those high on the pleasure–taste factor showed a sharp drop in the number of cigarettes smoked, but those low on the factor did not (Leventhal and Avis 1976). When asked to monitor their smoking by filling out a card for each cigarette smoked, habit smokers significantly reduced their smoking, whereas pleasure–taste smokers did not (Leventhal and Avis 1976). Finally, there was more smoking during and after a fear-arousing film for smokers who used smoking for anxiety reduction (Ikard and Tomkins 1973). Both studies also found that addicts suffered the most during periods of deprivation.

Findings such as these could have important implications for clinical therapy. For example, therapy aimed at a smoker whose main motive in smoking is to reduce anxiety would have to differ from that aimed at someone who smokes out of habit. However, in a review of studies that related individual smoking motives to cessation processes, Shiffman (1993b) found little evidence 'that smoking typology classifications substantially affect cessation processes or inform treatment decisions' (p. 736). Furthermore, Shiffman claimed that the motives for smoking inferred from typology measures showed little relationship with actual smoking patterns in the natural environment assessed by self-monitoring.

Smoking attitudes and intentions

According to the theories of reasoned action and planned behaviour, attitudes, subjective norms, perceived control, and intentions are important determinants of smoking behaviour (Ajzen 1988). These models further assume that attitudes, subjective norms and perceived control are all based on beliefs.

That smokers differ from non-smokers with regard to their evaluative beliefs about the consequences of smoking has been demonstrated in numerous studies conducted nearly exclusively on student samples (for a review, see Sutton 1989). It is interesting to note that smokers differed from non-smokers mainly in their evaluation of the social consequences (e.g. causes bad breath, is offensive) rather than the negative health impact of smoking (Budd 1986). Although the young age of the respondents may have contributed to this pattern, it is mainly due to the fact that even smokers have accepted by now that smoking impairs their health.

Consistent with expectations from the model of reasoned action, numerous studies have indicated that smoking intentions are closely linked to positive attitudes towards smoking, and subjective norms (e.g. Sutton 1989). That intention is a good predictor even of the onset of smoking behaviour has been demonstrated in prospective studies in the USA and Europe (e.g. Chassin *et al.* 1984; de Vries *et al.* 1995). Because smoking is addictive, it is difficult to execute the intention to stop smoking. One would therefore expect that intentions to stop smoking would be a good predictor of attempts to give it up, but a poor predictor of long-term abstinence. As discussed below (p. 92), this assumption has been supported by empirical evidence (e.g. Borland *et al.* 1991).

Addiction

According to the nicotine regulation model developed by Schachter and his colleagues, individuals smoke to regulate the level of nicotine in the internal milieu (Schachter 1977, 1978; Schachter *et al.* 1977b). Smoking is stimulated when the nicotine level falls below a certain set point. Thus, Schachter (who was a lifelong smoker himself) conceptualized smoking essentially as an escape–avoidance response. Smokers smoked to escape the aversive consequences of nicotine withdrawal. By implication, pleasurable aspects of smoking are considered incidental (Pomerleau and Pomerleau 1989).

Schachter and his colleagues tested this hypothesis in a series of innovative studies (Schachter 1977; Schachter *et al.* 1977a, b). In their first study, they lowered the level of nicotine in cigarettes and found that long-time, heavy smokers increased their smoking by 25 per cent, but light smokers only by 18 per cent (Schachter 1977). To examine whether these changes reflected a need to maintain an optimal level of nicotine in the blood, Schachter *et al.* (1977a) compared smoking levels in respondents who were chemically induced to excrete nicotine either at a very high or a very low rate. Most of the nicotine absorbed by an individual is chemically broken down, but a fraction of nicotine which escapes this process is eliminated as such in the urine. The rate of excretion of unchanged nicotine (an alkaloid) in the urine depends on the acidity of the individual's urine. During different weeks, respondents in this experiment took either substantial doses of placebo or of drugs that acidify the urine (e.g. vitamin C = ascorbic acid). The fact that respondents who took vitamin C increased their average cigarette smoking by roughly 15 to 20 per cent supported Schachter's hypothesis.

Smokers are not only convinced that smoking reduces stress, they also smoke more in stressful situations like examinations, colloquia, stressful seminar presentations or when being administered painful electric shocks (Schachter *et al.* 1977b). Schachter and his colleagues reasoned that this behaviour is induced by the fact that stress makes the urine more acidic and thus lowers the blood-nicotine level. Thus, cigarette smoking under stress serves the function of regulating serum nicotine. To test this assumption, Schachter *et al.* (1977b) conducted an experiment which independently manipulated level of stress and acidity of urine. Consistent with the nicotine regulation model, exposure to a painful rather than a weak electric shock increased smoking in respondents who had been given a placebo, but not in respondents who had been given a pill that prevented their urine from acidifying.

Does smoking help smokers to reduce stress, to calm down or to improve their performance? It does indeed, but only if they are compared to smokers who are deprived of nicotine. Thus, smokers who are smoking high-nicotine rather than low-nicotine cigarettes can take more painful electric shocks, are less irritated by aeroplane noise and do better at motor performance tasks (Schachter 1978). However, when the mood or performance of smokers who are permitted to smoke as much as they want is compared with the mood or performance of control groups of non-smokers, a remarkable fact emerges: smoking only improves the mood of smokers or their performance to the level customary for non-smokers (Schachter 1978). In other words, 'the heavy smoker gets nothing out of smoking. He smokes only to prevent withdrawal' (Schachter 1978: 106).

The conclusion that smokers only smoke to prevent nicotine withdrawal symptoms has been criticized by Pomerleau and Pomerleau (1989). These authors argued that an addiction interpretation cannot explain the fact that many stimuli which reliably increase the probability of smoking are unrelated to the time since the last cigarette was smoked. Thus, the temptation to smoke is increased at the end of a meal, when drinking a cup of coffee, or when put under intellectual demands (Shiffman 1982). Thus, many cigarettes smoked have no clear connection with nicotine deprivation or time since last cigarette and cannot therefore serve the function of preventing nicotine withdrawal.

From a review of the pharmacological effects of inhaled nicotine, Pomerleau and Pomerleau (1989) concluded that nicotine exerts direct and indirect effects upon several neuroregulatory systems. Many of the endogenous substances whose synthesis, release, and turnover in the central nervous system are affected by nicotine have been shown, independently of nicotine, to influence behaviour and subjective states. Because nicotine alters the availability in the organism of such substances, it is reasonable to suppose that smokers learn to 'use' the drug to regulate the body's normal adaptive mechanisms. Thus, smoking can be used as a pharmacological 'coping response' resulting in temporary improvements in affect or performance.

Genetics and smoking

Since everybody is exposed to smoking and most people are likely at some point in their lives to experiment with smoking, it is reasonable to assume that nicotine-dependent smokers are not only behaviourally but also biologically different from individuals who never smoked (Pomerleau and Kardia 1999). The first scientific evidence on the heritability of smoking was reported by Fisher (1958), who found that monozygotic twins had higher concordance rates than dizygotic twins. Greater concordance of a trait or behaviour among monozygotic twins is an indication of a genetic influence, because monozygotic and dizygotic twin pairs are exposed to the same family environment, but differ in the extent to which they share genetic material (i.e. monozygotic twins share all, dizygotic half). These findings have been frequently replicated in large studies of twins, with the magnitude of the genetic influence estimated around 50 per cent of the total variance in smoking behaviour (for reviews, see Hughes 1986; Heath and Madden 1994). It has also been established that genetic factors contribute not only to the initiation but also to the maintenance of smoking habit (Heath and Martin 1993). Given that smoking is an addiction, it is interesting to note that the magnitude of the genetic influence on smoking is comparable to that of alcoholism (Heath and Martin 1993).

Stopping smoking

In view of this substantial genetic influence on the persistence of smoking, it is gratifying to learn that the overwhelming majority of smokers who stop do so without professional help (Carey et al. 1993). It would appear plausible to use the success rates of these individuals as a baseline against which to compare the efficacy of all types of interventions. However, such a comparison would only be valid if one could assume that the two groups were identical at the outset. This is unlikely to be the case. It seems plausible that smokers try at first to stop by themselves and will only seek professional help if they cannot manage to stop on their own. However, the success rates of individuals who give up smoking without professional help are interesting in their own right.

Success rates

Early studies of unaided smoking cessation based on interviews with smokers who had stopped reported that 60 per cent had done so without outside help (Schachter 1982; Rzewnicki and Forgays 1987). More recently it has even been estimated that 90 per cent of the 44 million Americans who had stopped smoking at that time had done so without professional help (Fiore et al. 1990). To avoid raising unrealistic optimism in smokers who want to stop, it should be emphasized that these lifetime reports of successful stopping reflect success as a result of multiple attempts which have been made over the years. Success rates on individual trials of persons who stop unaided are rather low. According to a study by Cohen and colleagues (1989), abstinence rates of smokers at 12 months after the attempt to stop unaided are 13 per cent if one uses the standard criterion for abstinence, namely that individuals are not smoking around the time when the follow-up measurement is taken (*point prevalence abstinence*). Abstinence rates are reduced to just over 4 per cent if *continuous abstinence* since the stop attempt is used as the criterion.

Predictors

Who tries to stop smoking and who is ultimately successful? These are questions which can best be addressed in longitudinal studies of the natural history of smoking in which smokers are assessed before and after their attempts at giving up smoking. One such study followed a young community sample from 1987 to 1994 (Rose *et al.* 1996). A second study involved a smaller sample of adult smokers assessed before and six months after the introduction of a mandated smoking ban at their workplace (Borland *et al.* 1991). A third longitudinal study by Carey *et al.* (1993), for which respondents were recruited on the basis of their intention to stop, only provides information on the predictors of success.

According to stage theories of behaviour change discussed earlier (p. 44), one would expect that the factors which motivate individuals to stop may no longer be helpful in attempts at maintaining abstinence. In line with this assumption, Borland and colleagues found that the desire to stop smoking was the best predictor of making an attempt, but was unrelated to success. Similarly, the belief that smoking was damaging to their own health was strongly related to attempts to stop but not to success in doing so in the young sample of Rose and colleagues (1996). However, this differential pattern could also be a methodological artefact reflecting reduced variance: if most of the individuals who stop smoking believe that smoking is dangerous, this factor can no longer differentiate between successful and unsuccessful quitters.

It is interesting to note that whereas the fear of the negative health consequences of smoking only motivated individuals to stop smoking but did not appear to help them to maintain abstinence, strongly valuing a healthy lifestyle increased the likelihood of both stopping and abstaining. The differential effect of such apparently similar constructs could be due to the fact that keeping a healthy life involves much more than the mere avoidance of illness. Whereas the fear of smoking-related illnesses will have abated once people have stopped, the wish to keep fit and to feel healthy is likely to be a continuing concern which should help individuals not only to maintain abstinence but also to engage in health-enhancing activities such as eating a healthy diet and exercising.

With regard to social support, one has to distinguish between support for stopping and support for continuing to smoke. Experiencing support for stopping from family and friends increased the motivation to stop as well as the success in stopping in the sample of workers (Borland *et al.* 1991). However, the study of the young adolescents suggests that if social support for stopping is perceived as social pressure, it can become negatively associated with successful cessation (Rose *et al.* 1996). This finding may indicate that behaviour change that can be attributed to external causes by the individual is less likely to be maintained than change attributed to internal causes (Harackiewicz *et al.* 1987). In the course of this study these young individuals moved out of the sphere of influence of their parents who may have exerted the social pressure, and this could also have contributed to this finding. Surprisingly, support for continuing to smoke, such as having close friends who smoke, was no barrier to making attempts to quit. However, it did increase the opportunity for relapse for those who attempted to stop.

Self-efficacy with regard to stopping smoking should be related to both the motivation to stop and success rate. Smokers who feel that they have no control over their smoking behaviour should be less likely to try to stop than smokers who feel very much in control. Given that their perception of control is somewhat realistic, smoking self-efficacy should also be a predictor of success rate. Support for this last assumption comes from a longitudinal study by Carey and colleagues (1993). These authors reported that smokers who had stopped successfully and were abstinent at the end of the 12-month period had significantly higher smoking self-efficacy at intake than those who had failed to stop.

The extent to which smokers are addicted is also likely to affect the success in maintaining abstinence. Cohen and colleagues (1989) found lighter smokers to be approximately twice as likely as heavy smokers to succeed in their cessation attempts. Other studies support this association (e.g. Borland *et al.* 1991; Carey *et al.* 1993). How long people smoked, on the other hand, was unrelated to success in stopping (Carey *et al.* 1993; Rose *et al.* 1996). Educational status was positively associated with motivation to stop as well as to success (Rose *et al.* 1996; Jeffery *et al.* 1997).

Weight concerns have typically been considered as a factor that negatively affects both the decision to give up smoking and the success rate in doing so (Perkins 1993; Meyers *et al.* 1997). The belief that smoking controls weight is much stronger among high school students who smoke regularly, especially girls, than among those who do not (Perkins 1993). Furthermore, a substantial proportion of high school smokers state that they use smoking to control weight (Perkins 1993). Similarly, among adult smokers self-reports of weight control as a reason for smoking are associated with lack of intention to stop (Weekley *et al.* 1992). And yet, studies of the association of weight concerns and smoking cessation report conflicting results. In two prospective studies of unaided smoking cessation no association was observed between weight concerns and either serious attempts to quit or the likelihood of smoking cessation (French *et al.* 1995; Jeffery *et al.* 1997). In contrast, a study of participants in community-based smoking cessation intervention found that weight-concerned smokers were significantly less likely to be abstinent after 12 months than smokers who were not concerned about their weight (Meyers *et al.* 1997). The reasons for these inconsistencies remain unclear.

One promising way to address the problem of weight concerns in smoking cessation interventions would be to combine smoking treatment with weight gain prevention programmes. However, the two studies to date which followed this line found that the weight gain programmes included in smoking treatment programmes were not only ineffective in preventing weight gain, but that they also appeared to interfere with the success of the smoking treatment (Hall *et al.* 1992; Pierie *et al.* 1992). One reason for this finding could be that smokers who seek clinical treatment for their smoking might find it difficult enough to cope with stopping smoking without being distracted by having to pay attention to strategies that prevent weight gain.

Helping smokers to stop

Clinical intervention programmes

Most clinical approaches to smoking cessation are based on a mixture of behavioural and cognitive behavioural approaches. The techniques used include classical conditioning (aversion therapy), operant procedures (stimulus control, contingency management), self-management procedures and nicotine fading. Most recent work relies on multi-component programmes that combine several of these techniques (for reviews, see Glasgow and Lichtenstein 1987; Schwartz 1987; Hall *et al.* 1990; Shiffman 1993a; USDHHS 1996a). The use of nicotine replacement therapy (i.e. nicotine chewing gum or patches) has proved effective in the treatment of the more nicotine-dependent patients (for reviews, see Cepeda-Benito 1993; Hughes 1993; Fiore *et al.* 1994; Silagy *et al.* 1994).

Three kinds of stimuli have been used in *aversion therapies*: electric shock, imaginal stimuli, and cigarette smoke itself. *Shock aversion* has been consistently ineffective and the efficacy of imaginal aversion or *covert sensitization* has also been fairly low (Schwartz 1987). In this latter procedure, smokers have first to imagine themselves preparing to smoke and then to experience nausea. As an escape–relief dimension, they then imagine themselves feeling better as they turn away and reject their cigarettes.

Cigarette smoke as an aversive stimulus is used in *rapid smoking*, a clinical procedure in which individuals are instructed to smoke continually, inhaling every six to eight seconds, until tolerance is reached. This results in a nicotine satiation, and an irritation of the mucous membrane and throat passages which reduces smoking pleasure. It is expected that this unpleasant experience will be cognitively rehearsed and thus have a long-term effect. In recent years, rapid smoking has been successfully combined with other intervention techniques (Schwartz 1987). The clinical practice guidelines on smoking cessation written by a panel of experts for the USDHHS (1996a) specifically recommend including some kind of aversive smoking procedure in multi-component interventions. A meta-analysis of nine studies suggested that inclusion of this procedure resulted in a doubling of the success rate and was thus the most effective single content category analysed in that report (USDHHS 1996a). However, because rapid smoking affects the heart–lung system and results in increases in heart rate, carboxyhaemoglobin, and blood-nicotine levels, the health of the patients should be carefully assessed before rapid smoking is selected as a treatment procedure (Lichtenstein 1982).

Operant procedures

These are designed to detect the environmental stimuli that control the smoking response (stimulus control) or to manipulate the consequences of this response (e.g. contingency contracting). *Stimulus control* techniques are based on the assumption that smoking has become linked to environmental and internal events which trigger the smoking response (e.g. finishing a meal and drinking coffee or alcohol). The effectiveness of traditional stimulus control approaches to smoking *cessation* has not been impressive (Lichtenstein and Danaher 1975; Schwartz 1987). However, a novel method of reducing stimulus control called 'scheduled smoking' has recently been found effective in studies conducted by Cinciripini and colleagues (e.g. 1995). All smokers in these studies received behaviour therapy. However, in addition, smoking schedules and smoking reduction were manipulated in a factorial design during a period of three weeks before

Table 4.1   Percentage of smokers abstinent after one year

		Smoking reduction	
		Reduced	Non-reduced
Smoking	Yes	44%	32%
schedule	No	18%	22%

Source: Adapted from Cinciripini *et al.* (1995).

the agreed-upon stop date (Cinciripini *et al.* 1995). Scheduled smokers who were only allowed to smoke at specific times of the day were more likely still to be abstinent one year later than smokers who had been allowed to smoke freely before they stopped. The effectiveness of smoking schedules is probably due to the fact that scheduled smokers learn to break the pattern of nicotine self-administration. It is interesting to note that smoking schedules were most effective when combined with a planned progressive reduction in smoking frequency (Table 4.1), but that non-scheduled progressive reductions, where smokers could decide when to smoke the reduced number of cigarettes, was least effective. This latter finding is in line with the results of a meta-analysis of 18 studies on monitored nicotine fading, a procedure by which smokers are asked to monitor their daily tar and nicotine intake and try a progressive reduction, which found little evidence that the procedure was effective (USDHHS 1996a).

In *contingency contracting*, smokers agree with some agency (usually the therapist) on a set of rewards/punishments that will be enacted contingent on their behaviour. For example, smokers may pay a sum of money to the therapist and have it returned when they succeed in cutting down. Schwartz (1987) reviewed 13 contingency contracting studies reported between 1967 to 1985, and concluded that contracting was quite successful during treatment or until the deposit is returned. However, once the contract has ended, many individuals regress because no techniques for maintenance have been provided. A meta-analysis of nine studies found no evidence for the long-term effectiveness of contingency contracting (USDHHS 1996a). The failure of these contracts to have long-term effects could be due to the fact that individuals who abstain from smoking because they feel bound by a contract attribute their *not* smoking to this agreement. They may therefore be less likely to develop the sense of self-efficacy and feeling of control over their smoking behaviour that is necessary to maintain their abstinence at the end of therapy (Bandura 1986). They might also not be motivated to engage in the kind of negative re-evaluation of smoking that is likely in people who have to justify the stopping to themselves.

Self-management procedures

Self-management procedures which are also implemented under professional supervision include many behavioural techniques, such as:

1 The monitoring and recording of one's own smoking behaviour.
2 Changes in the antecedent conditions and consequences of one's smoking.
3 Developing awareness of and changing the environmental conditions that elicit smoking responses (Hall *et al.* 1990).

The most effective use of self-management procedures seems to be as part of multi-component programmes.

These self-management procedures which form part of professional therapy should not be confused with *self-help materials* (pamphlets/booklets/manuals) which are used without professional help. Self-help manuals do not increase the cessation rates relative to no self-help materials and the same seems to be true for video and audiotapes when used alone (USDHHS 1996a). For example Curry *et al.* (1995) found no significant difference in cessation rates at 12 or 21 months in a population-based non-volunteer sample who received a self-help booklet as compared to no treatment at all.

Hotlines or helplines allowing patient-initiated telephone calls for counselling or aid increase smoking cessation rates relative to no self-help materials even when used alone (USDHHS 1996a). This may indicate that supportive human contact (social support) is essential for successful interventions. However, the greater efficacy of telephone counselling could also be due to the fact that smokers could be given information tailored to their specific condition. There is empirical evidence that self-help materials which are tailored to the specific situation of individual smokers on the basis of questionnaire information can be effective (Dijkstra *et al.* 1998a). Smokers who had signed up for a 'research project on minimal interventions for smoking cessation' were randomly assigned to one of four conditions, namely 'only information of outcomes of smoking cessation', 'only self-efficacy-enhancing information', 'both kinds of information', and a 'no information' control condition. The information participants received was tailored by a computerized expert system on the basis of the pre-test responses of participants to a smoking questionnaire. After 14 months, 4.8 per cent in the combined condition were (continuously) abstinent, compared to 1.6 per cent of the individuals in the control group. This was the only significant difference between conditions. These findings demonstrate that self-help information can be effective. It remains unclear, however, whether this effect can be attributed to tailoring, because the study lacks control conditions in which the same information was given but without tailoring.

Most recent behavioural treatments of smoking use *multi-component treatment* and include a variety of methods. In addition to aversive smoking procedures, the clinical practice guidelines recommend interventions which help smokers to recognize and cope with problems encountered in stopping (problem solving/skill training) and provide social support as part of the treatment. Examples of danger situations given are being around other smokers, being under time pressure, getting into an argument, experiencing urges and negative moods, and drinking alcohol. Coping skills should include strategies which help the smoker to anticipate and avoid danger situations, to reduce negative moods, to accomplish lifestyle changes that reduce stress, and to distract attention from smoking urges. Thus, the clinical guidelines are in fact recommending the teaching of relapse prevention strategies (Klesges *et al.* 1991; Caroll 1996; see also p. 77). According to Schwartz (1987), the more successful multi-component programmes have used a greater number of treatment sessions, stronger maintenance components, and manuals that guide and instruct the subject on how to use self-control procedures. The clinical practice guidelines also conclude that the greater the number of weeks over which person-to-person counselling or treatment is delivered, the more effective is the treatment. Person-to-person treatment delivered over four to seven sessions appears to be especially effective (USDHHS 1996a).

In view of the important role of nicotine dependence in smoking, it would seem useful to provide *nicotine replacement therapies* to abate withdrawal symptoms. Once people have overcome the initial withdrawal symptoms and managed to stop smoking, the nicotine replacement can be gradually tapered off to avoid further withdrawal. The first type of nicotine replacement which became widely available was nicotine chewing gum. In a meta-analysis of 33 studies of the efficacy of nicotine chewing gum in smoking treatment programmes which employed random assignment of respondents to gum treatment groups or to either placebo or no-gum control groups, Cepeda-Benito (1993) concluded that nicotine gum consistently improved the efficacy of smoking cessation therapy that used nicotine gum as an additional component in a more comprehensive therapy, and that it was more effective among heavier smokers. The superiority of therapy plus nicotine gum over mere therapy was illustrated by the greater mean abstinence rates at long-term follow-up (approximately 12 months) displayed by the nicotine gum groups (35 per cent) vs the control groups (22 per cent). Thus, nicotine gum improved the overall effectiveness of therapy in the studies samples by 56 per cent (Cepeda-Benito 1993). However, approximately 20 per cent of individuals who use nicotine gums to stop smoking appear to become dependent on them. Furthermore, some minor side effects have been reported (Hughes 1993). Most of these problems can be avoided with the transdermal nicotine patch that has to be applied only once per day.

The effectiveness of treatment with nicotine patch has been assessed in a meta-analysis of 17 studies which used random assignment of respondents to active patch or placebo control groups (Fiore *et al.* 1994). The placebo control groups were unaware that they were in the placebo condition and received the same patch as the experimental groups, except that this patch did not contain any nicotine. Nicotine patch was demonstrated to be an effective aid to smoking cessation. With the active patch individuals were more than twice as likely to quit smoking (22 per cent) than were individuals wearing the placebo patch (9 per cent). There was also little evidence that patients became dependent on the nicotine replacement.

Can cognitive behaviour therapy help smokers to maintain long-term abstinence? The answer seems to be a qualified 'yes'. Although there is considerable variability in outcomes across studies, two-thirds of 17 multi-component programmes reviewed by Schwartz (1987) achieved at least a 33 per cent cessation rate at one year, with a median success rate of 40 per cent. There is also evidence that the effectiveness of intensive therapy can be improved by adding nicotine replacement therapy as a pharmacological element. However, because nicotine patch (unlike gum) appears to be effective even without added psychological treatment, it has been suggested that this treatment should be tried as a first step and that therapy should be added only if and when this pharmacological approach has failed (Fiore *et al.* 1994). In contrast, there is little evidence to date that written self-help materials used by themselves or in combination with mass media programmes are effective.

Community interventions

In spite of the substantial decline in cigarette smoking observed in the years after the US Surgeon General's report which received wide coverage in the mass media, one cannot be confident that this decrease in rates was caused by this communication, rather than some other reason (Figure 3.1). To demonstrate the effectiveness of mass communication in inducing smoking cessation, one needs *experimental* studies, in which one group of people is exposed to the communication while an otherwise comparable group is not. If it can be shown that the experimental group has an advantage in cessation rates over the control group, this difference can be attributed to the communication. Fortunately, such data are available from several major community studies which aimed at a reduction in smoking rates as part of their campaign to reduce the risk of coronary heart disease.

Probably the most successful community intervention was achieved in the North Karelia project described in the preceding chapter (e.g. Puska *et al.* 1985). As part of this project, an intensive educational campaign was implemented for the reduction of cigarette smoking. The neighbouring province of Kuopio was selected as a control group not exposed to the campaign. Self-reported numbers of cigarettes smoked per day fell by more than one-third among the men in North Karelia, compared to only a 10 per cent reduction among men in the control community. The campaign had no effect on smoking rates of women. Because self-reports of smoking rates could be distorted by social desirability effects, it is encouraging that a 24 per cent decline in cardiovascular deaths among men was observed in North Karelia as compared with a 12 per cent decline in other parts of the country (Puska *et al.* 1985). Similar effects on smoking reduction have been observed in two community studies conducted in Australia (Egger *et al.* 1983) and Switzerland (Autorengruppe Nationales Forschungsprogramm 1984). On the basis of these studies, the US Surgeon General (USDHHS 1984) concluded that the absolute reduction in smoking prevalence in intervention sites was about 12 per cent greater than the reduction in comparison communities.

Recent community studies conducted in the USA have reported more moderate effects (e.g. Farquhar *et al.* 1990), or no effect at all (e.g. Carleton *et al.* 1995). Typical of these modest effects are the findings of the COMMIT study, the largest community trial for smoking intervention to date, launched in 1989 (COMMIT Research Group 1995). In this study one of each of 11 matched community pairs was randomly assigned to the intervention. The four-year community-based intervention used methods similar to those of earlier community trials (e.g. Farquhar *et al.* 1990) to encourage smokers, particularly heavy smokers, to achieve and maintain abstention. It was therefore disappointing that the intervention had no effect on heavy smokers (those who smoked more than 25 cigarettes per day). The percentage of the members of the cohort of heavy smokers who stopped smoking in the period between 1988 and 1993 and had smoked no cigarettes for at least the preceding six months at the end of the trial was 18 per cent for the treatment and 18.7 per cent for the comparison communities. However, for the group of light-to-moderate smokers a small but significant difference emerged. The proportion of light-to-moderate smokers who stopped in the intervention communities (30.6 per cent) was 3 per cent higher than the proportion of smokers who stopped in the control communities (27.5 per cent). Although this is a very modest effect, an extrapolation to the community level would imply that more than 3000 smokers were induced to stop in the intervention communities beyond the naturally occurring secular trend. Nevertheless, the reduction is much smaller than the 12 per cent average suggested in the report of the Surgeon General.

One can only speculate about the reasons for this apparent reduction in the impact of more recent interventions. A likely reason is the vast improvement in knowledge about the health-impairing nature of smoking that occurred during the last few decades. Community interventions still rely heavily on the dissemination of information about the deleterious consequences of smoking and thus have little impact on the large proportion of smokers who are well aware of the damage they are doing to their health. These smokers need help to stop and this help is less easily provided in community settings. However, the fact that the impact of health education could not be demonstrated in these community studies should not be taken as evidence that health education is no longer important. Data from the 1985 National Health Interview Survey (Kenkel 1991) demonstrate that while smoking knowledge is fairly widespread, the remaining differences in knowledge are still significantly related to smoking.

Interventions at the worksite

The place of work is an excellent setting for health promotion programmes because large numbers of people can be reached on a regular basis. Therefore, many large firms have introduced health promotion programmes (for reviews, see Klesges and Glasgow 1986; Fisher *et al.* 1990). A meta-analysis of studies of worksite smoking cessation published through 1988 combined data from 28 controlled studies which assessed cessation rates (i.e. the number of employees stopping smoking to the number of employees who started the intervention) on average 12 months after the intervention (Fisher *et al.* 1990). Fisher and colleagues found interventions to have a modest but significant overall effect. The average cessation rate was 13 per cent. Effects were somewhat stronger in smaller than in larger worksites. Surprisingly, it was the heavier smokers who profited most from these worksite interventions (average rate 16 per cent).

Since then, a number of large worksite smoking cessation trials have been published which had rather mixed results. The smoking intervention of the largest study, the Working Well Trial (Sorensen *et al.* 1996), was conducted by three centres in 84 worksites (mean number of workers per site: 316). Half of the worksites were randomly assigned as control conditions. The intervention consisted of a two-year health promotion at the worksite focusing on smoking and eating behaviour. The study used a 'participatory model' with employee advisory boards to 'incorporate employee input and concerns'. Core interventions included 'kickoff events, interactive activities, posters and brochures, self-assessments, self-help materials, campaigns and contest, direct education through classes and groups' (1996: 940). Overall, there was only a negligible and non-significant difference in abstinence rates between intervention and control sites. However, treatment effects were significant for one of three centres, incorporating 24 worksites. Here 17.3 per cent of smokers stopped in the intervention sites as compared to 12.7 in the control sites. No explanation has been provided as to why the intervention worked for one of the centres but not for the other two. Even more disappointing findings were reported from two similar large-scale intervention studies, Take Heart I and II (Glasgow *et al.* 1995, 1997). In both studies, the interventions did not result in any significant effects on smoking behaviour.

The reasons for the failure of these large-scale, low-intensity worksite interventions to influence smoking behaviour are probably similar to those for the community interventions. Most smokers who still smoke in the USA today would like to stop (USDHHS 1990). Providing them with information about the health risk of smoking is therefore ineffective. What they need is skills training and social support, which may not have been supplied in these interventions.

That intensive anti-smoking interventions can still be effective at worksites has been demonstrated in several worksite intervention studies conducted in the USA (e.g. Salina *et al.* 1994) and Europe (e.g. Willemsen *et al.* 1996). In a study conducted in the Netherlands two interventions of varying intensity instituted at eight worksites were compared (Willemsen *et al.* 1996). Participants were 498 smokers (out of more than 10,000 workers in the participating firms) who volunteered to participate in an anti-smoking programme. All participants were sent self-help materials, but in the intensive intervention they also took part in self-help groups led by trained advisers. At 14 months follow-up, 16 per cent of the participants in the intensive intervention had stopped smoking, compared to 12 per cent in the minimal programme condition, again demonstrating the greater effectiveness of intensive over minimal anti-smoking interventions. It is interesting to note, however, that the difference in effectiveness only emerged for heavy smokers (average of 23 cigarettes per day). Of the heavy smokers, 15 per cent stopped after the intensive intervention, as compared to 8 per cent following the minimal intervention. The corresponding percentages for light smokers (average of 13 cigarettes per day) were 18 per cent and 17 per cent. Since the study did not include a non-intervention control group, it is difficult to tell whether the minimal intervention had any impact. What one can conclude from these results, however, is that for the light smokers, participation in the self-help groups appears to have been superfluous.

In conclusion, there is evidence that intensive anti-smoking worksite interventions can be effective, particularly for heavy smokers who are likely to be nicotine addicted. At a time where most smokers are well aware of the health consequences of smoking and are also likely to have failed already in attempts to stop smoking, merely providing participants with information about health consequences no longer appears to be sufficient.

Physicians' advice

Physicians can be important agents in health promotion. There is evidence that even minimal advice from physicians can be effective in changing smoking behaviour. A classic study was conducted by Russell and colleagues (1979) in five group practices in London. During a four-week period 2138 cigarette smokers attending the medical practice of 28 general practitioners were assigned to one of four groups:

1 Follow-up only.
2 Questionnaire assessing their smoking behaviour and follow-up.
3 Physician's advice to stop smoking plus questionnaires and follow-up.
4 Advice to stop plus a leaflet helping them to stop and follow-up.

Outcomes were assessed at one and 12 months and were biochemically validated.

The minimal intervention was quite effective. Compared to the non-intervention groups, more patients in the groups that received advice were successful in stopping after one year. In the two non-intervention groups the proportion of patients who gave up smoking during the first months and were still not smoking one year later were 0.3 per cent and 1.6 per cent. In comparison, 3.3 per cent of the patients who merely had been told to give up smoking and 5.1 per cent of patients who in addition had received a leaflet with advice were still not smoking a year later. These differences are small but, as the authors argued, if all general practitioners in Great Britain were to adopt this procedure, the yield would exceed half a million ex-smokers within one year.

In a meta-analysis of 39 controlled trials of smoking interventions in medical practice, Kottke and colleagues (1988) reported an average success after 12 months (i.e. the difference in the proportions of participants who stop in intervention vs control conditions) of 5.8 per cent. The interventions included in this analysis ranged from counselling or advice to the handing out of written material or the prescribing of nicotine gum. It may be comforting to medical practitioners that the authors concluded that these effects were not due to some particularly effective intervention strategy but that it was 'the repeated help and advice to stop smoking' (p. 2888) which did the trick. These effects could probably be increased if nicotine patch treatment was added in the case of heavy smokers.

It is interesting that the advice to stop smoking appears to have much greater impact when given by physicians than when provided as part of a community intervention. This is probably due to the fact that physicians are health experts and that the advice is personalized. Because individuals who visit their physician often seek remedy for some health problem, they may also be in a particularly receptive mood on such occasions. Thus, although the effects of smoking interventions in medical practice are modest, their advantage is that they are cost-effective and reach smokers who might not be reached by any other programme.

Primary prevention

School-based health education

In view of the serious difficulties smokers experience when they try to stop smoking, school-based anti-smoking programmes aimed at preventing young adolescents from starting the habit would appear most promising. After all, teenagers are most at risk of starting to smoke. A recent survey in the United States indicated that the probability of starting to smoke at a given age for individuals who have not started previously (the hazard rate of starting smoking) increases to a peak of 15 per cent at age 19, then declines quickly to two per cent at age 24 (Douglas and Hariharan 1993: Figure 4.1). Furthermore, a longitudinal study of the natural history of cigarette smoking by Chassin and colleagues (1990) suggested that even infrequent experimentation in adolescence was associated with a substantial increase in the probability that the individual would smoke as an adult. Regular adolescent smoking appeared to raise the risk of adult smoking by a factor of 16 compared to non-smoking adolescents. Furthermore, there was a positive linear relationship between the grade in which adolescents began to smoke and adult smoking. These findings underline the importance of primary prevention programmes directed at adolescent populations.

Unfortunately, most of the early programmes, which were conducted in health education courses and emphasized long-term health risks of smoking, were ineffective in persuading children not to smoke. The likely reason for this failure is that children are already familiar with the health consequences of smoking and in any case are not yet very much concerned about health issues. The more recent programmes developed by Evans and his collaborators therefore avoided the health and threat-oriented

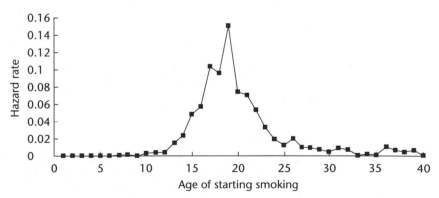

Figure 4.1 The probability of starting to smoke at any given age (US sample).
Source: Douglas and Hariharan (1994).

approach that was predominant in earlier programmes (e.g. Evans 1976; Evans *et al.* 1978). Instead, they emphasized the socially undesirable aspects of smoking to motivate individuals not to smoke (e.g. cigarettes smell bad). They also included the development of specific action plans and social skills to resist pressures to try cigarettes. Thus, individuals were trained in skills needed to reject offers of cigarettes without alienating peers.

In a review of four generations of school-based anti-smoking studies, only moderate reductions in the number of students who start smoking have been found. Cleary and colleagues (1988) estimated that on average 5 to 8 per cent of students who might otherwise have started to smoke were prevented from doing so. Similar conclusions were drawn in a more recent meta-analysis of 90 studies published from 1974 to 1991 (Rooney and Murray 1996). The studies included in this meta-analysis were school-based, took place in the 6th to 12th grade (ages 11 to 17), had some quantitative measure of tobacco use, included a control or comparison group, and were 'social' or 'peer-type' programmes. Although most of these programmes included information about the health consequences of smoking, they mainly focused on providing training, modelling, rehearsal, and reinforcement of techniques to resist social pressure to smoke, and to resist smoking messages in advertisements and the media. Some programmes also included public commitments not to smoke, cognitive strategies to improve self-efficacy and methods for coping with anxiety. These types of prevention efforts translated into a 5 per cent reduction in smoking assessed one year after the intervention. Similar intervention effects have been reported in the Netherlands (Dijkstra *et al.* 1992).

Given the serious health consequences of smoking and the difficulty smokers have in stopping once they have become addicted, interventions which reduce the number of young people who start the habit by 5 per cent should be regarded as quite effective. However, Rooney and Murray (1996) stressed that with the most effective programmes the impact could be as high as 19 to 29 per cent. To be most effective, programmes should be delivered relatively early (e.g. 6th grade), include same-age peers as programme leaders, be part of a multi-component health programme rather than focus on tobacco use only, and incorporate booster sessions to be given in subsequent years. Following a suggestion by Leventhal and colleagues (e.g. Hirschman and Leventhal 1989), when interventions are conducted at a somewhat later age, one might also incorporate measures which are aimed at slowing or reversing the progress from experimental to regular smoker in order to be effective with adolescents who already had experimented with cigarette smoking.

Legal and economic measures

A second strategy of primary prevention could involve further restrictions in the sales of cigarettes (e.g. stricter age limits) as well as increases in taxation. On average, teenagers have less disposable income than adults, and are therefore more likely to be deterred from smoking by marked increases in the price of cigarettes, particularly if they have not yet started the habit or are still in a period of experimentation. The price elasticity of demand for cigarettes varies from -1.40 in adolescents to -0.42 in adults (Lewit and Coate 1982). Thus, a 10 per cent increase in the price of cigarettes would result in a 14 per cent decrease in the demand for cigarettes in adolescents but only in a 4 per cent decrease in adults.

Recent economic models distinguish addictive consumption from other consumption by recognizing that for addictive goods such as cigarettes or heroin, current consumption depends on past consumption. Such models predict that the impact of price increases would increase over time (e.g. Becker et al. 1994). Heavy smokers are likely to continue smoking heavily and will not respond readily to increases in price. However, they might be able to reduce their smoking slowly in response to price increases. Furthermore, price increases will also reduce the probability of adolescents picking up the habit. The combined impact of such effects should result in a reduction in smoking in the long run.

These analyses suggest that legal and economic measures are effective means of reducing consumption among current smokers as well as smoking initiation. Because adolescents have less disposable income, tax increases would seem a promising strategy to prevent young people from being recruited into smoking, particularly if these are combined with the various educational programmes described earlier. Another promising strategy would be restrictions on tobacco advertising. There is persuasive evidence that restrictions on the advertising of tobacco products reduce consumption (e.g. Laugesen and Meads 1991).

Conclusions

Smoking has been identified as the single most important source of preventable morbidity and mortality and nowadays this fact is accepted by smokers and non-smokers alike. Most smokers admit that they would like to stop. However, only about 13 per cent of smokers who try to stop by themselves really manage to be abstinent a year later, and this rate is further reduced if one takes continuous abstinence as the criterion. And yet the majority of smokers who stop smoking do so without professional help. Those smokers who seek therapy are likely to be the most problematic cases. The 30 to 40 per cent success rates of multi-component treatment programmes are therefore quite impressive.

With the war against smoking having been waged continuously since the mid-1960s, most smokers in Western industrialized nations are now aware of the negative health consequences associated with smoking. This may be the reason why community or worksite interventions which rely mainly on educating smokers about health consequences are less and less likely to have a measurable impact. However, more intensive interventions which provide social support and skill training are still effective. Furthermore, nicotine replacement therapies have also been demonstrated to be effective even when not accompanied by therapy.

Giving up a long-established habit like smoking is difficult. The most promising strategy for smoking prevention therefore involves inducing people not to start smoking. For this reason school-based programmes are very important, as are all measures which increase the price and reduce the availability of tobacco products. These measures should be complemented by a restriction on tobacco advertising. Finally, the fact that the large educational components of community anti-smoking interventions do not appear to have a demonstrable impact should not be taken as evidence that health education is no longer important. It merely demonstrates that education is not effective for people who are already well informed. However, to keep people well informed the war against smoking has to be continued.

ALCOHOL AND ALCOHOL ABUSE

Alcohol and health

There is widespread consensus among health professionals that the inappropriate or excessive use of alcohol leads to an increased risk of morbidity and mortality (Bruun *et al.* 1975; Ashley and Rankin 1988; Hurley and Horowitz 1990). Ashley and Rankin (1988) even claimed that 'in the United States in 1977, total alcohol-related health costs ranked a close second to heart and vascular disease, as the prime health cause of economic loss, well ahead of cancer and respiratory disease' (p. 234). In recognition of these health risks, any alcoholic beverage that is bottled for sale in the USA now has to carry the following health warning:

> Government Warning: According to the Surgeon General, women should not drink alcoholic beverages during pregnancy because of the risk of birth defects. Consumption of alcoholic beverages impairs your ability to drive a car or operate machinery, and may cause health problems.

Morbidity and mortality

Heavy drinkers suffer an increased risk of liver diseases (particularly cirrhosis), elevated blood pressure, and various forms of cancer, even breast cancer (Hurley and Horowitz 1990; Longnecker 1994). Furthermore, the use and abuse of alcohol increases the risk both of being involved in accidents and of being seriously injured as an accident victim (Committee on Trauma Research 1985).

In the USA only about 3 per cent of the recorded deaths are officially attributed to causes directly linked to alcohol. However, epidemiologists suspect that there is a substantial under-reporting of alcohol-related conditions, particularly as contributing causes of death, and that the actual number is much higher (Hurley and Horowitz 1990). One strategy to trace the relationship between mortality and excess alcohol consumption has been to demonstrate that the mortality rate of alcoholics for a given cause is in excess of that for moderate drinkers or abstainers (Bruun *et al.* 1975). However, in order to attribute a difference in mortality between these groups to the difference in alcohol consumption, one has to be certain that differential consumption was the only risk factor in which the two groups differ. This assumption is often unfounded, because people who are heavy drinkers or alcoholics usually engage in other habits that are deleterious to their health. For example, a review of studies on the relationship between alcoholism and smoking found that an average of 90 per cent of the men and women in the alcoholic groups were smokers, a proportion that is much higher than that in the general population (Istvan and Matarazzo 1984). In interpreting findings that alcoholics suffer from an excess mortality from certain forms of cancer, one has therefore to separate the impact of alcohol from that of smoking. For example, the excess in the development of cancer of the oral cavity, pharynx, larynx and oesophagus among alcoholics must be attributed to the combined effects of both alcohol consumption and smoking (Bruun *et al.* 1975).

Alcohol and liver cirrhosis

A second strategy for investigating the health risk of alcohol abuse has been to focus on mortality from specific causes that are likely to be related to excess alcohol consumption. Not surprisingly, the most clear-cut evidence comes from mortality due to cirrhosis of the liver. Cirrhosis is a disorder of the liver in which healthy liver tissue has been damaged and replaced by fibrous scar tissue. In 1964 cirrhosis of the liver was the eleventh leading cause of death in the United States, and the fifth leading cause for men in the productive years from 25 to 64 (Terris 1967). There is evidence of a positive correlation between per capita consumption of alcoholic beverages (measured in litres of absolute alcohol during a given year) and deaths due to liver cirrhosis (per 100,000 population aged 25 years and older). The data presented in Figure 4.2 show a correlation of .94 between these two variables across different nations (Helzer 1987).

There is also evidence that imposed restrictions in alcohol consumption are accompanied by a drop in death due to liver cirrhosis (Ledermann 1964). For example, in Paris there was a sharp drop in cirrhosis death rates coincidental with the two World Wars. The data for World War II are particularly instructive, because cirrhosis deaths dropped from 35 in 1941 to a low of six in 1945 and 1946. They began to rise again in 1948, the year when wine rationing was discontinued. Obviously, there were other factors present during this period that are likely to have at least contributed to the drop in liver cirrhosis mortality.

Alcohol and violent deaths

Alcohol has also been implicated in death from injuries. According to some estimates, a third to a half of adult Americans involved in accidents, crimes, and suicides had been drinking alcohol prior to the event (Hurley and Horowitz 1990). In 1982 the US National Highway Transportation Safety Administration estimated that 57 per cent of all fatal car crashes were alcohol-related and even though the estimated proportion had dropped substantially by 1996, it was still high at 41 per cent (DeJong and Hingson 1998).

One major problem with research in this area is that it often lacks appropriate control groups. For example, in a very thorough study of the

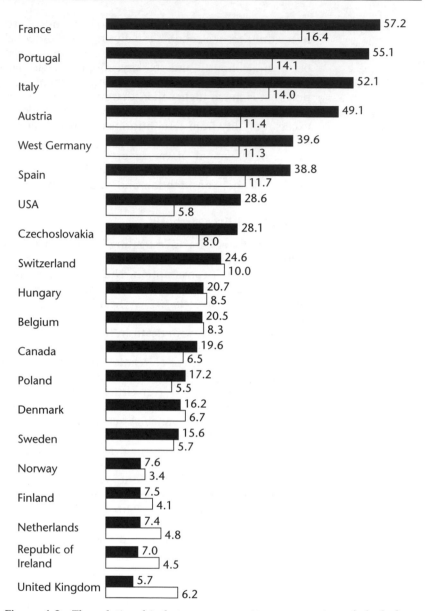

Figure 4.2 The relationship between per capita consumption of alcohol (in litres of absolute alcohol) (□) and death from cirrhosis of the liver (per 100,000 population aged 25 and older) (■). $r = .94$.
Source: Schmidt (1977).

role of alcohol in violent deaths, Haberman and Baden (1978) give estimates of alcohol presence at the time of death for a sample of unnatural deaths that occurred in New York City between August 1974 and August 1975. Table 4.2 indicates the percentage of individuals in each event

Table 4.2 Blood or brain alcohol concentration for suicide, homicide and accident victims[a]

Casualty	Sample size (n)	Per cent BAC = 0.10 and above	Per cent positive BAC
Suicide	247	16	32
Homicide	499	27	42
Motor vehicle			
driver	61	38	52
passenger	25	16	24
pedestrian	61	21	30
Fall	54	41	48
Fire	28	46	54
Drowning	19	53	68

[a] Data collected between 1974 and 1975.
Source: Adapted from Haberman and Baden (1978).

category for whom the presence of alcohol in the bloodstream could be demonstrated or who were intoxicated (Blood-Alcohol Concentration of more than 0.10 per cent).

Nevertheless, the fact that 52 per cent of the drivers killed in car accidents had previously consumed some alcohol is difficult to interpret unless one knows the percentage of drivers of the same age and sex and with the same amount of alcohol at the same time and weekday who were not involved in accidents. If 52 per cent of those drivers had also consumed alcohol, there would be no case to argue that alcohol consumption increases the risk of traffic accidents. However, the evidence from studies that employed adequate control groups suggests that alcohol consumption significantly increases the risk of injuries from all types of accidents. In a study of drivers who were killed in car accidents in New York City, McCarroll and Haddon (1962) found that 50 per cent of these drivers had Blood Alcohol Concentrations (BAC) at or above the 0.10 per cent level (i.e. were fairly intoxicated), as compared to less than 5 per cent of drivers tested at the site of the accident a few weeks later. These tests were conducted on the same day of the week and at the same time of day at which the accident had occurred, with drivers who moved in the same direction. Similarly, a study of fatally injured adult pedestrians that used the same type of control group reported that 74 per cent of the injured pedestrians had consumed some alcohol, as compared to 33 per cent of the control group (Haddon *et al.* 1961). Taken together, these studies strongly suggest that people who have consumed alcohol are at an increased risk of accidental injuries and violent death.

Is there a protective effect of moderate consumption?

In view of the high proportion of smokers among alcoholics, it is surprising that studies of the impact of alcohol consumption on coronary death often find no relationship (e.g. Dawber 1980), or even that moderate drinkers have lower mortality rates than abstainers (e.g. Hennekens *et al.* 1979).

The existence of an apparently protective association between light to moderate alcohol consumption and coronary heart disease has recently been questioned by Shaper *et al.* (1988). These authors concluded from a prospective study of more than 7000 middle-aged men that the apparently positive health impact of moderate drinking is a selection artefact: men who have health problems reduce their drinking and thus move into the non-drinking or occasional drinking category. However, a large case-control study conducted in New Zealand compared the risk among light and moderate drinkers with that of *lifelong* abstainers and found that drinking up to five to six drinks a week was associated with a reduced risk of myocardial infarction (Jackson *et al.* 1991). Further research is needed to reconcile these contradictory findings.

Foetal alcohol syndrome

Aristotle was probably the first to observe that drunken women often bore children who were feeble-minded. The advice of the US Surgeon General that women should not drink alcohol during pregnancy is based on more recent observations suggesting that prenatal exposure to alcohol is associated with a distinct pattern of birth defects that have been termed the foetal alcohol syndrome (FAS). A number of physical malformations have been reported, for example, head circumference and nose are smaller, the nasal bridge is lower, and there is a growth deficiency. However, the most serious aspect of the foetal alcohol syndrome is mental retardation. Although the exact number of children born with this syndrome is not known, it is estimated that in the USA one to three live births per 1000 are afflicted (Hurley and Horowitz 1990). In Germany approximately 2200 children per year are born with the foetal alcohol syndrome (Jonas 1995).

Although the description of the foetal alcohol syndrome is non-controversial, its causes, and particularly the level of alcohol consumption during pregnancy that is considered safe, are highly disputed. Current estimates place the foetus at risk for the physical signs of foetal alcohol syndrome if maternal drinking during pregnancy is six glasses of wine per day (450 ml of wine or approximately 60 ml of absolute alcohol) (Abel 1980). However, the frequency of alcohol-related birth defects is much lower than the frequency of abusive drinking among pregnant women (Hurley and Horowitz 1990). This suggests that other factors may modify the impact of alcohol on prenatal development. Women who drink excessively during pregnancy are also likely to do a number of other things that are unhealthy to the foetus, such as smoking, not eating properly, and taking drugs. For example, nutritional deficiencies during pregnancy may be responsible for the low birthweight of the children born with foetal alcohol syndrome. One extensive study of factors which increase the risk of FAS for women who abuse alcohol during pregnancy has identified four variables, namely number of previous births, history of alcohol problems, greater proportion of drinking days, and race (Sokol *et al.* 1986). However, even though being black has been found to be associated with an increase in the risk of FAS, studies around the globe have shown that no racial group is immune. Furthermore, FAS represents only the most severe type of foetal damage that can be produced by prenatal alcohol exposure. Lower levels of maternal drinking also have measurable effects on the foetus (Hurley and Horowitz 1990).

Behavioural and cognitive consequences of alcohol consumption

Although many of the health effects of alcohol are directly caused by the pharmacological properties of alcohol, others are likely to be mediated by the impact alcohol has on decision-making processes. These effects have often been attributed to disinhibiting effects of alcohol, assumed to decrease temporarily the impact of societal norms on individual behaviour. Steele and colleagues (e.g. Steele and Josephs 1990) have recently suggested an alternative explanation, based on the fact that consumption of alcohol decreases cognitive capacity and thereby limits the amount of information to which one can attend. As a consequence, intoxicated individuals are particularly impaired when complex deliberations about conflicts between competing instigating and inhibiting cues are demanded. They are unable to pay attention to any but the most salient aspects of a situation. This 'alcohol myopia' will prevent individuals who deliberate under alcohol influence about potential courses of action from considering the more subtle or remote consequences of their alternatives. As a result, the impact of the most salient immediate aspects of experience on emotions and behaviour will increase, whereas the effect of the more remote and subtle aspects will decrease.

MacDonald et al. (1995) have applied this theory to the factors which affect decisions to drive under the influence of alcohol. When people are deciding whether to drink and drive, they are likely to be confronted with inhibiting cues which discourage them from drinking and driving and instigating cues that encourage this behaviour. Inhibiting cues are the knowledge that one might be involved in accidents or caught by the police, whereas instigating cues may include the fact that one is tired, does not want to leave one's car, or that public transport is very cumbersome. Whereas a sober person is able to weigh all these pros and cons in arriving at a decision, an intoxicated person might be disproportionately influenced by the most salient cues, such as that one is tired, and that using the train would take hours.

MacDonald and her colleagues (1995) reasoned that intoxicated individuals might decide to drive in situations in which cues that tend to instigate driving are more salient than cues which normally inhibit driving under the influence. They tested this hypothesis in a series of laboratory and field studies in which individuals who were either intoxicated or sober were asked questions about drinking and driving. For half the respondents, these questions were straightforward. They were simply asked whether they would drive after having consumed alcohol. For the other half, the questions were formulated in a conditional way so that an impelling reason to drive was made salient. Thus, half of the respondents were merely asked whether they would drink and drive the next time they are out at a party, whereas the other half were asked whether they would drink and drive, if they were out at a party and 'only had a short distance to drive home', or 'had promised their friends that they would drive'. In line with predictions derived from alcohol myopia theory, respondents who had ingested alcohol before responding to the questionnaire were equally (or even more) negative about drinking and driving than sober individuals when the questions were unconditional, but much less negative when the questions were formulated in a conditional way. These effects occurred even though intoxicated individuals realistically perceived their ability to drive as rather poor.

MacDonald and colleagues (1995) derived suggestions for interventions aimed at reducing drinking and driving from the alcohol myopia theory. They argued that efforts to persuade people not to drink and drive may be best implemented in contexts in which people are intoxicated (i.e. bars and restaurants) because these are the contexts in which people make decisions. Such interventions could consist of providing salient reminders of the possible costs of drinking and driving (e.g. signs which say that drinking and driving kills). However, an alternative strategy could involve persuading individuals to decide on whether or not to drive before they start their evening. Thus, mass communication campaigns in the States have successfully aimed at persuading groups of people who go out together to designate a driver beforehand who would then not drink (DeJong and Hingson 1998). However, the effectiveness of this strategy depends on the actual abstention of the designated driver. If a designated driver drinks despite being designated as driver, alcohol myopia makes it more likely that this person will finally drive even if intoxicated.

Hazardous consumption levels and alcoholism

What level of consumption is hazardous to the health of men or non-pregnant women? This is largely a matter of conjecture. Clark and Midanik (1982) defined a heavy drinker as one who ingests 30 ml or more of pure alcohol a day (one ounce or more). Thus somebody who drinks three or more drinks would already be considered a heavy drinker. It should be noted that three glasses of wine per day at 75 ml of wine per glass contain approximately 30 ml of pure alcohol.

Approaching the problem from the standpoint of the lower limit of consumption of clinical alcoholics, Schmidt and de Lint (1970) found that the reported consumption of 96 per cent of the alcoholics in their sample was a daily intake at or above 150 ml of pure alcohol, the quantity of alcohol contained in one litre of Burgundy. There is reason to doubt the accuracy of such self-reports, however, because representative surveys done in the United States, Finland and Canada on self-reported consumption account for only 40 to 50 per cent of total alcohol sales when projected to the whole population (Furst 1983).

However, even if accurate, measures of the quantity of drinking are of little help in diagnosing alcoholism. As Vaillant (1983) pointed out, 'a yearly intake of absolute alcohol that would have represented social drinking for the vigorous 100-kilogram Winston Churchill with his abundant stores of fat would spell medical and social disaster for an epileptic woman

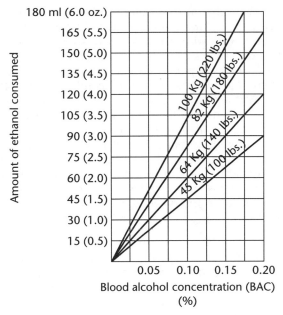

Figure 4.3 Nomogram of ethanol (pure alcohol) intake, body weight and blood alcohol concentration.
Note: To approximate the BAC, trace horizontally to the right to intercept the diagonal line representing body weight. Then trace downward to find the peak BAC. This process can be reversed to estimate the amount of alcohol consumed. The BAC falls consistently at 0.015 per cent per hour.
Source: Mooney (1982).

of 60-kilogram or for an airline pilot with an ulcer' (pp. 21–2). Thus the percentage of pure alcohol in an individual's blood (Blood Alcohol Concentration), which is used by governments all over the world to determine safe driving limits, depends very much on body weight (Figure 4.3).

A more promising approach to the definition of alcohol abuse, and one that is also more in line with the common view of alcoholism, is to combine reported consumption and reported problems related to drinking. Thus, the Diagnostic and Statistical Manual of Mental Disorders (DSM-IV; APA 1994) defines *alcohol abuse* as a maladaptive pattern of alcohol use leading to clinically significant impairment or distress, as manifested by one (or more) of the following problems occurring within a 12-month period:

1 Failure to fulfil major role obligations at work, in school, or home due to recurrent alcohol use (e.g. repeated absence, poor performance, neglect of children or household).
2 Recurrent alcohol use in situations in which it is physically hazardous (e.g. driving).
3 Legal problems due to recurrent alcohol use.
4 Recurrent alcohol use despite having persistent social or interpersonal problems caused by drinking (e.g. arguments with spouse about drinking, physical fights).

The DSM-IV also distinguishes alcohol abuse from *alcohol dependence*, the latter being the more serious form of alcoholism. The alcohol dependent person is one who, in addition to some of the above symptoms of alcohol abuse, shows evidence that he or she has tolerance to the effects of alcohol or has experienced withdrawal symptoms. Using the similar DSM-III criteria, a community study conducted from 1981 to 1985 in the United States indicated that about five per cent of the population had alcohol abuse and eight per cent had alcohol dependence at some time in their lives. Approximately 6 per cent had alcohol abuse or dependence during the preceding year (APA 1994: 202).

A number of screening instruments have been developed which can be used in health care and community settings to detect individuals with drinking problems (for a review, see Cooney *et al.* 1995). One of the standard screening interviews for clinical practice, CAGE (Ewing 1984) assesses the following four areas related to lifetime alcohol use:

1 Have you ever felt a need to cut down on your drinking?
2 Have you ever felt annoyed by someone criticizing your drinking?
3 Have you ever felt bad or guilty about your drinking?
4 Have you ever had a drink first thing in the morning to steady your nerve and get rid of a hangover?

Two positive responses are considered sufficient indication for the existence of an alcohol problem. The weakness of the CAGE is that it does not include questions about the frequency of drinking and intensity of drinking. Such questions should be added to identify current problems, levels of alcohol consumption, or binge drinking. If determination of a formal clinical diagnosis is necessary, individuals identified through screening should undergo a structured clinical interview to determine whether the DSM diagnostic criteria are met.

There are also biological indicators of alcohol abuse based on laboratory analyses of blood samples. The best known indicators are plasma gamma glutamyl tranferase (GGT) and mean corpuscular volume (MCV). Both reflect cellular injury to the liver (Cooney *et al.* 1995).

Theories of alcohol abuse

Theories of alcohol abuse can be divided into two groups: those that view it as an identifiable unitary disease process, and those that conceive of it in terms of behavioural models. This section will discuss both these approaches.

The disease concept of alcohol abuse

Of the various disease conceptualizations of alcoholism which have appeared in the literature over the past 40 years (e.g. Alcoholics Anonymous 1955; Jellinek 1960), the one developed by Jellinek has become most widely known. Jellinek (1960) presented a typology of alcoholism, specifying two types of alcoholic disease, which he called the 'gamma' and the 'delta' syndromes. Gamma alcoholism, which is said to be the predominant type of alcoholism in North America, is characterized by:

- acquired increased tissue tolerance to alcohol;
- adaptive cell metabolism;
- physical dependence on alcohol (craving); and
- loss of control.

Once a person with gamma alcoholism begins to drink, he or she is unable to stop. The social damage is general and severe. In delta alcoholism, which is said to be the predominant type of alcoholism in France and other wine-drinking countries, the gamma alcoholic's inability to stop is replaced by inability to abstain. Delta alcoholics drink great amounts of alcohol on a regular basis. There is little social or psychological damage, but there may be physical damage, such as liver cirrhosis.

It has been hypothesized that the difference between alcoholics and non-alcoholics is based on a psychological predisposition, an allergic reaction to alcohol, or some nutritional deficits which may or may not be genetically influenced. One major implication of this approach is that treatment must emphasize the permanent nature of the alcoholic's problem and that the disease can only be arrested by lifelong abstinence.

Despite a great deal of research, there is no reliable empirical evidence for a psychological predisposition (Vaillant 1983) or for the physiological processes assumed by the disease model to lead to alcoholism (George and Marlatt 1983). Furthermore, there is now evidence that, rather than having to give up alcohol altogether, some alcoholics (the less severely dependent ones) can be taught to return to controlled social drinking through therapy (Heather and Robertson 1983; Rosenberg 1993). Definitions of controlled drinking have varied but have usually included some limit on the amount and frequency of consumption (e.g. a maximum of 30 ml alcohol per day) and the condition that drinking results in neither signs of dependence nor social, legal or health problems (Rosenberg 1993).

Most damaging to Jellinek's conception, however, have been studies examining the 'loss of control' hypothesis using balanced placebo designs (Marlatt *et al.* 1973; Maisto *et al.* 1977; Berg *et al.* 1981). These studies examined the hypothesis that the apparent 'loss of control' after alcohol consumption is due to the *knowledge* that one has consumed alcohol rather than to the pharmacological effects of alcohol. The knowledge that they have drunk alcohol probably provides individuals with an excuse to consume more alcohol. The balanced placebo design allows one to manipulate independently expected and actual beverage content.

For example, social drinkers and alcoholics who participated in a study of Marlatt and colleagues (1973) were either led to believe that their drinks would contain vodka and tonic, or that it would contain only tonic. In fact half the respondents in each of those conditions received a drink containing vodka, the other half received tonic water only. Following this drink, participants had to participate in a taste-rating of alcoholic beverages. Participants who believed that their 'primer' drink had contained alcohol drank significantly more than those who thought that they only drank tonic. The amount consumed was unaffected by the actual alcohol content of these drinks, thus disconfirming the loss of control hypothesis.

Furthermore, studies using the balanced placebo design suggest that many of the behavioural consequences of alcohol are due to expectations about the effects of alcohol rather than its pharmacological impact (Marlatt *et al.* 1973; Marlatt and Rohsenow 1980; Hull and Bond 1986). In particular, the knowledge that one has consumed alcohol appears to disinhibit enjoyable but illicit behaviour (such as sexual behaviour, or further alcohol consumption) by providing an excuse for what would otherwise be considered inappropriate acts (Hull and Bond 1986).

Genetics and alcoholism

It is ironic that at a time when Jellinek's disease model seemed to have been thoroughly discredited, research into the heredity of drinking habits and into biological markers for alcoholism produced evidence suggesting some form of biological vulnerability to alcoholism (for reviews, see Devor and Cloninger 1989; Hurley and Horowitz 1990). Although it had long been known that susceptibility to alcoholism runs in families, it seemed reasonable to attribute this relationship to socialization rather than heredity. However, twin and adoption studies have made it possible to disentangle the influence of genetic and environmental factors on alcoholism. For example, if *adopted* children whose biological parents have alcohol problems also have a higher risk of alcoholism than do adopted children whose biological parents have no alcohol problem, this increase in risk is likely to be due to genetic factors. In line with this assumption, studies have shown that biological sons of alcoholics adopted away at birth were several times more likely to become alcoholics than were the sons of non-alcoholics (e.g. Goodwin *et al.* 1973, 1974; Cloninger *et al.* 1981; Sigvardsson *et al.* 1996).

Twin studies have also been used to assess the extent to which alcoholism is determined by genetic factors. Because twins share the same family environment, regardless of whether they are monozygotic or dizygotic, a greater similarity in alcohol problems among monozygotic than dizygotic twin pairs would be an indication of a genetic influence on alcoholism. In line with this assumption, a twin study of nearly 200 twins of individuals with alcohol dependence found concordance in the alcohol dependence of twin pairs to be 76 per cent for monozygotic twins and 53 per cent for dizygotic twins (Pickens *et al.* 1991). This difference in concordance was even greater when only male twins with an early onset of alcohol problems (i.e. before age 20) were considered. These findings were replicated with an extended sample of 392 twins (McGue *et al.* 1992). That it is particularly the early onset of alcoholism among men which was found to be heritable is in line with the assumption that there are two types of alcoholism which differ in the extent to which they are influenced by genetic factors. The more genetic type occurs only in men. This male type of alcoholism is characterized by an early onset of problem drinking and is often associated with antisocial personality traits. Hurley and Horowitz (1990) estimated that this type of alcoholism accounts for 25 per cent of all male alcoholics found in the population.

It is now generally agreed that biological inheritance can be a major factor in the development of early onset alcoholism in men. It is less clear, however, whether the same is true for women. The twin study of McGue and colleagues (1992) found no evidence for heritability among the female twins. However, Bohman *et al.* (1981) reported maternal inheritance of alcoholism for women. They found a threefold excess of alcohol abusers among women who were born to alcoholic mothers but adopted during the first few months of their lives by non-relatives. In contrast, alcohol abuse by the biological father had no impact on the drinking habits of daughters who were adopted away. Finally, a population-based twin study of alcoholism in women reported substantially higher concordance rates among monozygotic than dizygotic twins which would indicate strong genetic influence (Kendler *et al.* 1992). It is unclear why the findings of this latter study differ from that of most previous research. The major difference was that the twins in this study were selected from the general population and not from treatment facilities. It seems plausible that the genetic loading for alcoholism in the modest proportion of women who seek treatment may not be typical of that found in the entire population of women with alcoholism.

In assessing the impact of environmental factors, genetic studies allow us to distinguish two types, namely those shared by all the family members and those which are non-shared. Examples of shared conditions are social class, modelling by parents and child rearing practices. Examples of unshared environmental influences are damage to the embryo before birth, accidents, or peer relations. For alcoholism, most but not all studies suggest that environmental effects are due to shared rather than unshared experiences. Although the precise nature of these environmental risk factors have not yet been identified, there is evidence that it was not the alcoholism of adopted parents which increases the risk for the development of alcoholism in these adopted children (for a review, see Hurley and Horowitz 1990). This may seem puzzling at first. But it has to be considered that having an alcoholic parent may also serve as a salient and very effective reminder of the negative consequences of excessive drinking.

Behavioural models of alcohol abuse

Behavioural approaches to understanding the causes and development of alcohol abuse subsume a number of diverse conceptual models that share a common emphasis on learning processes. According to this approach, alcoholism is fundamentally a manner of drinking alcohol that has been learned either through conditioning (classical, operant) or through observational learning. Because I cannot do justice to the whole range of behavioural theories of alcoholism in the context of this chapter, I will focus on the best known learning theory of alcohol use and abuse, namely the Tension Reduction Hypothesis of alcohol consumption (Cappell and Greeley 1987). Some cognitive modifications of this model will also be discussed (e.g. Marlatt 1976; Hull 1981, 1987). The reader interested in a more extensive review and evaluation of psychological theories of alcoholism is referred to the excellent volume edited by Blane and Leonard (1987).

The basic assumption of the tension reduction hypothesis is that alcohol is consumed because it reduces tension. According to this model,

- increased tension constitutes a heightened drive state;
- by lowering tension and thus reducing this drive state, alcohol consumption has reinforcing properties; and
- such drive-reducing reinforcement strengthens the alcohol consumption response.

Research conducted with animals and humans to test the original model has produced rather inconclusive findings (for reviews, see George and Marlatt 1983; Cappell and Greeley 1987). The major problem with the tension reduction hypothesis is the assumption of a linear relationship between alcohol consumption and tension reduction. Contrary to this assumption, experimental evidence indicates that alcohol produces a biphasic response, with small amounts leading to a state of arousal that is experienced by the drinker as a euphoric high. With continued consumption, this phase gives way to a suppressive effect accompanied by tension and depression (George and Marlatt 1983). This could explain most of the inconsistencies in research results.

More recently, two cognitive models have been developed which may be able to account for most of the inconsistencies in research that has tested the tension reduction hypothesis with human participants (George and Marlatt 1983; Hull 1981, 1987). George and Marlatt (1983) argued that because the relaxing and euphoric effect associated with small amounts of alcohol immediately follows the initiation of drinking, it has a much more potent associative tie to drinking behaviour than the delayed negative effect. Thus, people may drink to have this positive effect. George and Marlatt suggested that it is the expected rather than the actual tension-reducing properties of alcohol that are most influential in determining alcohol consumption. People drink because they expect that it will relax them.

In developing their cognitive model George and Marlatt (1983) drew on the findings of McClelland and colleagues (1972) showing that the consumption of alcohol leads to increased fantasies of personal 'power'. George and Marlatt reasoned that if alcohol produced an increase in both physiological arousal and fantasies of personal power or control, drinking would increase in situations in which the drinker feels deprived of personal control. Lack of control is one of the major features that characterizes stressful situations (Seligman 1975).

George and Marlatt (1983) predicted that the probability of excessive or inappropriate drinking would vary as a function of the following variables:

- the degree to which individuals exposed to a particular situation feel that they are helpless and have no control over their outcomes;
- the availability of an adequate coping response as an alternative to drinking in such a high-risk situation; and
- the person's expectation about the effectiveness of alcohol as an alternative coping response in the situation.

Thus, if a drinker experiences a loss of personal control in a stressful situation and has no other adequate coping response available, the probability of drinking will increase. Under these conditions alcohol consumption has the function of restoring the person's sense of personal control. George and Marlatt (1983) argued that this model offered a coherent explanation for most of the research testing tension reduction hypothesis with human research participants.

Whereas Marlatt and colleagues see helplessness and the need for personal control as an important motive underlying problem drinking, Hull (1981, 1987) suggested that individuals consume alcohol to lower their level of self-awareness following failure, in order to avoid negative self-evaluation. Self-awareness is a state of self-focused attention in which individuals compare their real and their ideal self. When such comparisons lead to unfavourable results (i.e. when the real self does not measure up to the ideal), negative affect is created. This motivates the individual either to reduce the self-ideal discrepancy or to avoid self-awareness. There is empirical evidence that alcohol interferes with encoding processes fundamental to a state of self-awareness, and thereby decreases the individual's sensitivity to both the self-relevance of cues regarding appropriate forms of behaviour and the self-evaluative nature of feedback about past behaviour (Hull *et al.* 1983). By lowering the individual's level of self-awareness, alcohol consumption decreases negative self-evaluation following failure.

Both Marlatt (1976; George and Marlatt 1983) and Hull (1981, 1987) emphasized that their models offer only a partial explanation of alcohol use and abuse. Thus, drinking is also likely to be affected by such factors as observational learning and social reinforcement in situations that are not stressful. There is also overlap in the conditions which should encourage problem drinking according to these two models. However, whereas failure situations tend to be stressful, not all stressful situations involve failure. Thus, the husband whose spouse died of cancer may experience (universal) helplessness but not failure. And yet, bereavement has been found to be associated with an increased risk of alcohol abuse at least for men (for a review, see Stroebe and Stroebe 1987).

Clinical treatment of alcohol problems

Virtually all approaches to the treatment of alcoholism include some cognitive–behavioural treatment procedures. Since excellent reviews of behavioural treatment procedures are available (e.g. Riley *et al.* 1987; Hurley and Horowitz 1990; Heather 1995; Hester and Miller 1995), only a brief overview will be given here.

Treatment goals

With the increased acceptance of behavioural approaches to alcoholism, the goals of treatment have also changed. Although the proponents of Jellinek's disease concept believed that the only cure for alcoholism is complete abstinence, some behaviour therapists felt that at least the less severely dependent alcoholics could be taught to drink moderately. Several factors seem to be important in predicting which problem drinkers may succeed at controlled drinking rather than complete abstinence (for reviews, see Miller and Hester 1986; Rosenberg 1993). Individuals who have the best prospects are relatively young, married and are employed, have had a relatively brief history of alcohol abuse, and believe that the goal of controlled drinking is attainable. Controlled drinking training does not seem to be an effective method for chronic alcoholics who are severely dependent. Once severe dependence has occurred, the alcoholic no longer has the option of returning to social drinking (Hurley and Horowitz 1990). Thus complete abstinence still appears to be the preferred goal for most patients who need clinical treatment.

Detoxification

Before the initiation of therapy, alcoholics frequently have to be 'dried out'. In severe cases they may need medication to counteract alcohol withdrawal symptoms, which include anxiety, tremors and hallucinations. There are basically two approaches to detoxification. One method employs the substitution of alcohol with another more easily controlled drug in this category (usually barbiturates or benzodiazepines). Slow reduction of the medication minimizes withdrawal symptoms (Mooney and Cross 1988). An alternative approach uses minimal medication in the hope that severe withdrawal symptoms will help patients to recognize the severity of their condition. Obviously, the second approach requires very close medical supervision.

Aversion therapies

These therapies aim to reduce the patient's desire for alcohol by pairing the sight, smell, or taste of alcohol with a variety of unpleasant experiences. If successful, these alcohol stimuli should then elicit the unpleasant experiences and patients should acquire a conditioned aversion to alcohol (Rimmele *et al.* 1995). Depending on the noxious stimulus employed, three kinds of aversion therapy can be distinguished. *Electrical aversion therapy* pairs alcohol cues repeatedly with electric shock until a conditioned response (anxiety) is developed in response to these alcohol cues. Anxiety should then trigger alcohol avoidance which is presumably reinforced by anxiety reduction. In *chemical aversion therapy* patients who have been given an emetic (vomiting-inducing) drug are then administered alcohol a few minutes before nausea and vomiting occurs. Again it is hoped that the nausea response becomes associated with the alcohol cues. Finally, in *verbal aversion therapy* (covert sensitization), the noxious stimulus consists of aversive imagery which is repeatedly paired with alcohol-related imagery. The initial procedure involves pairing drinking stimuli with vivid imagination of nausea or other uncomfortable consequences of drinking. At a later phase, non-drinking alternatives, such as pouring out the drink, or leaving the drinking setting will be added. Results of empirical evaluations have been somewhat more encouraging for chemical and verbal aversion than for electrical aversion therapy (Miller *et al.* 1995).

Disulfiram

Disulfiram is a drug which induces nausea and vomiting if one drinks alcohol in the days following ingestion of the drug. Because under ideal circumstances disulfiram should deter clients from ever drinking alcohol and thus from experiencing conditioning, it should not be classified as an aversion therapy. When disulfiram was first introduced, the practice was to have the patient experience the disulfiram–alcohol reaction. This practice has now been replaced by vividly describing this reaction. Fuller (1995) recommends the use of disulfiram only as part of a multi-component treatment and, because of its numerous side effects, only for alcohol dependent patients who have relapsed. Because the effectiveness of disulfiram is dependent on patients taking the drug, this type of treatment is mainly effective if the drug is administered by someone at the clinic or a family member (Fuller 1995).

Operant treatment

Contingency management involves arranging the individual's environment so that positive consequences follow desired behaviour and either negative or neutral consequences follow undesirable behaviour. Crucial to the planning of therapeutic strategies based on contingency management is the identification of reinforcers that maintain drinking behaviour as well as the rewards that may be manipulated to modify the drinking. Because marital partners are important sources of reinforcement in everyday life, they have been included in designing therapy. Thus partners of alcohol abusers have been taught basic principles of behaviour modification (Cheek et al. 1971) or have been involved in behavioural contracting with the alcohol abuser (Miller 1972). Other interesting applications of contingency management techniques have used behavioural contracting to increase participation in treatment programmes or aftercare (e.g. Bigelow et al. 1976; Pomerleau et al. 1978).

Self-management procedures

These procedures accept that individuals can arrange their own reinforcement contingencies in order to make certain behaviour more likely (e.g. Miller and Munoz 1976; Hester 1995). For example, they can reward themselves for doing something which is unpleasant or punish themselves for transgressing predetermined rules. Hester (1995) suggests the following components of a self-management programme:

1 Setting limits on the number of drinks per day and on peak BACs.
2 Self-monitoring of alcohol consumption.
3 Changing the rate of drinking.
4 Setting up a reward system for achievement of goals.
5 Learning which antecedents result in overdrinking and which in moderation.
6 Practising refusing drinks.
7 Learning alternative coping skills as an alternative to drinking.
8 Learning to avoid relapse back into heavy drinking.

Self-monitoring of drinking usually reveals some regularities in the individual's drinking behaviour. Individuals can reorganize their environments to avoid circumstances associated with heavy drinking. Goals may be negotiated which set precise limits to alcohol consumption (Miller and Munoz 1976). Although these techniques are typically used to pursue the treatment goal of moderation, they can also be used to achieve abstinence. Research has shown that these techniques are effective with problem drinkers if employed by a therapist or used with a self-help manual (Hester 1995).

Skill training procedures

These are based on the assumptions that alcoholics *lack certain skills* for dealing with their environments, and that they use alcohol as an *alternative coping strategy*. Coping skills can be divided into intrapersonal skills and social skills. Intrapersonal skills enable the individual to deal with urges and emotional states that may increase the risk or severity of drinking. Social skills help the individual to interact with the important people in his or her social environment. For example, alcohol abusers frequently seem to drink as a coping response to stressful interpersonal situations (Monti *et al.* 1995). By teaching these coping skills to problem drinkers, one should increase their ability to deal with difficult situations without having to drink alcohol. An even more extensive approach, the Community Reinforcement Approach, includes problem-solving training, behavioural family therapy, social counselling and – for unemployed clients – job-finding training (Hunt and Azrin 1973; Azrin 1976). The importance of this type of skill training follows from the cognitive theories of George and Marlatt (1983) and Hull (1981), who conceive of stress and failure experiences as potent motivators of alcohol consumption. Both social skills training and the community reinforcement approach have been shown to be effective in well-controlled studies (Miller *et al.* 1995).

The effectiveness of behavioural and non-behavioural treatment of alcohol abuse has been extensively assessed (e.g. Emrick 1975; Riley *et al.* 1987; Miller *et al.* 1995; Süß 1995). Emrick (1975) evaluated 45 alcoholism treatment studies published between 1952 and 1973 with follow-up periods of at least six months: he reported an average abstinence rate of 28 per cent as compared to 13.4 per cent for alcoholics who had not received systematic treatment. More recently, Miller and colleagues (1995) conducted a careful analysis of 219 controlled studies of therapy effectiveness. However, rather than using modern methods of meta-analysis, their analysis is essentially based on box-scores, that is a summing up of positive and negative results. This type of analysis is problematic for a number of reasons: it treats all positive results the same, independent of the size of an effect. Similarly, it combines all negative results, regardless of whether an effect was in the right direction, but non-significant, or in the wrong direction and perhaps even significant.

A much more limited meta-analysis of outcome studies by Süß (1995) was based on 23 experimental and 21 non-experimental studies conducted in the USA, Canada, Great Britain and Germany. These 44 studies were selected from 310 studies on the basis of clearly defined criteria. Only the outcome calculation based on the strictest criterion, namely success rate as a proportion of all patients (those who finished the therapy and those who stopped) will be reported here. Patients who could not be reached at

Table 4.3 Differential effectiveness of alcohol therapies[1]

% (n Groups)	Abstinence	Improvement
Minimal therapy	21.2	25.1
Disulfiram	23.2	28.6
Eclectic therapy	33.0	44.5
Behavioural–cognitive multi-component therapies	44.5	54.2

[1] Only in-patient treatments.
Source: Adapted from Süß (1995).

follow-up were counted as failures. The average abstinence rate over groups and over all follow-up periods was at 34 per cent. The average rate for substantial improvements in drinking behaviour is 6 per cent higher than the abstinence rate.

This review also assessed the differential effectiveness of therapy programmes. Treatments were classified into four categories:

1 Minimal therapy (placebo, short counselling).
2 Disulfiram without any added treatment.
3 Eclectic standard therapy (therapy programme without a particular theoretical orientation).
4 Multi-component treatment based on cognitive behavioural therapy concepts.

The majority of treatments were conducted with in-patients either in general hospitals or addiction clinics. The average abstinence and improvement rates (over groups) are reported in Table 4.3. These results indicate that the success rates of behavioural therapies was approximately 10 per cent higher than that of eclectic therapies and both therapies were better than Disulfiram or minimal therapies. The difference between the behavioural therapies on the one hand, and Disulfiram and minimal therapies on the other, was also statistically significant.

Does behavioural treatment improve people's chances of overcoming their alcohol problem? One way to address this question is to compare the treatment outcomes reported for multi-component therapies with those of minimal therapies (Süß 1995). The average success rate of multi-component therapies is 44.5 as compared to 21.2 per cent for minimal therapies. Thus, if one makes the conservative assumption that minimal therapies are at least not harmful, then using a state of the art multi-component therapy more than doubles the chance of success.

Similar conclusions can be drawn if one compares the success of treatments with the remission rates of untreated alcoholism. Only limited data are available on the rates of spontaneous remission (Kendell and Staton 1966; Imber *et al.* 1976; Polich *et al.* 1981). Polich and colleagues (1981) reported that of the untreated alcoholics in their study 16 per cent had been abstinent for at least six months at the time of the interview four years after the first assessment. Imber and colleagues (1976), who conducted a follow-up study of 83 alcohol abusers who did not receive any treatment other than simple detoxification, reported an abstinence rate of 19 per cent for the one-year and 11 per cent for the three-year follow-up.

The comparison of treated and untreated alcoholics is problematic for two reasons. On the one hand, individuals who enter therapy are likely to have more severe alcohol problems than those who do not. On the other hand, those who enter therapy may also be more motivated to stop drinking. However, the comparison does suggest that even though not all alcoholics require formal treatment for alcoholism in order to recover, those who enter clinical treatment have a much better chance of recovery, particularly if they receive behaviourally-oriented multi-component treatment.

Who profits most from treatment? Research on patient characteristics has demonstrated that patients who are married, in stable employment, free of severe psychological problems, and of higher socio-economic status respond most favourably to treatment (Hurley and Horowitz 1990). In one of the few studies of social psychological predictors of treatment success, Jonas (1995) assessed the extent to which the determinants of the model of planned behaviour measured during therapy predicted relapse one year later in a sample of alcoholics undergoing therapy. When intention and perceived control were used as predictors of behaviour, only perceived control emerged as an independent predictor, accounting for 16 per cent of the variance in relapse behaviour. Thus, whether or not these alcoholics managed to abstain from drinking was unrelated to the strength of their intentions to abstain. It was solely related to their own estimate of how much control they perceived over their drinking. This suggests that, once people have agreed to undergo therapy, it might be more effective to work on the factors which determine the patients' perceived control rather than further strengthening their intention to abstain.

Community-based interventions for alcohol problems

General hospitals or medical practices offer convenient settings in which to screen individuals for alcohol problems and to apply short interventions. The most basic intervention consists of about five minutes of advice from a physician following the assessment of drinking and drinking-related problems (Heather 1995). Individuals identified as excessive drinkers on the basis of screening are told by the physician that they drink too much. The physician then discusses with them their drinking-related problems which the client has described during the screening assessment. The physician finally gives advice about 'sensible drinking limits' for those who choose non-abstinent drinking. Heather (1995) recommends three to four drinks per occasion for men, and two to three drinks for women. In addition one should advise two or three days of abstinence per week. If available, this brief intervention can be backed up with an information booklet.

Advice by a general practitioner can be effective in reducing drinking among clients with a drinking problem, as demonstrated in several studies (e.g. Wallace et al. 1988; Anderson and Scott 1992). For example, in a randomized controlled trial using 47 group practices, the proportion of men with excessive consumption had fallen at one-year follow-up by 44 per cent for men and 48 per cent for women in the treatment group, compared to 26 and 29 per cent in the control group (Wallace *et al.* 1988). Anderson and Scott (1992) reported similar treatment effects for men but did not find any difference for women.

Chick and colleagues (1985) assessed the impact of a brief intervention in a general hospital. They selected 156 male problem drinkers on the basis of screening of hospital in-patients. These men, who did not have previous treatment for alcoholism and had a good social support network, were randomly assigned to an intervention group or a control group. The intervention group received a single one-hour session of counselling given by an experienced nurse. The control group received only routine medical care. At one-year follow-up both groups showed significant decreases in consumption but the intervention group had fewer alcohol-related problems and also showed a significant improvement in terms of physiological measures (GGT).

Finally, Heather *et al.* (1986) sent either a self-help manual based on behavioural principles of self-management or a general information and advice booklet to individuals who had responded to a newspaper advertisement offering free help in cutting down drinking. At the six-month follow-up the self-help manual group showed a significantly greater improvement in mean alcohol consumption and greater improvement on self-report measures of physical health. These differences were maintained at a second assessment 12 months after treatment. Similar results were reported by Heather *et al.* (1990) and Spivak *et al.* (1994).

That self-help pamphlets are successful in the treatment of drinking problems even when used alone and not as part of a clinical therapy is surprising, because they do not appear to work for smokers. One of the reasons for their differential impact may be that, unlike most smokers, problem drinkers often seem to be unaware that they are having a problem. They are often surrounded by friends with similar drinking habits and therefore think that what they are doing is perfectly normal and not unhealthy. To induce in these people the self-realization that they have a drinking problem by giving them the information that they drink much more than others, that the amount they drink is unhealthy, and that they have drinking-related problems is likely to motivate them to change their behaviour. That many of them seem able to succeed is due to the fact that these individuals are typically not alcohol-dependent. Although even alcohol-dependent individuals are sometimes able to stop drinking by themselves, they are likely to need more extensive therapy, and therapy that aims at abstinence as a drinking goal rather than at the controlled reduction in alcohol consumption.

No discussion of alcohol problems would be complete without a brief consideration of self-help groups, in particular the largest network of self-help groups in the world, namely Alcoholics Anonymous (AA). This network has approximately 87,000 groups in 150 countries, and over 1.7 million members (McCrady and Delaney 1995). As Heather (1995) succinctly puts it, the AA is more a way of life than a form of treatment. Best known about the AA is that its members believe in the disease concept of alcoholism. Since the disease cannot be cured, the only solution is total abstention.

The code of AA principles are reflected in 12 steps, through which new members have to move, typically with the help of other more established members. The first step is an admission of powerlessness. The frequent reference to a higher power in the 12 steps indicates the strong spiritual element in AA teaching.

There are very few controlled outcome studies on the AA or other self-help groups. Reviews of this research (e.g. Heather 1995; McCrady and Delaney 1995) indicate that only two studies have succeeded in assigning problem drinkers randomly to AA or other forms of treatment. Neither study showed any advantage of the AA. However, both studies used court-referred problem drinkers who had been forced to attend for treatment and were thus poor prospects for any type of treatment. Outcome studies that assess the impact of the AA on those who attend voluntarily suffer from selection effects (e.g. Morgenstern *et al.* 1997). The positive correlation between increased attendance and better outcome found in these studies could be due to the decision of those who relapse to stop attending AA meetings. There is still a need for a controlled study using random assignment of clients to AA or no self-help group following treatment.

Primary prevention

Since the late 1960s the attention of those concerned with public health aspects of alcohol has shifted from individuals suffering from alcoholism to the general overall consumption of alcohol in a given society and the factors that affect this consumption (Ashley and Rankin 1988). This change of approach was motivated by research conducted by Ledermann (1956, 1964). According to Ledermann, the frequency distribution of drinkers in a population is continuous, unimodal and positively skewed (Figure 4.4). The fact that there is no separate peak at the high end of the distribution for alcoholics suggests that

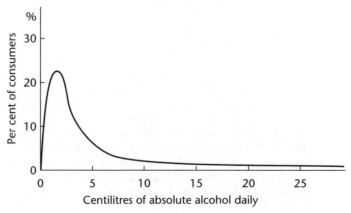

Figure 4.4 Frequency distribution of alcohol consumption. *Source*: de Lint (1976).

- the proportion of heavy drinkers in a given population can be estimated from knowledge of the mean per capita consumption; and
- that this proportion can be decreased by reducing the mean per capita consumption by means of fiscal and legal measures.

Consistent with Ledermann's position, there is convincing evidence that per capita consumption and excessive drinking (inferred from the rates for death from liver cirrhosis) are closely related (see Figure 4.2). Although one cannot infer causality on the basis of purely correlational evidence, the finding described earlier, that restrictions imposed on alcohol consumption led to a drop in deaths from liver cirrhosis, suggests that measures reducing the per capita consumption are likely to result in a decrease in alcohol problems. There are two main strategies of primary prevention which have been employed to reduce drinking problems, namely health education to persuade people not to engage in harmful drinking, and health protection measures aimed at controlling the availability of alcohol.

Health education

Health education programmes have been shown to affect public knowledge about, and attitudes towards, alcohol, but it has not been demonstrated convincingly that such programmes have resulted in behaviour change leading to a reduction in per capita consumption (Ashley and Rankin 1988). Such education programmes are likely to be counteracted by the pervasive efforts of the alcohol industry in promoting alcohol consumption. For example, in 1981 an estimated two billion US dollars were spent on alcoholic beverage advertising in the USA (Ashley and Rankin 1988). There is some evidence that alcohol advertising not only affects brand choice, but increases overall alcohol consumption. In an analysis of data from 17 countries for the period 1970 to 1983, Saffer (1991) demonstrated that countries with bans on the advertising of spirits (i.e. hard liquor) have about 16 per cent lower alcohol consumption than countries with no bans.

However, the success of brief therapy interventions described above tends to suggest that interventions which target problem drinkers should be effective. Such interventions should provide information which helps to identify problem drinkers and which recommends sensible drinking goals. After all, unlike most smokers, many heavy drinkers are still unaware that they are damaging their health. Making them aware of this fact might motivate them to change their behaviour. In view of the widespread desire of people to diet and lose weight, such anti-alcohol campaigns might also stress the fact that the consumption of alcoholic beverages results in weight gain.

That school-based health education can be effective has been demonstrated in a major alcohol use prevention programme that was conducted in 24 school districts in north-eastern Minnesota using random assignment to the intervention or control conditions (Perry et al. 1996). The intervention programmes were implemented during sixth, seventh and eighth grade for three school years. The intervention consisted of social–behavioural curricula in schools, peer leadership and parental involvement. Students were trained in skills to communicate with their parents about alcohol and to deal with peer influence and normative expectations. The project was more successful with students who had not used alcohol at the beginning of sixth grade than among students who had begun drinking. Students who had not used alcohol at the beginning of the study showed lower onset rates in the intervention than the control groups and also reported lower alcohol use for the past year and past month at eighth grade. There were no significant differences in the alcohol use between intervention and control groups for those students who had already begun to drink alcohol at the start of the study. This might indicate that alcohol use is difficult to reverse, even as early as the beginning of sixth grade. But it would also seem plausible that adolescents who begin drinking alcohol early live in a social context that supports drinking and thus dampens the effect of educational programmes.

Health protection

Health protection measures include legislative and regulatory controls of the price of beverages, numbers and locations of outlets, hours and days of sale, and minimum legal drinking age. Studies spanning several decades have indicated that price control via taxation can be effective in reducing alcohol consumption (Ashley and Rankin 1988; Hurley and Horowitz 1990).

It has been demonstrated that the demand for alcoholic beverages responds to changes in price and income. For example, Johnson and Oksanen (1977), who used data on the relationship between changes in price of alcoholic beverages and consumption for 10 Canadian provinces for 15 years (1956–70), estimated the elasticity for beer at –0.29, for spirits at –1.70, and for wine at –1.36. According to these estimates demand for spirits and wine was more likely to respond to changes in price than that for beer. A 10 per cent increase in price should result in a 2.9 per cent decrease in beer consumption, as compared to a 17 per cent decrease for spirits and a 13.6 per cent decrease for wine.

On the basis of a quasi-experimental design, Cook (1981) came to very similar estimates of the elasticities in demand for spirits in the USA. He compared changes in the consumption of liquor in 39 US states before and after a significant rise in excise taxes with changes in the consumption for the same period in comparable states in which taxes had not been increased. In 30 of the 39 states, there was a decrease in consumption following the increase in taxation as compared to the comparison states. The price elasticity was estimated at –1.6. Cook (1981, 1982) argued that a doubling of federal tax on liquor in the United States would lead to a 20 per cent reduction in the nation's mortality from liver cirrhosis.

It is unclear, however, whether price increases also affect the drinking behaviour of heavy drinkers. A study of individual drinkers conducted in Scotland before and after a substantial increase in tax on alcoholic beverages (Kendell *et al.* 1983a, b) found that alcohol consumption fell by 18 per cent after the tax increase and that this effect was at least as strong for heavy as for more moderate drinkers. However, a recent study which used data on alcohol consumption of more than 20,000 individuals from the 1983 National Health Interview Study in the United States concluded that both light and heavy drinkers are much less price elastic than moderate drinkers (Manning *et al.* 1995).

Minimum legal drinking age laws which forbid the sale of alcohol to individuals below a certain minimum age are key measures for reducing alcohol availability among youth. States in the USA which increased the minimum drinking age to 21 in the late 1970s and early 1980s experienced a 10 to 15 per cent decline in alcohol-related traffic death among drivers in the targeted age groups, compared with states that did not adopt such laws. Furthermore, there is evidence that people aged 21 to 25 who grew up in states with an age 21 law drink less alcohol compared to those who grew up in other states (DeJong and Hingson 1998). It is not surprising therefore that in 1984 the federal government passed a law which induced all states to increase the minimum drinking to age 21.

Summary and conclusions

Alcohol abuse and dependence are widely recognized to be a serious public health problem. Alcohol abuse is characterized by a long-standing pathological pattern of daily alcohol consumption, and an impairment of social or occupational functioning. Alcohol dependence is in addition characterized by increased tolerance to alcohol and the experience of withdrawal symptoms. Although there is a biological vulnerability to alcohol, drinking patterns are learnt and can be influenced by changes in reinforcement contingencies. However, given the damage that alcohol abuse can do to the lives of alcoholics, and given the high costs and moderate success rates of treatment techniques, strategies of health protection and health education that aim to prevent alcoholism would appear to be a necessary additional approach to reduce alcohol problems in society.

EATING CONTROL, OVERWEIGHT AND OBESITY

Obesity is a medical problem that, like alcoholism, carries a social stigma. Society has a strong bias against people who are obese, a bias that can even be found in young children (Maddox *et al.* 1968). But unlike people with physical handicaps, obese persons not only suffer the stigma of their obesity; they are also blamed for it. The common view holds that people are obese because they eat too much and that it is up to them to slim down. And yet, the evidence on differences in food intake of obese and normal weight individuals is less than conclusive (Wooley *et al.* 1979; Brownell 1983; Striegel-Moore and Rodin 1986). Furthermore, results of treatment outcome studies suggest that obese individuals have great difficulty in reducing their weight even if they want to do so, and only very few manage to maintain their weight loss in the long term.

Overweight, obesity and body weight standards

The concepts of overweight and obesity imply a standard of normal or ideal weight against which a given weight is judged. Because height and

Table 4.4 Percentage of obese persons in several European countries

	Year	Ages	% obese[1] Men	% obese[1] Women
England	1991	16–64	13	15
Germany	1990	25–69	17.2	19.3
Netherlands	1993	20–59	8	10

[1] BMI of 30 kg/m² or more.
Source: Adapted from Seidell and Rissanen (1998).

weight are highly correlated, such a standard has to be height-specific. One index defines normal weight in terms of the average weight of representative samples of men and women, stratified by age and height. A second index (Metropolitan Relative Weight) uses the ideal weight for a given height as a reference point. The ideal weight is defined as the weight associated with the lowest mortality for persons of a given height in insurance statistics. The Metropolitan Relative Weight is computed for each subject by forming the ratio of his or her body weight and the ideal weight for his or her height. Overweight is defined as a body weight that is between the upper limit of normal and 20 per cent above that limit. A body weight that is more than 20 per cent above that limit would be considered obese. Obesity has been further classified into mild (20 per cent–40 per cent), moderate (41 per cent–100 per cent), and severely obese (> 100 per cent), depending on the extent to which the body weight exceeds the normal weight (Stunkard 1984).

A third index uses the Body Mass Index (BMI), obtained by dividing weight in kilograms by height in metres squared (kg/m²). This index has a very high correlation with body fat (as estimated from body density), particularly when age is taken into account (Simopoulos 1986). In terms of this index, overweight has been defined as a BMI of 25 to 30 kg/m². A BMI above 30 kg/m² constitutes obesity. Table 4.4 presents the percentages of obese men and women in a number of European countries. In the United States, 22.5 per cent of the population is currently obese according to this standard, nearly one-third more than in 1980 (Taubes 1998b).

It is important to note that all these indices are affected by secular trends. Not only have the average weight and the average BMI been increasing substantially in Europe and the United States over the last few decades, but, more troublesome for these indices, US data suggest that even estimates of the weight associated with the lowest mortality have shifted upwards (Andres 1995; Seidell and Rissanen 1998). As a result, the recommended ranges of BMI have been adjusted upwards (see below).

Obesity and health

The association between obesity and ill health has been well documented. Sources of evidence have been studies conducted by life insurance companies (Society of Actuaries 1960; Society of Actuaries and Association of Life Insurance Medical Directors of America 1979) and longitudinal studies such as the Framingham Study (Dawber 1980), the Gothenburg Study (Larsson et al. 1981) or the American Cancer Society Study (Lew and Garfinkel 1979). The causes of excess death associated with overweight are cardiovascular disease, stroke and diabetes mellitus (Willett and Manson 1996). However, there appear to be different types of obesity which differ in health risk. There is evidence from prospective studies that the health risk associated with obesity is affected by the distribution of body fat (e.g. Larsson et al. 1989; Lapidus 1990). Fat distribution in these studies was measured as the waist over hip circumference ratio (WHR). It emerged that men and women whose fat depots were mainly concentrated around the abdomen were at particularly high risk of ill health and mortality (e.g. Larrson et al. 1989; Lapidus 1990). This relationship remained significant even when the association between the outcome measures and BMI was statistically controlled.

Scientific opinions about the shape of the association between body weight and mortality have changed during the last decade. Whereas earlier reports based on the insurance data assumed a J-shaped function, with an optimal BMI around 20 and the rate of mortality increasing with increasing degrees of overweight (e.g. Bray 1986), more recent cohort studies of populations which include also non-insured individuals have suggested that being underweight is as unhealthy as being overweight (Andres 1995; Troiano et al. 1996). Furthermore, the estimate of the BMI that is associated with minimal mortality has been shifted upwards. The new dietary guidelines for Americans jointly published by the US Departments of Agriculture and Health and Human Services (reported by Andres 1995) recommend as healthy a BMI range from 19 to 25 for individuals between the ages of 19 and 34 and from 21 to 27 for individuals of 35 and older. These recommendations are in line with conclusions from a recent meta-analysis of 22 cohort studies on the association between body mass index and all-cause mortality. This quantitative review found the relationship between the BMI of men who were aged 50 at entry and mortality over a 30-year period to be U-shaped. Mortality was lowest at a BMI of 24 and increased with lower as well as higher BMI values, with a recommended range from 23 to 28 BMI (Troiano et al. 1996). BMI values below 23 and above 28 were found to be associated with a significantly increased mortality risk.

How can one account for the fact that these cohort studies of populations which also include non-insured individuals found underweight as well as overweight to be associated with increased mortality risk? Two potentially confounding variables have been suggested, namely cigarette smoking and undetected illnesses. First, smokers weigh less than non-smokers and also have a higher mortality. Second, undetected illnesses at the time of entry into the study might have the same effect.

The explanation in terms of smoking has been tested by analysing data separately for smokers and non-smokers, or more elegantly, by including smoking as a factor in the analysis. Although smoking had substantial impact on mortality risk, it had very little impact on the outcome of these analyses. The potential impact of undetected illnesses at baseline measurement has been minimized by two procedures: medical examination of all respondents at baseline (in order to detect and exclude cases of illness), or by excluding all cases of mortality in the first two to five years after baseline measurement (assuming that these may have been due to illnesses that were already present at baseline). Again, the use of these procedures has not altered the U-shaped association between BMI and mortality.

Troiano and colleagues (1996) suggested that the increased mortality risk of underweight individuals could be due to differential access to health care services. This explanation would not only be consistent with the fact that such increases were not found in samples of individuals who carried health insurance but with the fact that the effects of underweight were less strong in studies conducted in Northern Europe where nearly everybody is insured or where access to public health services is free.

The social consequences of obesity

Obese individuals, and particularly obese women, not only suffer adverse effects on their health, but are also likely to be the target of prejudice and discrimination, because in present-day Western industrialized countries people view fat as unattractive and unhealthy. Obesity seriously lowers women's chances of marrying. Gortmaker *et al.* (1993) found that young obese women were far less likely to marry during a seven-year period than were non-obese women who differed from them only in body weight. If obese women did finally marry they were far more likely to drop in social class than were non-obese women.

The discrimination against the obese is not restricted to the interpersonal domain. A study conducted in 1964 and 1965 found that obese high school students were less frequently accepted into prestigious 'Ivy League' colleges than were non-obese students, even though obesity is unrelated to intelligence or school performance (Canning and Mayer 1966). Again, the effects were more marked for women than for men. The relation of non-obese vs obese male high school students who were accepted by an 'Ivy League' college was 53.3 per cent vs 49.9 per cent. The comparable difference in acceptance rate for women was 51.9 per cent (non-obese) vs 31.6 per cent (obese). Thus, many more of the non-obese women went to one of the high-prestige colleges, even though a comparison of application rates showed that both weight groups were equally interested in attending a high-ranking college (Canning and Mayer 1966).

Because these colleges require an interview before accepting students, the lower admission rates of obese women are likely to be due partly to the anti-fat stereotypes of the interviewers. However, there is also evidence that greater unwillingness of parents to pay college fees for obese children exacerbates this difference. Crandall (1991) found that fatter female students were less likely (53 per cent) to rely on their parents for financial support than were thinner women (74 per cent), even when controlling for parents' socio-economic status and level of education. Discrimination is likely to continue when obese individuals enter the job market. In one study

16 per cent of the employers surveyed said that they would not hire obese women under any circumstance (Stunkard and Sobal 1995).

Given this evidence, it is particularly surprising that the stigma attached to being obese does not appear to result in emotional damage. Cross-sectional studies comparing obese to non-obese samples suggest that obesity is not associated with general psychological problems (Friedman and Brownell 1995). Findings from a longitudinal study of weight loss and regain suggest that even a 40 kg cycle of loss and gain did not significantly affect depressive symptomatology (Foster *et al.* 1996). However, even though being overweight does not appear to increase the risk of depression, it does seem to lower self-esteem. A recent meta-analysis of 71 studies of the association between body weight and self-esteem reported a correlation of −.12 between actual weight and self-esteem and of −.33 for self-perceived weight (Miller and Downey 1999). The association was somewhat higher for women (r = −.23) than for men (r = −.19) and for samples containing mainly individuals of high socio-economic rather than low socio-economic status (−.31 vs −.16). All these associations as well as the differences between them were statistically significant. These findings suggest that body weight, and particularly self-perceived body weight, has a substantial impact on the self-esteem of certain sections of the population such as women, or individuals of high socio-economic status for whom anti-fat attitudes are particularly negative.

Genetics and weight

There is ample evidence from twin and adoption studies that body weight is strongly influenced by genetic factors. An extensive review of behaviour-genetic studies of weight and obesity suggested heritability to be approximately 70 per cent for weight and 60 per cent for BMI (Grilo and Pogue-Geile 1991). These estimates are similar in magnitude to those for intelligence. Somewhat lower values were suggested by Bouchard and Pérusse (1993) based on measurement of the BMI obtained in a Norwegian sample of approximately 75,000 individuals. These data, which were used to compute familial correlations in a large number of first- and second-degree relatives, suggested a heritability of 40 per cent.

Such estimates still allow for a substantial influence of environmental factors on body weight. Because the food one eats and the extent to which one exercises are the most important environmental influences on weight and because meals are typically shared within a family, it would appear plausible to expect the shared family influences to be more important than the non-shared effects. It is therefore surprising that Grilo and Pogue-Geile (1991) concluded on the basis of their review that 'experiences which are shared within a family do not play an important role in determining individual differences in weight, fatness, and obesity' (p. 534). This conclusion was based on convincing evidence from different types of studies. First, there was no correlation between the weight of adoptive siblings living in the same family. Second, the correlation between the weight of children and their biological parents was the same for those who lived with these parents and those adopted away. Third, monozygotic twins who were reared together were as similar in their weight as monozygotic twins who were reared apart. Fourth, spouses who lived together were no more similar in their weight than engaged couples who did not yet live together. These data suggest that practically all the environmental influences on weight are due to experiences which are not shared by family members.

The physiological regulation of eating behaviour

Many of our physiological systems are regulated by set points familiar from the thermostats used in central heating systems, refrigerators or air conditioning. If one adjusts the thermostat of one's central heating system to a given temperature, the system will switch on whenever the sensors register that the temperature has dropped below this set point. Whereas it is plausible that body temperature is regulated according to a set point, the fact that there is such a wide variation in body weight seems to rule out such regulation. However, even though there is wide interpersonal variability, the body weight of most adults remains remarkably stable over time. Keesey (1986) therefore suggested that different people may have different set points and that for some, their biological weight is set far above culture's ideal.

The most important derivation of the set point theory is that the organism will defend its body weight against pressure to change. This would certainly explain why most obese individuals have such trouble in achieving and maintaining a normal weight. There is evidence from animals as well as humans that is consistent with this assumption. Thus, laboratory animals adjust food intake and physical activity to compensate for starvation or forced feeding (for a review, see Koopmans 1998). Adult humans seem to respond similarly to weight displacement. Thus, during World War II, a group of conscientious objectors was maintained on a starvation diet for several months (Keys *et al.* 1950). Their body weight fell at first, but eventually stabilized at 75 per cent of the previous values. This equilibrium was reached partly by a decrease in basal metabolic rate and partly by a comparable decrease in amount of metabolically active tissue. Furthermore, most returned to their previous weight once food restrictions had been removed. Similarly, when Vermont prisoners agreed to a considerable increase of their daily caloric intake, they achieved weight gains of 15 to 25 per cent during the half-year period. However, when the experiment terminated, these respondents soon returned to their normal weight (Sims and Horton 1968).

It would seem from this evidence that some obese individuals might be fighting a battle against relentless biological forces. As Keesey (1980) stated:

> If we view such (obese) individuals as different not in how they regulate body weight but rather in terms of the set point each is prepared to defend, we might better understand why most of us remain at essentially the same body weight without so much as trying, while others remain obese no matter how hard they try to change.
>
> (Keesey 1980: 163)

The work by Björntorp, Sjöström and collaborators at the University of Gothenburg in Sweden suggested that fat cells may play an important role in the regulation of body weight (e.g. Sjöström 1980; Björntorp 1986). This work stimulated the popular view that the number of fat cells is determined in childhood and remains fairly stable in adult life. Increases in fat mass in adult life appear to be mainly due to an enlargement of existing cells, even though the number of fat cells can increase in cases of extreme obesity (Ailhaud and Hauner 1998).

The regulation of food intake and energy homeostasis is accomplished by a variety of integrated neurohumoral systems which I cannot even attempt to discuss adequately in the context of this book. However, it is interesting to note that there is evidence for the existence of hormones which regulate food intake in inverse proportion to fat mass. Of particular importance in this regulatory process appears to be the hormone 'leptin'. It is secreted by fat cells and direct administration of leptin into the central nervous system potently reduces food intake. If deficiencies in leptin regulation play a role in the development of obesity, it would have to be an insensitivity in leptin receptors rather than a deficiency in the secretion of leptin by fat cells. There is ample evidence that obese individuals have elevated levels of leptin which are in line with their increased fat stores (Fried and Russell 1998). If leptin insensitivity were to play a role in the development and maintenance of obesity, then one would expect the obese to consume more food than normal weight individuals. This assumption would appear to be inconsistent with reviews of studies on eating behaviour in normal weight and overweight individuals which typically conclude that there was no clear difference. However, findings that obese tend systematically to underreport their intake of energy relative to energy expenditure to an even greater degree than do normal weight individuals raise doubts about the validity of these conclusions (for a review, see Blundell and Stubbs 1998).

The cognitive regulation of eating behaviour

Early cognitive theories

The earliest psychological theory of eating behaviour, the so-called externality hypothesis of Schachter and colleagues (Goldman *et al.* 1968; Nisbett 1968), derived from an observation reported by Stunkard and Koch (1964) that gastric contractions and reported hunger correlated highly for normal weight but not obese respondents. Schachter and colleagues suggested that obese people differ from normal weight individuals in the cues that trigger their eating behaviour. They argued that normal weight individuals respond mainly to internal factors, that is to the visceral and physiological states that vary with food deprivation such as gastric motility and blood sugar concentration. Eating behaviour in overweight individuals, on the other hand, was said to be strongly influenced by external factors such as the sight and smell of food, social stimuli and habit. Despite the plausibility of this 'externality hypothesis', numerous studies failed to demonstrate these effects (for a review, see Rodin 1981). It is now widely accepted that across all weight groups there is only a weak relationship between the degree of overweight and the degree of internal or external responsiveness (Nisbett 1972; Rodin et al. 1977).

The construct of 'dietary restraint' developed by Herman and Polivy (1984) offers an explanation for why there is only a weak relationship between obesity and externality. They argued:

- that obese people frequently try to diet in an attempt to conform to social prescriptions regarding body weight; and
- that it was the conscious restraint of eating that was responsible for the relationship between externality and obesity (e.g. Herman and Mack 1975).

When restrained individuals force themselves to ignore or override internal demands in their attempt to diet, an insensitivity to internal hunger cues and an over-reliance on external cues is likely to develop. Although overweight is one of the determinants of dietary restraint, the fact that many individuals of normal weight are also restrained eaters may explain why the relationship between externality and overweight is weak. Herman and Mack (1975) developed the Restraint Scale to assess the degree of self-imposed restriction of food intake and weight fluctuations. The Restraint Scale was later revised to a 10-item questionnaire with two sub-scales, measuring weight fluctuations and concern for dieting (Polivy et al. 1988).

The boundary model of eating

More recently, Herman and Polivy (1984) incorporated their hypotheses regarding restraint into a 'boundary model' of the regulation of eating which has become the dominant psychological theory of eating behaviour (Figure 4.5). They proposed that biological pressures work to maintain food intake within a certain range. The aversive qualities of hunger keep consumption above a minimum level and the aversive qualities of satiety keep it below some maximum. Between these two zones, there is a zone of biological indifference, where eating is regulated by non-physiological, social and environmental influences. Restrained eaters or dieters are assumed to differ from non-restrained eaters (or non-dieters) in two respects: first, restrained eaters impose a 'diet boundary' within their zone of biological indifference. This boundary consists of a set of cognitive rules construed to limit food intake in order to maintain or achieve a desirable weight. Thus, in contrast to unrestrained eaters whose eating is regulated via bodily feedback, restrained eaters are assumed to regulate their food intake cognitively. Second, restrained eaters are assumed to have a larger zone of biological indifference. Due to their frequent dieting and overeating, they have become somewhat insensitive to hunger and satiation cues: they can take much more food deprivation than unrestrained eaters before they experience hunger, and they can eat much more before feeling really full.

According to the boundary model, the diet boundary is both the strength and the Achilles heel of restrained eaters' attempts to achieve or maintain a desirable weight. It allows restrained eaters to keep their weight down if they monitor it. But if they cross this boundary, due either to circumstances outside their control or to lapses in attention, then a goal violation effect

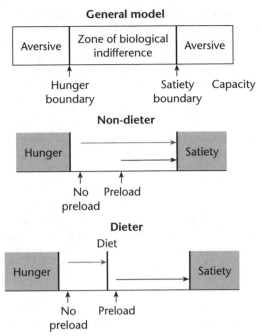

Figure 4.5   The boundary model of eating regulation.
Source: Herman and Polivy (1984: 149).

sets in, and they eat until they are full. This disinhibited reaction, termed
'counter-regulation', has been attributed to the 'all or none' thinking of
restrained eaters. Once they have crossed their diet boundary, they see no
point in further restraint.

There are two sets of factors assumed to induce overeating in restrained
eaters, namely the impairment of cognitive resources and actual or perceived dietary violations. Factors that interfere with cognitive control are
assumed to disturb the regulation of food intake in restrained eaters,
because they impair the ability of restrained eaters to monitor their food
intake. Thus, the experience of emotional distress should result in overeating either because individuals need cognitive resources to cope with their
emotions or because the goal of achieving a desirable weight loses its
importance when compared to the problems which induce distress.

This 'emotion hypothesis' has been tested in experiments which compared the eating behaviour of restrained and unrestrained eaters after the
induction of negative mood or in a neutral situation. Most of these studies found that the induction of negative emotions in the laboratory (e.g.
via a film or a failure experience) led to overeating among restrained
eaters (e.g. Baucom and Aiken 1981; Schotte *et al.* 1990; Heatherton *et al.*
1991). Similar effects have been observed for the induction of stress on
eating (for a review, see Greeno and Wing 1994). The consumption of
alcoholic beverages under laboratory conditions has resulted in less reliable
effects (e.g. Polivy and Herman 1976).

Table 4.5 Number of grams of ice cream consumed by restrained and unrestrained subjects under different preload conditions

	Preload (number of milk shakes)		
	0	*1*	*2*
High restraint	97.17	161.09	165.90
(> 8.5)	(9)	(11)	(10)
Low restraint	205.20	130.12	108.22
(< 8.5)	(10)	(8)	(9)

Source: Herman and Mack (1975: 656).

A second set of factors which disturbs dietary restraint is actual or perceived dietary violation. The effects of dietary violation on subsequent eating behaviour of restrained and normal eaters have been examined by inducing respondents to 'preload' with some rich (and therefore normally forbidden) food at the beginning of what was apparently a food-tasting experiment (e.g. Herman and Mack 1975; Hibscher and Herman 1977). In the first study on the effects of preload by Herman and Mack (1975), normal weight female respondents were asked to taste different flavours of ice cream after having been given either no preload or a preload of one or two milk shakes. Respondents were divided into restrained and non-restrained eaters on the basis of the Restraint Scale. It was expected that non-restrained eaters would eat less ice cream after a large rather than no preload. Restrained eaters, on the other hand, would 'binge', once they realized that their calorie intake already exceeded their daily ration. Consistent with these expectations, the intake of non-restrained respondents varied inversely with preload size, whereas that of restrained respondents showed a direct relationship (Table 4.5).

Critique of the boundary model

Although the boundary model still dominates psychological research on eating regulation, it has attracted a great deal of criticism on both empirical and theoretical grounds (e.g. Heatherton and Baumeister 1991; Lowe 1993; Boon 1998). For example Boon (1998) pointed out that in contrast to the emotion hypothesis for which there was consistent support, there was scarce evidence for counter-regulation in response to preload-induced dietary violations. Preload experiments usually assess counter-regulation by testing whether restrained or non-restrained eaters react differently to having eaten a preload (i.e. preload x restraint interaction). However, there are different patterns which can result in a significant interaction between preload and restraint on eating and not all of these are consistent with predictions from the boundary model. For example, the interaction between preload and restraint might be significant because non-restrained eaters eat less with, than without, a preload whereas restrained eaters eat the same under both conditions (i.e. show non-regulation). As Boon (1998) pointed out, of the 11 studies which manipulated preload, only three found significant evidence for counter-regulation (Herman and Mack 1975; Herman *et al.* 1987; Polivy *et al.* 1988).

A second criticism focused on the evidence for the assumed mediating role of cognitions (Boon 1998). According to the boundary model, restrained eaters overeat following a preload because of 'disinhibitive thoughts' (i.e. 'what-the-hell' cognitions). Jansen *et al.* (1988) examined this hypothesis in a study in which respondents' 'self-talk' (of preloaded and non-preloaded restrained and non-restrained eaters) was taped during and after a standard ice cream 'taste test'. There was no indication of an increase in disinhibitive thoughts in restrained eaters.

A third criticism focused on the discrepancy between the theoretical concept of dietary restraint and the way restraint is measured by the Restraint Scale. As Lowe (1993) argued, the boundary model conceptualizes dietary restraint as current dieting and often uses the two terms synonymously. However, the Restraint Scale measures chronic rather than current dieting. Although most current dieters score high on the Restraint Scale, not all restrained eaters are currently on a diet. In fact, Lowe (1993) reported findings to suggest that only 37 per cent of normal weight restrained eaters were currently on a diet.

Lowe (1993) argued persuasively that weight cycling (i.e. chronic dieting) and current dieting affect eating behaviour via different pathways. Repeated cycles of dieting and overeating result in an acquired insensitivity to bodily feedback and extended range of physiological indifference. As a consequence, restrained eaters who are not on a diet and are therefore not carefully monitoring their food intake are at risk of overeating. If one adds to this the fact that their basal metabolic rate might have decreased in response to dieting, it is not surprising that these individuals are likely to regain quickly any weight they might have lost during their diet.

Currently being on a diet could have several effects. First, these individuals will be motivated to restrict their food intake and monitor it closely. Second, due to 'the psychological frustration or the physical deprivation (or both) associated with their diets, dieters should have difficulty in resisting the temptation of tasty food' (Lowe 1993: 111). Third, because keeping to the diet boundary becomes an important goal during dieting, transgression of their dietary boundary should evoke strong goal violation effects in current dieters. This would suggest that current dieters are not only permanently running the risk of violating their diet boundary to reduce their hunger, but that, if they do, they should also respond with stronger goal violation reactions to this transgression.

Studies which tried to separate the effects of chronic dieting and current dieting on eating behaviour found no evidence that restrained dieters reacted with more counter-regulation to preloads than restrained individuals who were not currently on a diet (Lowe 1993). In fact, there is evidence to the contrary. In a study in which restrained dieters, restrained non-dieters and non-restrained individuals tasted ice cream with or without a preload, Lowe *et al.* (1991) found that, in the conditions without any preload, restrained eaters who were currently on a diet ate significantly more than non-dieters did. In contrast, after having been given a preload, restrained eaters on a diet sharply reduced their intake whereas non-dieting restrained eaters showed evidence of counter-regulation. These findings tend to suggest that although restrained eaters on a diet are tempted by tasty food and may indulge momentarily, they are quickly able to re-establish control. It appears to be the restrained non-dieters who are most prone to counter-regulation.

The boundary model reformulated: an ironic process theory of eating regulation

To resolve these inconsistencies, Boon and her colleagues (e.g. Boon, 1998; Boon et al. 1997, 1998a, b) have drawn on dual processing theories (e.g. Shiffrin and Schneider 1977; Bargh 1996) and ironic process theory (Wegner 1994) to modify the boundary model. They argue that the difference in the way non-restrained and restrained eaters are assumed to regulate their eating behaviour closely parallels the distinction made between automatic and controlled processing in dual process theories. The boundary model is a theory of the regulation of eating behaviour and not of the instigation of eating. Once the process of eating has been set into motion, non-restrained eaters are assumed to rely on internal hunger and satiety cues in regulating their eating in a way which has all the characteristics of an automatic process: it is unintentional, occurs outside awareness, is uncontrollable, and uses few attentional resources. In contrast, the regulation of eating behaviour is assumed to be effortful and non-automatic for restrained eaters who cognitively monitor their food intake and relate it to some diet boundary.

Restrained eaters appear to be reasonably able to control their eating behaviour when they can focus their cognitive resources on keeping to their diet. However, as research on the induction of negative emotions or stress has demonstrated, when restrained eaters are distracted from monitoring their food intake because they have to cope with their emotions, they tend to overeat. As Boon and her colleagues pointed out, these effects are similar to those demonstrated by Wegner (1994) in tests of his ironic process theory. Wegner showed that individuals who were given the instruction to control a mental state or a behaviour were able to do so when they could concentrate on this task. However, when they were distracted, the opposite state or behaviour of that intended would typically be displayed.

Ironic process theory accounts for these findings by assuming that two cognitive processes are responsible for mental control: an intentional operating process and an ironic monitoring process. The operator works to produce a desired state of mind by searching consciously and effortfully for items consistent with this state. The monitor, on the other hand, checks continuously for 'mistakes', that is sensations and thoughts which are inconsistent with this state. The latter process is unconscious and requires little cognitive effort. Since the monitoring process is much less liable to be impaired by distraction than the more effortful operating process, Wegner's theory can explain why impairment of cognitive capacity ironically and often results in a mental state which is opposite to that desired.

If one incorporates the ironic process theory into the reformulated boundary model, one would predict that any reduction in cognitive resources should lead to overeating in restrained but not non-restrained eaters. This reduction in cognitive resources can be due to either an impairment in ability or a lack of motivation. Whereas Wegner (1994) only manipulated cognitive load to reduce cognitive capacity (i.e. ability to monitor), I would argue that motivational variables can have the same effect. Thus, restrained eaters are defined as individuals who chronically aim at restricting their dietary intake. However, whether they will be motivated to put all their cognitive resources at the disposal of this goal will depend on whether or not they are currently on a diet.

There is empirical evidence to support this reformulation of the boundary model. For example, Boon *et al.* (1998a) found in a study, in which respondents listed their thoughts following an ice cream taste test, that the thoughts about eating control entertained by restrained eaters on a diet were negatively related to their eating. Thus, the more they thought about controlling their eating, the less they ate. In contrast, restrained eaters not on a diet ate more ice cream the more they thought about controlling their eating. We would argue that restrained eaters who are not currently on a diet are not putting their full cognitive resources at the disposal of their dieting goal. They are therefore particularly liable to the impact of ironic processes.

In a more direct test of their reformulated boundary model, Boon and colleagues (1998b) had restrained and non-restrained eaters taste ice cream which was either described as particularly high or particularly low in calories. One would expect that restrained eaters would be more intent on controlling their eating when the ice cream was described as rich, creamy and highly calorific, rather than as low in calories. Furthermore, restrained eaters could be expected to succeed in acting according to their intentions when not under any cognitive load. However, when distracted, ironic processes should set in and induce overeating. In line with these predictions, restrained eaters in the high-calorie condition ate slightly less than non-restrained eaters when not distracted, but considerably more when distracted.

Unresolved issues

One of the questions which needs to be addressed with regard to the regulation of eating behaviour is how the concept of restrained eating is related to the determinants of behaviour implied by the social psychological models. Theories and research on eating regulation and dieting have developed relatively independently from social cognitive theories of behaviour. This is surprising in view of the dominance of social cognition theories in other areas of health behaviour and given the fact that restrained eaters are characterized by a strong motivation to lose weight.

From the perspective of the theory of planned behaviour, the intention to go on a diet to lose weight would be the immediate determinant of dieting behaviour. The intention would in turn be assumed to be a function of three conceptually independent variables, namely the attitude towards losing weight, the subjective norm with regard to losing weight, and the perceived control over one's body weight. These assumptions have been tested in a study of a small sample (86 women) of college students recruited on the basis of their intention to lose weight (Schifter and Ajzen 1985). Attitudes, intentions, subjective norms, perceived control and body weight were measured at intake. Body weight was measured again six weeks later. No measure of eating restraint was administered. Attitudes (r = .62), subjective norms (r = .44) and perceived control (r = .36) were significantly correlated with the intention to lose weight, jointly accounting for 55 per cent of the variance in intention. Actual weight loss was related to intention (r = .25) and perceived control (r = .41), accounting for 19 per cent of the variance in weight, with perceived control rather than intention accounting for the major share.

It is unfortunate that Schifter and Ajzen (1985) did not measure eating restraint. One can therefore only speculate about the relationship between eating restraint and the determinants of eating behaviour in the model of planned behaviour. One would assume that restrained eaters have a strong and persistent intention to lose weight and have positive attitudes towards weight loss. Because they are typically dissatisfied with their body weight, they might also feel that important others expect them to lose weight. The association between eating restraint and perceived control over body weight is more difficult to predict, because restrained eaters often manage to lose weight in the short run, but typically fail to maintain their weight loss in the long run. Thus, one would probably assume that the impact of eating restraint on weight loss would be mediated by the intention to lose weight and the perceived control over body weight.

A second issue which has rarely been addressed in the literature on restrained eating is why restrained eaters have such difficulties in keeping to their good (diet) intentions. With regard to other substances such as alcohol and smoking, users get addicted and therefore find it difficult to abstain. But what is it about eating which makes it so difficult for restrained eaters to maintain a calorie-reduced diet? It cannot be a deficiency in their physiological feedback loops, because they are assumed to regulate their eating cognitively. It is also unlikely to be heightened sensitivity to hunger sensations, because the boundary model expressly assumes that they have become insensitive to hunger and satiety signals.

I suspect that one major reason is that restrained eaters enjoy the taste of good food. Support for this assumption can be found in the early work of Nisbett (1968, 1972) who argued that obese individuals are particularly discriminating with regard to the taste of food. Nisbett drew on the findings of a study by Hashim and van Itallie (1965) who fed hospitalized patients a nutritive formula characterized by an unappetizing taste. Whereas obese patients reduced their energy intake to 400 to 500 calories, normal weight individuals on the same formula maintained a normal caloric intake. Nisbett (1968) conducted an experimental study in which obese and normal weight individuals were asked to taste ice cream which was either good-tasting or adulterated with quinine. He summarized the findings of his study as follows: '. . . overweight respondents did not merely eat more ice-cream than normal subjects. They ate more ice-cream than normal subjects if they liked it and they ate roughly the same amount if they did not. It appears that responsiveness to the taste cues is indeed a positive function of weight' (p. 112). A similar pattern was reported by Rodin et al. (1977). Discussing differences between obese and normal weight individuals in his review of research on restrained eating and externality, Ruderman (1986) concluded that the 'only variable that has consistently produced obese– normal differences in amount eaten is palatability. Overweight people's consumption is more affected by their perceptions of palatability than is that of normal weight people' (p. 248).

Nisbett (1968, 1972) assumed that the responsiveness of restrained eaters to the taste of food was a *consequence* of their restrained eating. In our view, an equally plausible explanation could be that the heightened responsiveness to taste cues of restrained eaters is one of the *causes* contributing to the development of their eating restraint. Individuals who enjoy the taste of good food are vulnerable to weight gain. Particularly the women, but also some of these men, will respond to the social pressure towards slimness and begin a diet to lose weight. Due to the fact that they tend to overeat when they are hungry and exposed to tasty food, they experience difficulties in losing weight or, if they have lost weight, in maintaining their weight loss. As a result they become weight cyclers and develop the syndrome which characterizes restrained eaters. Some support for the assumption that heightened responsiveness to weight cues may precede the development of eating restraint comes from a study by Milstein (1980) who found that infants of overweight parents were significantly more responsive to differences between the taste of water and the taste of sweet solution than were infants of normal weight parents.

Conclusions

The early work on externality by Schachter and his colleagues promised to lead to a psychological theory of obesity. This theory attributed obesity to the fact that the eating behaviour of obese individuals was mainly controlled by external cues. However, more recent findings suggest that externality may merely be a side effect of individual battles against the physiological mechanisms of weight regulation. With the development of the boundary model, Herman and Polivy (1984) shifted the theoretical focus from obesity to eating disorders such as anorexia and bulimia. Based on a physiological explanation of obesity, the boundary model explains why eating disorders develop among individuals who try to suppress their weight below their biological set point.

Empirical support for the boundary model is mixed. Although evidence on the impact of dietary violations on eating behaviour is not very supportive of the boundary model, there is a great deal of support for the assumption that the impairment of cognitive resources results in overeating among restrained eaters. The boundary model would attribute this type of overeating to the greater zone of biological indifference of restrained eaters due to repeated weight cycling. Our reformulation of the boundary model offers an alternative explanation in terms of ironic processes. We argue that the chronic dieting intention of restrained eaters increases the risk of overeating under conditions where the individual is either unable (i.e. through distraction) or unmotivated (i.e. no current diet) to commit all cognitive resources to the dieting goals. We also suggest that a heightened sensitivity to the taste of food may contribute to the development of the weight problems motivating eating restraint.

Clinical treatment of obesity

Behavioural approaches

The basic assumption underlying behavioural treatment of obesity is that eating and exercise are learned behaviours and, like any other learned behaviour, can be modified. It should therefore be possible to reduce body weight by achieving a reduction in the quantity of food eaten and by increasing exercise behaviour (Wadden and Bell 1990; Wing 1998). The starting point for a successful behavioural treatment of obesity is the functional analysis of behaviour. This analysis tries to identify the association between eating and exercise behaviours and environmental events such as time of day, presence of other people, or other activities. The data for the functional analysis are provided by the client who is asked to self-monitor his or her eating and exercise behaviours. This allows the therapist to determine specific problem areas which can then be targeted in treatment. For example, the self-monitoring record might indicate that a large proportion of the patient's calories are consumed in the form of snacks between meals or in the form of alcoholic beverages. Alternatively, the individual may eat sensibly, but lead too sedentary a lifestyle. Different interventions would be designed to target the different problem areas.

The behavioural approach assumes that environmental cues are important in eliciting behaviour. Weight control patients are therefore taught to restructure their home environment in order to elicit the desired behaviour. Thus, they may be asked to stop buying high-calorie desserts, to store high-calorie foods in difficult-to-reach places, and to buy more fruit and vegetables. Therapists also try to provide new reinforcers to replace the reinforcement value of the forbidden foods. Weight loss would constitute one such potent reinforcer. Therapists also use reinforcers such as praise and positive feedback.

Sometimes more formal reinforcement systems such as contingency procedures are used (for a review, see Bellack 1977). With *financial contingencies*, participants are typically required to deposit a sum of money with the therapist before treatment begins. This money is then returned at weekly meetings contingent on the participant's fulfilling a pre-set criterion (e.g. loss of a given amount of weight). The application of *self-reinforcement* relies on *self-monitoring*. Patients will reward themselves when they have reached a given criterion (e.g. lost a given amount of weight, kept to a set daily calorie input). Both financial reward and self-reinforcement presuppose some kind of *goal setting*. Most of these rewards are no longer present after therapy or during the maintenance period, which may be one of the factors contributing to the poor maintenance typically observed in the weight loss achieved by obese individuals.

Effectiveness of behavioural approaches

A survey of data from controlled trials of behaviour therapy conducted between 1970 and 1990 indicates that the average weight loss for participants in such programmes was 8.5 kg in 1988–90, as compared to 3.9 kg lost in therapy programmes conducted before 1974 (Table 4.6). Data for

Table 4.6 Summary analysis of selected studies from 1974 to 1990 providing treatment by behaviour therapy and conventional reducing diet

	1974	1978	1984	1985–7	1988–90
No. of studies included	15	17	15	13	5
Sample size	53.1	54.0	71.3	71.6	21.2
Initial weight (kg)	73.4	87.3	88.7	87.2	91.9
Initial % overweight	49.4	48.6	48.1	56.2	59.8
Length of treatment (weeks)	8.4	10.5	13.2	15.6	21.3
Weight loss (kg)	3.8	4.2	6.9	8.4	8.5
Loss per week (kg)	0.5	0.4	0.5	0.5	0.4
Attrition (%)	11.4	12.9	10.6	13.8	21.8
Length of follow-up (weeks)	15.5	30.3	58.4	48.3	53
Loss at follow-up	4.0	4.1	4.4	5.3	5.6

Source: Wadden (1993).

the years 1990 to 1995 suggest a further increase in the average weight loss at the end of treatment, to 8.7 kg (Wing 1998). These differences do not appear to be due to the greater effectiveness of more recent programmes (i.e. at 0.5 kg per week, the average weight loss per week has remained unchanged) but to an increase in the average length of these programmes from 8.4 weeks before 1974 to 27 weeks in the years from 1990 to 1995.

Although the weight loss of 5.3 kg which is typically observed at follow-up is substantial for somebody who is slightly overweight, it is quite insufficient for really obese individuals who may need to shed 20 kg or more. Furthermore, many researchers in this area are pessimistic about the long-term effectiveness of clinical weight loss treatments. Although there are few studies with follow-up periods of more than a year, the results of these studies are not very encouraging. For example, one study recontacted 55 women who had successfully participated in 18-month treatment programmes that combined mostly very low-calorie diets with behaviour therapy (Foster *et al.* 1996). Five years later, most of these women averaged 3.6 kg above their weight before starting therapy. Only 17 per cent had been successful in maintaining at least part of their weight loss. However, more research is needed in which larger groups and groups who participated in a greater variety of weight loss programmes are followed before definite conclusions can be drawn.

In contrast to the outcomes with adults, behavioural treatment of childhood obesity has yielded promising results. In a report of 10-year treatment outcomes for obese children in four randomized treatment studies, Epstein *et al.* (1994) reported that 30 per cent of these children were not obese 10 years after the treatment. These changes were substantially greater than those of various control groups included in these studies. The children had been between 20 per cent and 100 per cent overweight when 6 to 12 years old at intake. Treatment was family-based and included weekly meetings for eight to twelve weeks, with monthly meetings continuing for six to twelve months from the start of the programme.

Consistent with findings reported earlier, the obese parents who were treated in the same programme showed initial weight loss, followed by relapse. After five years all had regained their baseline weight and after 10 years, parents in all groups were more heavily overweight than they had been at the beginning of the study.

Why is behavioural treatment so much more effective with children than with adults? One reason could be that the set point for weight is more malleable in children. There appears to be a peak for accelerated growth of fat tissue between the ages of 9 and 13 (Ailhaud and Hauner 1998). Reduction in overweight before this age may therefore prevent a proliferation in the number of fat cells which would later be difficult to reverse. It also seems plausible that children are not yet as fixed in their eating habits as adults. Finally, the eating of children is very much under the control of adults who may be more effective in controlling the diets of their children than they are in controlling their own. By the time these children grow up to manage their own diets, they may have internalized the pattern of eating learned at home.

Pharmacotherapy

Before the widespread acceptance of behaviour therapy, appetite suppressant (anorectic) drugs were the most popular treatment for obesity. These drugs were widely used because they led to substantial and effortless weight loss. Nevertheless, this type of pharmacotherapy had two major disadvantages: some of these drugs (especially the amphetamines) were likely to be abused, and the weight loss achieved with drug therapy could rarely be maintained.

Anorectic drugs have now become safer (though not really safe). Pharmacotherapy would therefore be useful in cases of severe obesity, if the problem of the maintenance of weight loss could be solved. Because the maintenance of drug-induced weight loss requires some change in lifestyle, the combination of anorectic drugs with behaviour therapy would seem to constitute an optimal therapy. The use of drugs would achieve a fast and effortless weight loss while the techniques of behaviour therapy would lead to the required changes in lifestyle.

To test this hypothesis, Craighead and her colleagues (Craighead et al. 1981; Craighead 1984) conducted two studies to compare the combined effects of drug and behaviour therapy with the impact of drug or behaviour therapy used alone (Figure 4.6). Although participants who received pharmacotherapy alone or in combination with behaviour therapy had significantly greater weight losses than those under only behaviour therapy (14.5 kg and 15.3 kg vs 10.9 kg), a one-year follow-up showed a striking reversal in the relative efficacy of treatments. Behaviour therapy patients regained significantly less weight (1.9 kg) than respondents under pharmacotherapy (8.2 kg) or the combined treatment conditions (10.7 kg). The resulting trend in net weight loss now favoured the behaviour therapy alone (net loss of 9.0 kg) over the other two conditions (net loss pharmacotherapy alone: 6.3 kg; net loss combined treatment: 4.6 kg). Thus, somewhat surprisingly, therapy was not only ineffective in helping to maintain the weight losses due to pharmacotherapy, but the long-term

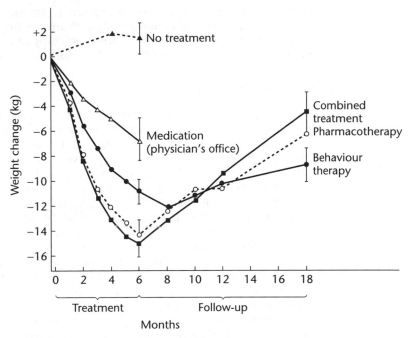

Figure 4.6 Weight change during six months of treatment and one-year follow-up.
Source: Craighead *et al.* (1981).

effects of behaviour therapy were actually poorer if patients had also received pharmacotherapy than if they had not.

It is interesting to speculate how the addition of medication could compromise the effectiveness of behaviour therapy (though note a failure to replicate, by Craighead 1984). It seems possible that the reduction in appetite caused by the anorectic drug prevented individuals from learning the behavioural techniques in the presence of competing hunger cues. Thus, when the drug was stopped, they might have been unprepared to cope with the resulting increase in hunger. However, this interpretation was not supported by findings of a second study conducted by Craighead (1984) in which she used pharmacotherapy during either the first or the second half of a 16-week behaviour therapy programme. Long-term results of these two sequences were no different from those of a combined treatment in which medication was administered for the total 16 weeks of behaviour therapy.

A second interpretation could be derived from theories of cognitive control (e.g. Bandura 1997). Patients who received the combined treatment may have attributed their weight loss to medication and may thus have failed to develop the feeling of control over their weight that is important for the maintenance of weight loss. The validity of this explanation could have been tested if Craighead and colleagues had included a condition in their studies that combined placebo medication with behaviour therapy. Even though some doubt may remain about the theoretical interpretation of these results, the practical implications are obvious: the long-term effects of behaviour therapy are not improved by pharmacotherapy. Thus, not only does pharmacotherapy carry a potential health risk (for a review, see Berg 1999); it also seems to be ineffective.

Very low-calorie diets

Although total fasting results in significant weight loss, much of the weight loss consists of lean body tissue as well as body fat. This protein malnutrition could have serious consequences for hepatic, renal and pulmonary functions (Blackburn *et al.* 1986). Very low-calorie diets are supplemented fasts that are designed to spare lean body mass through the provision of 70 to 100 grams of protein a day in a total of 300 to 600 calories. Very low-calorie diets produce average weight losses of 20 kg in 12 weeks (Blackburn *et al.* 1986). They appear to be relatively safe when undertaken under careful medical supervision and limited to periods of three months, even though there are some claims of severe health risks (e.g. Berg 1999). As with drug treatment, the major problem with very low-calorie diets is the rapid weight regain after the termination of treatment. On average, patients treated with this type of diet regain 35 to 50 per cent of their lost weight in the year following treatment.

Although there is some indication that the process of weight (re)gain can be slowed down by a combination of very low-calorie diet and behaviour therapy (e.g. Wadden and Stunkard 1986), the attempt to increase the effectiveness of very low-calorie diets by adding a weight maintenance therapy has not been successful. In a study conducted by Wadden *et al.* (1994), obese women were randomly assigned to either a 1200 kilocalorie-per-day balanced diet for 26 weeks or to a very low-calorie diet for the first four months followed by a 1200 kilocalorie-per-day diet. All patients attended treatment weekly for the first 12 months in which they received instruction in traditional behavioural methods of weight control. After that they received a bi-weekly maintenance programme for an additional six months. Figure 4.7 shows that patients who received the very low-calorie diet lost approximately twice as much weight during the first six months as those on the regular diet. However, in the year following the diet, they regained more than 50 per cent of their lost weight, even while attending weekly or bi-weekly weight maintenance sessions. Thus, at 18 months their mean weight was approximately the same as that of participants on a regular diet who hardly regained any weight under the maintenance schedule. Thus, very low-calorie diets are not only expensive (approximately $2500 for 26 weeks; Wadden 1995) and potentially unhealthy (Berg 1999), but also ineffective. Wadden (1995) has therefore suggested that these diets should be replaced by low-calorie diets which provide at least 800 kilocalories per day and may produce less of a maintenance problem.

Exercise

Most of the weight reduction techniques described earlier aim at the input side of the energy equation. But because overweight individuals consume

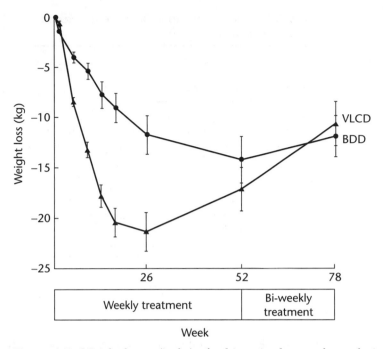

Figure 4.7   Weight losses (in kg) of subjects in the very low-calorie diet (VLCD) and balanced deficit diet (BDD) conditions during one year of weekly treatment and six months of bi-weekly maintenance therapy. *Source*: Wadden *et al.* (1994: 168).

more energy than they expend, increasing energy expenditure would offer an alternative or additional means of reduction. The neglect of exercise, particularly in the early weight control programmes, had been justified by the belief that exercise does not use up many calories (e.g. two miles of walking uses only about 200 calories) and that this minor effect is likely to be outweighed by the increase in appetite resulting from such exercise.

In contrast, studies that examined the impact of exercise alone and in combination with behavioural techniques have found that combination of diet plus supervised group exercise vs diet alone has resulted in greater weight losses in most cases (e.g. Stalonas *et al.* 1978; Dahlkoetter *et al.* 1979). There is therefore no longer doubt that the likelihood of long-term weight loss is increased in people who exercise. There is still discussion, however, about the different ways in which exercise contributes to weight control. The biological link between exercise and weight is relatively straightforward (USDHHS 1996b). Increases in fat mass and the development of obesity occur when energy intake exceeds daily energy expenditure for a long period of time. Theoretically, approximately one kilo of fat is stored for each 7700 kilocalories of excess energy intake. Unfortunately for weight control, the human body is a very efficient machine. Table 4.7 lists the duration of various activities to expend 150 kilocalories. As one can see, to work off the equivalent of eating a 150 g serving of creamy fruit

Table 4.7 Duration of various activities to expend 150 kilocalories for an average 70 kg adult

Intensity	Activity	Approximate duration in minutes
Moderate	Volleyball, non-competitive	43
Moderate	Walking, moderate pace (3 mph, 20 min/mile)	37
Moderate	Walking, brisk pace (4 mph, 15 min/mile)	32
Moderate	Table tennis	32
Moderate	Raking leaves	32
Moderate	Social dancing	29
Moderate	Lawn mowing (powered push mower)	29
Hard	Jogging (5 mph, 12 min/mile)	18
Hard	Field hockey	16
Very hard	Running (6 mph, 10 min/mile)	13

Source: USDHHS (1996b).

yoghurt, 30 g of salami or 200 ml white wine, an adult who weighs 70 kg has to walk at moderate pace for 37 minutes, jog for 18 minutes, or dance for 29 minutes.

There may be a second way by which exercise increases energy expenditure. There is evidence that the increase in metabolic rate produced by exercise is maintained for some time after a person has stopped exercising. Thus, exercise may use more calories than are needed for the physical movement *per se*. A recent meta-analysis of 22 studies examining the effects of diet and diet-plus-exercise on resting metabolic rate showed that exercise reduced but did not eliminate the drop in resting metabolic rate resulting from the diet (Thompson *et al.* 1996).

Most researchers in the area doubt, however, whether these metabolic effects can fully account for the substantial effects that have been observed in studies that assessed the added impact of exercise on weight control (Brownell 1995). They suggest that psychological mechanisms may contribute to the impact of regular exercise on weight loss. It would seem plausible, for example, that adherence to an exercise regimen increases people's feelings of self-efficacy. Such an increase in the sense of self-efficacy and the feeling of control over their weight might lead those who exercise to be more motivated in following a dietary instruction. This interpretation would also explain the finding that the impact of exercise on weight was even stronger at the long-term follow-up.

The assumption that the effect of exercise on weight control is mainly mediated by psychological rather than physiological or metabolic effects has implications for the type of exercise regimen one prescribes for obese individuals (Brownell 1995). Designs for exercise programmes have traditionally been guided by considerations of improving coronary fitness. For this purpose, exercise has to be done with sufficient frequency (three times a week) and at sufficient intensity to bring the heart rate to at least 70 per cent of maximum and of sufficient duration (i.e. 20 minutes per occasion). As Brownell (1995) has argued, these considerations, which may have discouraged generations of obese individuals from trying to exercise, are probably irrelevant for the type of exercise that should be recommended as part of weight loss diets. Dropping these requirements would allow us to prescribe exercise regimens which are more easily integrated into people's lifestyles (e.g. Perri *et al.* 1997).

Conclusions

The picture emerging from our review of clinical treatment of obesity is discouraging. Although behavioural diets are quite effective in the short run, the average weight loss at follow-up reported in these studies is not substantial enough for individuals who are seriously obese. Furthermore, the evidence available from the few studies which assess the long-term effectiveness of weight loss treatment suggests that five years later most individuals will have regained most, if not all, the weight they had lost during their treatment.

Self-help and self-help groups

It is plausible that, before going to a therapist, individuals who are overweight and want to lose weight will try one of the many popular weight loss diets. Self-help programmes by organizations such as TOPS (Take Off Pounds Sensibly), who offer classes throughout the United States and several other countries, should largely draw on those individuals who have failed to cure themselves but are not yet ready to undergo clinical therapy. The key element of TOPS is a weekly meeting to provide group support, with weigh-ins constituting the high point of these meetings (Stunkard 1986). Assessment of the effectiveness of this programme is difficult because of the high drop-out rate. According to Stunkard (1986), in one study nearly 67 per cent of members dropped out during the first year and these were persons who had been least successful in losing weight.

Commercial weight loss organizations such as Weight Watchers have added three important elements to the programmes pioneered by non-profit groups such as TOPS: behaviour modification, inspirational lectures drawn from successful members, and a carefully designed nutritional programme (Stunkard 1986). But they also suffer from the problem of attrition. Two prospective studies of a representative sample of the members of a large commercial organization found that approximately half the members dropped out during the first six weeks (Volkmar *et al.* 1981).

That self-help groups can be effective is suggested by a study conducted in Norway (Grimsmo *et al.* 1981). In this country, self-help organizations for weight control have grown into a nationwide movement with 80,000 people participating. They work in small groups (8–12 members), meeting once a week for eight weeks, monitoring body weight each time. Members are given dietary information, and are encouraged to do physical exercise and give up alcohol. The fee has to be paid in advance and the drop-out rate is less than 10 per cent.

In a prospective study Grimsmo and colleagues (1981) obtained data from the 'slim-club hostesses' on initial weight, weight at weekly intervals, and end results of 11,410 individuals who participated in a course during the spring of 1977. The average weight loss of the 10,650 participants (93.3 per cent) who completed the course was 6.9 kg. With drop-outs included it was still 6.4 kg. In a retrospective survey of the long-term effects of this self-help programme the authors found that the average weight remained stable for the first two years but then began to rise. After five years, participants had regained half of their initial weight loss.

Trying to lose weight without help

Most people who try to diet to lose weight do not join an organized weight loss programme. A national survey conducted in the USA in 1966 estimated that 46 per cent of all men and 70 per cent of all women had been on diets to lose weight at some time during their lives. Current dieting was estimated at 7 per cent for men and 15 per cent for women (reported in Jeffery *et al.* 1991). There is also evidence that dieting is strongly related to per cent overweight, with heavier individuals making more attempts to lose weight (Jeffery *et al.* 1991).

Unfortunately, the evidence on the effectiveness of these do-it-yourself diets is rather inconsistent. There is some indication that they are less effective than clinical treatment in the short run. For example, the college women who participated in the study of Schifter and Ajzen (1985) and who had on average expected to lose 4.5 kg during the six-week period of the study, only lost 0.76 kg. This is the amount the average participant in a clinical weight loss programme is expected to lose in 1.5 weeks. Data on weight loss from a telephone survey of a large sample of individuals who tried to lose weight compare more favourably with the effectiveness of clinical programmes. Average achieved weight loss was 0.634 kg per week for men and 0.5 kg per week for women, which is approximately the weekly weight loss achieved in clinical therapies. However, the authors of this study warned that these averages may reflect only the experience of those most successful at losing weight (Williamson *et al.* 1992). What is needed is long-term follow-up data on the success rate of a sizeable sample of obese men and women who are dieting to lose weight.

Can dieting be harmful?

It is a reflection of the changing attitude towards dieting that this question is being asked at all. However, concern has risen over the last decade that dieting, aside from the possibility of being ineffective, may also have potentially harmful effects (e.g. Brownell and Rodin 1994). There are two issues which have been discussed in this context, namely that weight cycling or yo-yo dieting has negative consequences for the physical and mental health of the dieters, and that weight concerns and dieting contribute to the development of eating disorders.

Because obesity appears to be unhealthy, it would seem plausible that losing weight should improve the health of obese individuals. In line with this assumption, it has been shown that weight reduction leads to changes in various health risk factors, including reductions in cholesterol (Thompson *et al.* 1979) and large decreases in blood pressure (e.g. Wadden and Stunkard 1986). However, it is unclear whether these reductions in risk factors are caused by the weight loss. They could also be the result of improvements in dietary habits or a reaction to mild starvation (Ernsberger and Koletsky 1999). In support of the latter explanation, Ernsberger and Nelson (1988) reported that the blood pressure reduction reported in weight loss trials showed a relationship to rate of weight loss but not to kilograms of weight lost. Finally, due to the poor long-term prognosis on the maintenance of weight losses, most individuals go through cycles of losing and gaining weight. These weight changes may be less beneficial to healthy functioning.

A recent review of studies on the association between weight loss and mortality by Williamson (1995) found only one study, the 1950 Metropolitan Life Insurance Study, reporting beneficial effects of weight loss. In this study, the life expectancy of individuals who had initially received substandard insurance because they were overweight, but who had subsequently lost weight, improved to that of insured people with standard risk. More recent epidemiological studies have typically found that weight fluctuation was associated with increased mortality (for reviews, see Brownell 1995; Williamson 1995). However, none of these studies allows one to separate the effects of intentional from unintentional weight loss. Unintentional weight loss can be due to factors such as severe illness, poverty, or certain eating disorders which could also result in health impairment. One therefore has to concur with both Brownell (1995) and Williamson (1995) who concluded that this evidence does not allow any firm conclusions to be drawn about the health consequences of intentional weight loss in the obese.

Do unsuccessful dieters get depressed? It appears plausible that individuals who chastise themselves into losing weight, only to regain it a few years later, react with depression. However, in a review of the findings of several cross-sectional studies of weight cycling, as well as of their own longitudinal study, Foster and colleagues (1996) found no evidence that individuals who had regained the weight they had lost reacted with increased depression.

Obese individuals who lose weight might even be at risk for depression if they succeed in maintaining their weight loss. According to set point theory (e.g. Keesey 1986), weight suppression can result in distress, because the body actively defends against changes in weight and attempts to return to its original weight or 'set point'. However, in a study of 629 women and 155 men who had lost at least 13.6 kg and maintained this loss for over a year, no evidence was found that long-term suppression of body weight was associated with psychological distress (Klem *et al.* 1998). In summary then, there is little empirical evidence to indicate that dieting increases the risk of depression.

There can be little doubt, however, that weight concerns contribute to the development of eating disorders. Prospective studies that followed samples of young girls found evidence for an association between weight concerns and shape concerns at the outset of the research and the development of partial syndromes of eating disorders (e.g. Killen *et al.* 1996). For example, Killen and his colleagues (1996) measured weight concerns and shape concerns in a sample of 877 ninth grade high school girls (average age 14.9 years). Eating disorder symptoms were assessed four years later in structured clinical interviews. To be classified as symptomatic, girls had to manifest bulimic episodes, compensatory behaviours such as the use of laxatives, diuretics or over-exercise, and over-concern with body weight. By age 17, 4 per cent of these girls had become symptomatic. Weight concern at entry was the best predictor of the development of the eating disorder syndrome: none of the girls in the lowest quartile of the weight concern scale had become symptomatic but 10 per cent of the girls who scored in the highest quartile had done so.

Conclusions

Obesity is associated with an increased risk of coronary heart disease, stroke, and adult-onset diabetes. Willett and Manson (1995) therefore concluded that for most adults, 'optimal health will be experienced if a lean body weight is maintained throughout life by means of regular physical activity and, if needed, modest dietary restraint' (p. 399).

It is less clear, however, what course of action one should recommend to those who become overweight or even obese. In the past, one would have recommended a diet to lose weight. These days one would hesitate in making such a recommendation. First, the evidence has become ambiguous as to whether the reduction of body weight is accompanied by a reduction in these health risks. Second, it is very doubtful whether dieting to lose weight will result in long-term weight loss. Although clinical weight loss therapies appear to be effective in the short run, the available evidence suggests that most of the weight which obese individuals manage to lose is regained within a few years after the end of these therapies. Furthermore, the resulting weight cycling may have a negative impact on health.

One of the reasons why attempts at dieting to lose weight often fail is that individuals who want to lose weight live mentally all day in the refrigerator as Wegner (1994) once aptly put it. Ironic process theory offers an explanation for this phenomenon. Therefore, instead of focusing individuals on trying to reduce the calorie content of their diets, one should persuade them to forget about calories and instead change the *composition* of their diet. There is evidence that overweight persons who eat a low-fat diet lose weight gradually over a long period even if they are allowed to consume as many carbohydrates as they want. Thus, recommendations aimed at lowering the fat content of a diet and increasing the consumption of fruit and vegetables are likely not only to have a positive health impact but also to result in slow weight loss in overweight individuals. This weight loss could be accelerated at further benefit to their health, if overweight individuals could be persuaded to become physically more active, or even to engage in regular exercise.

Obesity and eating disorders

Obesity does not by itself constitute an eating disorder. Eating disorders are characterized by a severe and persistent disturbance in eating behaviour that results in the altered consumption of food, and significantly impairs physical health or psychosocial functioning (Fairburn and Walsh 1995). Although the more extreme cases of obesity impair physical health or psychosocial functioning, they do not necessarily involve disturbances of eating behaviour or altered consumption of food. However, a substantial proportion of obese individuals engage in binge eating and those obese individuals would fall under the diagnosis of an eating disorder not otherwise specified according to the DSM-IV (APA 1994). The DSM-IV specifies two eating disorders, namely anorexia nervosa and bulimia nervosa. A third eating disorder which has only recently been described, the so-called 'binge eating disorder' is included in the category of 'eating disorder not otherwise specified'.

Anorexia nervosa is characterized by a refusal to maintain an even minimally normal body weight for age and height (i.e. BMI below 17.5 kg/m^2) combined with an intense fear of gaining weight or becoming fat. Anorexics also distort the way in which they perceive their body weight or shape. Some individuals feel globally overweight, even though they are underweight. Others realize that they are thin, but they find some parts of their body too fat (e.g. buttocks, stomach, thighs). This is particularly problematic because anorexics tend to judge self-worth nearly exclusively in terms of their body shape and weight. Weight loss is seen as great achievement and weight gain as totally unacceptable. Weight loss is accomplished mainly via a reduction in food intake. Additional methods of weight loss include purging (e.g. self-induced vomiting, misuse of laxatives) and increased or excessive exercise. Finally, anorectic women suffer from amenorrhea, the absence of at least three consecutive menstrual cycles. The DSM-IV distinguishes two kinds of anorexia, namely the restricting and the binge eating/purging subtypes.

Anorexia nervosa, as categorized by the DSM-IV, is relatively uncommon. Prevalence studies among females in late adolescence and early adulthood have found rates of 0.5 to 1.0 per cent. The incidence appears to have increased in recent years (APA 1994). Little is known about the prevalence of anorexia nervosa in men, but some authors estimate that 5 to 10 per cent of patients suffering from anorexia nervosa are male (Yanovski 1998). The mean age at onset for anorexia nervosa is 17 years, possibly with bimodal peaks at ages 14 and 18 (APA 1994). Studies of anorexia nervosa in twins have found significantly higher concordance rates for monozygotic than dizygotic twins which indicates that genetic factors contribute to the development of this illness (APA 1994).

Anorexia nervosa is treated through a combination of nutritional rehabilitation and psychotherapy. Nutritional rehabilitation is crucial and should be accomplished either before or alongside psychotherapy. Psychotherapies include cognitive behavioural therapy, which focuses mainly on the faulty cognitions regarding eating and weight, and psychodynamic or interpersonal psychotherapy, which explores the patient's current interpersonal relationships with others (Yanovski 1998). Medication is infrequently used in the treatment of anorexia nervosa.

The course and outcome of anorexia nervosa is highly variable, with some individuals recovering fully after one episode, some exhibiting a fluctuating pattern and others experiencing a chronically deteriorating course of illness. Of individuals admitted to university hospitals, the long-term mortality is 10 per cent, with death resulting from starvation, suicide, or electrolyte imbalance (APA 1994). Although long-term follow-up studies found that about half of all former patients reported normal weight over the long term, reproductive function, psychological well-being, and attitudes towards food and weight remain abnormal for more than half of these individuals.

Like anorexia nervosa, *bulimia nervosa* is characterized by a persistent over-concern with body shape and weight. In fact, bulimia was first investigated as a symptom of anorexia nervosa. Other essential features of bulimia according to the DSM-IV are binge eating, and inappropriate compensatory methods to prevent weight gain. To qualify for the diagnosis, both the binge eating and the compensatory behaviour must occur at least twice a week for three months. The DSM-IV distinguishes two subtypes of bulimics which differ in the kind of compensatory behaviour used, namely bulimics who purge and the non-purging type who rely on fasting or excessive exercise.

Episodes of binge eating are characterized by the rapid consumption of large quantities of food in discrete periods of time (e.g. within any two-hour period) and by a sense of lack of control over eating during the binge. Individuals have the feeling during these bulimic episodes that they cannot stop eating or control how much they eat. Afterwards, bulimics try to prevent weight gain through the use of compensatory behaviours such as self-induced vomiting or misuse of laxatives. Self-induced vomiting is employed by 80 to 90 per cent of individuals with bulimia who present in eating disorder clinics. Laxative misuse is less frequent, being presented in approximately one-third of bulimic patients. Patients with bulimia nervosa typically show no abnormalities when physically examined. Most are within the normal weight range, but a few are over- or underweight.

The prevalence of bulimia nervosa among high school and college age women has been estimated at 1 to 3 per cent, although a much greater percentage engage in bulimic behaviours that are not of sufficient frequency to meet the criteria for the disorder (Yanovski 1998). Again, only one-tenth of the patients suffering from bulimia are male. Bulimia nervosa usually begins in late adolescence or early adult life, with the binge eating frequently beginning after a period of dieting. The disturbed eating behaviour persists for at least several years in a high percentage of clinic samples (APA 1994).

The cognitive–behavioural approach to the treatment of bulimia nervosa is based on the assumption that the characteristic attitudes to body shape and weight are of primary importance in the maintenance of the disorder. In terms of the boundary model, bulimics have a very stringent diet boundary which, if it were consistently maintained, would make them indistinguishable from anorexics. Of course, bulimics do not always succeed in honouring the diet boundary. Binges arise from either actual or perceived transgressions of the diet boundary. This phenomenon is assumed to be analogous to the preload effect. A second, and perhaps more frequent, cause of binges is the elimination of the boundary by emotional agitation (Polivy and Herman 1987).

The cognitive–behavioural treatment of bulimia nervosa is generally conducted on a one-to-one basis and involves approximately 20 50-minute sessions over a period of four to five months. It involves a sequence of cognitive and behavioural procedures. The treatment has three stages. In the first stage, the emphasis is on enhancing control over eating using largely behavioural methods, such as self-monitoring and the prescription of patterns of regular eating. The second stage is more cognitively oriented and includes procedures designed to reduce the tendency to diet and cognitive restructuring focused mainly on the patients' attitudes to shape and weight. The third stage is concerned mainly with consolidating progress and includes a relapse prevention procedure.

The effectiveness of cognitive–behavioural treatment methods has been assessed in several studies (for a review, see Fairburn 1995). It appears that cognitive–behavioural therapy results in at least a 70 per cent reduction in the frequency of binge eating and purging, and between one-third and one-half of patients cease to binge altogether. One prospective study of a small sample of bulimics found that half the patients who had received cognitive–behavioural treatment six years earlier still showed 'abstinence' from the key behavioural features of bulimia nervosa (Fairburn *et al.* 1995). They had no objective bulimic episodes, no vomiting, and no laxative or diuretic misuse. However, approximately one-third of these individuals still suffered from either bulimia or an unspecified eating disorder six years after receiving treatment for bulimia.

Binge eating disorder is a newly described eating disorder characterized by frequent binge eating which is accompanied by emotional distress. But these individuals do not engage in the compensatory behaviours typical of bulimia. Binge eating disorder is the most common eating disorder affecting approximately 2 to 3 per cent of the general population (Yanovski 1998). It can be treated with the same kind of behavioural–cognitive therapy which has been used in the treatment of bulimia nervosa.

Although there are normal weight binge eaters, binge eating disorder is particularly frequent among the obese. According to some estimates, approximately 30 per cent of the obese who attend hospital-affiliated weight control programmes engage in this type of binge eating. Obese binge eaters experience greater levels of eating-related and general psychopathology, including earlier onset of obesity, dieting and weight concerns, great body dissatisfaction and preoccupation with thinness, and increase in cognitive distortions, depression, anxiety and personality disorder than obese individuals who do not binge eat (Goodrick *et al.* 1998).

GENERAL CONCLUSIONS

This chapter has presented evidence on the impact of smoking, alcohol abuse and excessive eating on health. Without doubt, the findings on health deterioration are strongest for cigarette smoking, which has been identified as the single most important source of preventable mortality and morbidity in each of the reports of the US Surgeon General produced since 1964. Although the empirical evidence on the health impact of *moderate* alcohol consumption is more ambiguous, there can be no doubt that alcohol *abuse* is also a very serious public health problem which impairs social and occupational functioning in addition to health. Finally, obesity is linked to increases in the risk of serious diseases such as diabetes and hypertension, and to increased mortality.

Once people smoke, drink too much alcohol or have a weight problem, these appetitive behaviours are difficult to change. Even though therapy might help individuals to act on their intentions to adopt more healthy habits, the strength of their intentions may be at least as important as the therapy for the eventual outcome. Because of the difficulties in changing these health-impairing habits, I argued that primary prevention is a more effective health strategy than behaviour change. I further suggested that programmes of primary prevention should rely not only on persuasion and health education but also on planned changes in the rewards and costs associated with these health behaviours. These latter strategies may be less applicable for weight control. However, there is evidence that cigarette consumption and alcohol abuse can be influenced by increases in the tax on tobacco and alcohol products, by instituting stricter age limits or by a reduction of availability through limiting sales.

FURTHER READING

Bray, G.A., Bouchard, C. and James, W.P.T. (eds) (1998) *Handbook of Obesity*. New York, NY: Marcel Dekker. This is the most authoritative and comprehensive treatment of obesity. The handbook contains an excellent collection of chapters by leading authorities in the field covering causes, health impact and treatment of obesity.

Hester, R.K. and Miller, W.R. (eds) (1995) *Handbook of Alcoholism Treatment Approaches: Effective Alternatives*, 2nd ed. Boston, MA: Allyn and Bacon. The chapters provide excellent reviews of a wide range of psychological treatment approaches. This book is an important sourcebook for anybody interested in issues of treatment of alcoholism.

Hurley, J. and Horowitz, J. (eds) (1990) *Alcohol and Health*. New York, NY: Hemisphere. Written by leading authorities in the field of alcoholism, the chapters in this edited book provide a comprehensive discussion of the epidemiology, health effects and treatment of alcoholism.

Macdonald, T.K., Zanna, M.P. and Fong, G.T. (1995) Decision making in altered states: effects of alcohol on attitudes towards drinking and driving.

Journal of Personality and Social Psychology, 68: 973–85. Presents laboratory experiments and field studies which demonstrated the effects of alcohol myopia, the notion that alcohol intoxication decreases cognitive capacity so that people are more likely to attend only to the most salient cues.

US Department of Health and Human Services (1996) *Clinical Practice Guidelines: Smoking Cessation*. Rockville, MD: AHCPR Publication No. 96-0692. An authoritative evaluation of the effectiveness of clinical techniques for smoking cessation by a panel of experts. Their evaluation is based on an extensive review and analysis (using meta-analysis wherever possible) of the scientific literature on outcomes of clinical smoking cessation interventions.

FIVE

BEHAVIOUR AND HEALTH: SELF-PROTECTION

This chapter will focus on health-enhancing or self-protective behaviours, such as eating a healthy diet, exercising, avoiding behaviours that are essential to the transmission of AIDS (unprotected sex, needle sharing) and protecting oneself against accidental injuries. The division of health behaviours into excessive appetites and self-protection is somewhat arbitrary. However, there is a difference between these two types of behaviour with regard to the extent to which they are under volitional control. Although people frequently need therapy to enable them to stop smoking, to give up alcohol or to lose weight, it would be rather unusual if people required therapy to reduce the salt content of their food, take up jogging, to practise safe sex or to fasten their seat belts.

HEALTHY DIET

Obesity is not the only health risk that is related to diet. There is growing evidence that important ingredients of our diet, when taken in excess, may have a deleterious effect on our health. Thus, an excessive fat consumption has been linked to an elevated morbidity and mortality from atherosclerotic heart disease and even cancer and a high intake of salt (sodium chloride) has been related to the development of hypertension and ultimately cardiovascular disease (Committee on Diet and Health 1989).

Cholesterol and coronary heart disease

Fat, cholesterol and coronary heart disease

Of all the dietary risk factors, the relation between excessive fat consumption and coronary heart disease has been studied most extensively. The hypothesis specifying the role of dietary fat in the development of coronary heart disease has been modified over the years with the emergence of new empirical evidence. This indicates that there are good and bad fats, just as there are good and bad cholesterols. Food fats can be divided into two categories, vegetable and animal fats. The latter may be further divided into three subcategories: dairy fats, land animal fats and marine fats, including the fats of fish and of marine mammals such as whales or seals. The properties of the fatty acid composition of these types of food fats are very different. Vegetable and marine fats are unsaturated and contain substantial amounts of polyunsaturated fatty acids, mainly linoleic acid. Dairy and meat fats are much more saturated and contain only small amounts of linoleic acid.

Cholesterol is a fat-like substance mainly produced by the liver. Contained in most tissues, it is also the main component of deposits in the lining of arteries. It is carried in the blood mainly by two proteins, namely low-density lipoproteins (LDLs) and high-density lipoproteins (HDLs). Low-density lipoproteins are considered bad cholesterols, because if they are increased to a high level they can be deposited on the walls of the blood vessels thereby helping the formation of 'plaques'. Plaque formation leads to a narrowing of the arteries and thus to atherosclerosis. As will be discussed below, there is evidence to suggest that excessive ingestion of saturated fats is a major cause of the elevation of low-density lipoproteins. In contrast, high-density lipoproteins are believed to be good cholesterols which protect against atherosclerosis. They serve as 'lipid scavengers', a means of transporting cholesterol from parts of the body where there is an excess to the liver where it can be disposed of (MAFF 1995). These modifications of the hypothesis have only been made during the last few decades. Therefore most of the early data available on population serum cholesterol or on food fats cannot be related to these distinctions. However, this poses no major problems because levels of low-density cholesterol are highly correlated with levels of total cholesterol, at least in population studies (Pasternak *et al.* 1996). Thus, averaged over groups, total cholesterol levels are a good indicator of levels of low-density cholesterol.

There is now wide consensus that, in industrial societies, the risk of coronary heart disease rises as serum cholesterol increases over most of the serum cholesterol range, with levels above 6 mmol/l (i.e. 238 mg/dl, 238 milligrams per 100 millilitres) being considered undesirable (Macpherson 1999). This consensus is based on population studies which compared dietary habits and serum cholesterol across different nationalities. These studies have consistently reported a strong relationship between dietary cholesterol and serum cholesterol (Blackburn 1983). For example, the so-called 'Seven Country Study' (Keys 1980), which was carried out in the USA, Japan, and five European countries, found a very high correlation between the ingestion of saturated fats and serum cholesterol levels (r = .89) and between the fat content of the diet and the incidence of coronary heart disease (r = .84).

Epidemiological studies which assessed the relationship between dietary cholesterol and serum cholesterol *within* a given culture at the individual level have typically failed to find an association. For example, 24-hour dietary recall interviews were conducted with a sample of approximately

2000 men and women residents in the community of Tecumseh (Michigan, USA) to determine the influence of diet on serum cholesterol levels. No relationship could be found between dietary variables and levels of serum cholesterol concentration for men or women. Similarly, in the Evans County, Georgia Study, 25 white males were selected whose serum cholesterol values were very low (160 mg/dl or less) and compared with 26 who had very high values (260 mg/dl or more). These two groups did not differ significantly in any of the dietary variables assessed (Stulb *et al.* 1965). There is also little evidence of a relationship between diet and coronary heart disease from these studies (Stallones 1983).

The failure of these studies to demonstrate a relationship between dietary cholesterol and serum cholesterol on an individual level has been used by proponents of a genetic perspective to argue that serum cholesterol levels are mainly determined by genetic levels and that diet has very little impact (e.g. Kaplan 1988). However, this claim would not only be difficult to reconcile with the outcomes of the population studies described earlier (e.g. Keys 1980), but would also be inconsistent with the evidence from dietary intervention studies which demonstrate that substantial reductions in dietary fat content result in reduction in serum cholesterol (e.g. Hunninghake *et al.* 1993; Schuler *et al.* 1992; Byers *et al.* 1995). I will therefore review these studies before discussing whether cholesterol-lowering interventions actually reduce mortality.

The effectiveness of dietary interventions

The impact of dietary interventions in community, worksite or primary health care settings in reducing cholesterol levels varies from 0 to 10 per cent. For example, in the large-scale community intervention conducted in Northern Finland described earlier (p. 72), Puska and his colleagues (1985) reported an average reduction in serum cholesterol of 4 per cent in men, and of 1 per cent in women, in the intervention as compared to the control communities during the period 1972–7. In contrast, none of the three community studies undertaken in the United States to reduce cardiovascular disease risks during the 1980s reported significant intervention effects on cholesterol levels (Luepker *et al.* 1994; Carleton *et al.* 1995; Winkleby *et al.* 1996).

Similar variability can be observed in the effects of worksite dietary intervention studies. Whereas two major dietary worksite interventions failed to have any impact on cholesterol levels (Glasgow *et al.* 1995, 1997), a worksite intervention on workers with cholesterol levels above 5.2 mmol or higher who had volunteered to participate in a screening and intervention study showed modest but significant effects (Byers *et al.* 1995). The control group received approximately five minutes of dietary education. The intervention group received in addition a total of two hours of nutrition education delivered in multiple sessions over the next month. Whereas the control group showed a reduction in their cholesterol level of 3 per cent 12 months later, the intervention group showed a reduction of 6.5 per cent. Since the change in the control group is well within the range of what might be expected due to a regression towards the mean, the authors concluded that their nutritional education programme resulted in a 3.5 per cent cholesterol reduction. One potential reason for the greater effectiveness of the intervention by Byers and colleagues (1995) is the fact that they focused on risk groups who should be more motivated to reduce their cholesterol levels.

The few school-based dietary interventions which have been conducted appear to have been quite successful in influencing dietary behaviour (Sorensen et al. 1998). One of the most extensive controlled school-based interventions was the Child and Adolescent Trial for Cardiovascular Health (CATCH), a randomized, controlled field trial with 56 intervention and 40 control elementary schools. Participants in this trial were a total of 5106 initially third grade students from ethnically diverse backgrounds in state schools located in four states of the USA. The intervention consisted of changes in the food served by the school food services and extensive classroom lessons emphasizing healthy eating habits. The outcome measures included an assessment of the dietary content of the food served by the school food service, and a self-report 24-hour dietary recall measure administered to a sub-sample of students at each school. At the school level, the percentage of energy intake from fat in the meals was significantly reduced in the intervention schools (from 38.7 per cent to 31.9 per cent) compared with the control schools (38.9 per cent to 36.2 per cent). Energy intake from saturated fats was also reduced in the intervention schools. Less marked but still significant effects of the intervention could also be found in the dietary recall measure which also reflects dietary changes outside the school setting. Thus, the CATCH intervention appears to have modified the fat content of school lunches and improved the eating habits of children in the intervention schools.

Studies of dietary counselling in primary medical care settings often show more powerful effects, particularly with patient samples who suffer from coronary heart disease. For example, in a 12-month study conducted in Germany, angina patients were randomly assigned to an intervention and a control group (Schuler et al. 1992). The control group was given the usual medical care. The intervention comprised intensive physical exercise in group training sessions (minimum two hours per week), home exercise periods (20 minutes daily), and a low-fat, low-cholesterol diet. Patients assigned to the intervention group stayed on a metabolic ward for the first three weeks of the programme. During this period they were taught how to lower the fat content of their regular diet to less than 20 per cent of total calories. Information sessions were conducted five times a year giving an opportunity for patients and their spouses to discuss dietary and exercise-related problems.

According to 24-hour dietary protocols, patients in the intervention group made considerable changes in their dietary schedule, reducing their total fat consumption by 53 per cent. This should have resulted in reduction in cholesterol levels of more than 20 per cent. However, the actual reduction was only 10 per cent. A similar discrepancy, and even less reduction in cholesterol, was reported by Hunninghake and colleagues (1993) who prescribed a lipid-lowering diet to more than 100 patients suffering from moderate hypercholesterolemia. These authors reported that the 5 per cent average reduction in the mean levels of total and LDL cholesterol produced by the low-fat diet was much less than the reduction anticipated

(Hunninghake *et al.* 1993). Again, dietary protocols completed by patients suggested good dietary adherence.

Additional information from the German study suggests that the discrepancy between reported fat reduction and the actual reduction in levels of cholesterol may have been due to the unreliability of the self-report data (Schuler *et al.* 1993). First, during the strict supervision of the metabolic ward in the first phase of the study, the fat-reduced diet resulted in the expected decrease of cholesterol levels of 23 per cent. Second, whereas patients' compliance in attending the supervised group exercise sessions was significantly correlated with average total cholesterol (r = −.51), the 24-hour dietary protocols were uncorrelated with any of the cholesterol measures. Although the unreliability of the dietary protocols could have been due to lapses in memory, or to the fact that patients show more adherence to their diets on days when they are completing their diaries, the most plausible explanation is that patients' dietary reports were influenced by the wish to be 'good patients'.

The main components of these interventions were nutritional education, combined with information about the health risk involved in eating diets high in saturated fats. Because information on health risks appears to be mainly effective for individuals who are unaware of these risks, one wonders whether persuasive messages which also increase eating-related self-efficacy or perceived control over eating behaviour would not have been more effective. A recent longitudinal study of the determinants of dietary intentions and behaviour based on the model of planned behaviour indicated that perceived behavioural control was a strong predictor of both intentions to eat healthily and actual behaviour (Conner in press). This would suggest that an intervention which, in addition to giving nutritional education, targeted respondents' confidence in being able to eat healthily would be more effective than these standard interventions.

However, findings from a controlled study using a computer-tailored nutrition intervention which also targeted self-efficacy were somewhat disappointing (Brug *et al.* 1996). In this study, respondents in the experimental group received computer-generated feedback letters tailored to their personal dietary intake levels, attitudes, and self-efficacy levels. Feedback messages aimed at reducing fat intake were tailored to dietary intake levels and to the individual's beliefs and awareness levels. Self-efficacy was targeted by providing respondents who held low self-efficacy expectations with information about how to recognize low-fat alternatives. Furthermore, suggestions were given on how to cope with situations reported by the respondents as difficult for sustaining low-fat diets. Respondents in the control group received general nutrition information which did not take account of their personal habits and beliefs. Although the tailored information had a more positive influence on attitudes and intentions towards reducing dietary fat, there was no tailoring effect on self-efficacy expectations. Furthermore, the impact of the intervention on actual fat consumption was somewhat disappointing. Three weeks after the intervention, participants with a fat consumption which was above the recommended guidelines (35 per cent of total calories) had reduced their consumption by 3 per cent in the control group and by 9 per cent in the intervention group. Although cholesterol levels were not measured, this change in fat consumption would probably have resulted in a 3.5 to 4.5 per cent change in levels of serum cholesterol.

There is one study, however, the Life-style Heart Trial, which suggests that a very intensive intervention can achieve quite dramatic lifestyle changes with groups of highly motivated patients (Billings *et al.* 1996). In this study the intervention group reduced their fat intake from 30.8 per cent of total calories at baseline to 7 per cent after one year, which means that they adopted a low-fat, totally vegetarian diet. This study was rather unusual in two respects: first, the 28 individuals suffering from coronary heart disease who formed the intervention group were very highly motivated. Some had at their own insistence been included in the intervention group, even though they had been originally been randomly allocated to the control group. 'This occurred in part because some of these patients did not have the option of coronary artery bypass surgery or angioplasty or assiduously wanted to avoid these invasive procedures' (Billings *et al.* 1996: 236). Second, the intervention was unusually intensive, beginning with a week-long retreat in a local resort hotel to acquaint patient and spouse or partner with the lifestyle-change programme. It apparently continued with group meetings twice a week for which patients and their spouses prepared food at home and brought it along. After dinner, participants gathered in groups with staff members present and spent an hour discussing the group process and specific problems. The dietary changes resulted in some improvements in coronary atherosclerosis in the intervention group. These findings suggest that if patients with atherosclerosis can be sufficiently motivated to adhere to a totally vegetarian low-fat diet and to exercise for three hours per week, their heart condition may improve even without surgery and/or drug treatment. It is more difficult, however, to identify the conditions necessary to achieve this level of motivation.

The effectiveness of cholesterol-lowering interventions

The most important issue from a public health perspective is, however, whether these types of intervention lower the risk of coronary heart disease and, even more importantly, decrease all-cause mortality. By early 1990, approximately 50 randomized clinical trials of cholesterol-lowering regimens by diet, drug, or surgical methods (i.e. ileal bypass; a bypass of the end of the small intestines) had been conducted. A review of several meta-analyses of the outcomes of these trials concluded that despite substantial reductions in cholesterol levels and even coronary mortality, none 'of the seven published meta-analyses reported an overall statistically significant effect of lipid lowering on all-cause mortality' (Furberg 1994: 1307).

None of these meta-analyses included trials of 'statins', a new generation of lipid-lowering drugs which block the endogenous synthesis of cholesterol in the liver to reduce the levels of low-density lipoprotein cholesterol. Recent large clinical primary and secondary prevention trials have shown these statins to be safe, well tolerated and effective. In a primary prevention trial conducted in Scotland, approximately 6000 men who had high plasma cholesterol levels, but no history of myocardial infarction, were randomly assigned to an intervention or a placebo control group (Shepherd *et al.* 1995). Both groups received dietary advice.

When the data were analysed for those who remained in the study for the full 5.5-year period, the statin treatment was found to have lowered plasma levels of cholesterol by 20 per cent, with LDL-cholesterol being lowered by 26 per cent and HDL-cholesterol being increased by 5 per cent. The cholesterol-lowering treatment also resulted in significant reduction in cardiovascular deaths (32 per cent) and in deaths from all causes (22 per cent).

Even more striking findings were reported from a secondary prevention study with more than 4000 patients with angina pectoris or previous myocardial infarction conducted in Scandinavia (Scandinavian Simvastatin Survival Study Group 1994). Again, the cholesterol-lowering drug treatment resulted in a 25 per cent reduction in total cholesterol levels, a 35 per cent reduction in LDLs, and an 8 per cent increase in HDLs. At the end of the 5.5 years clinical trial, coronary mortality in the treatment group was reduced by 30 per cent, and overall mortality by 40 per cent.

These findings indicate that the new cholesterol-lowering drugs (statins) achieve substantial reductions in low-density cholesterol which in turn result in a substantial reduction in mortality from coronary heart disease and from all causes. There is even evidence that these treatments can result in a slight improvement of coronary atherosclerosis (Brown et al. 1993). That these drugs not only reduce coronary mortality, but also all-cause mortality, can be attributed to two factors, namely their increased effectiveness in lowering cholesterol levels and the absence of the kinds of side effects of the early drugs which resulted in increases in non-coronary mortality (Jacobs 1993).

Conclusions

Although social psychologists may find ways to improve the effectiveness of public health interventions, it would be unrealistic at present to expect more than a 1 to 10 per cent reduction in cholesterol levels as a result of normal public health interventions involving dietary education delivered via mass media, at the worksite or in primary care settings. The effectiveness of mass media campaigns will probably be at the lower end of this range, with the effect of primary care settings being somewhat higher. These effects are unlikely to be sufficient when dealing with patients with a history of hypercholesterolemia and coronary heart disease. However, there are other important reasons why dietary education via the mass media (as well as legal measures relating to disclosure of the fat content of food products) are important and likely to have a major public health benefit. First, like all cut-off points, the cut-off point for what constitutes dangerous vs non-dangerous levels of cholesterol is somewhat arbitrary. Therefore, the effects on the cardiovascular system of a low-fat diet should be beneficial for many people, even if their cholesterol levels are not especially high. However, for individuals with very low cholesterol levels (< 160 mg/dl), lowering of cholesterol further might have adverse effects (Jacobs 1993). But then, such individuals are unlikely to eat a high-fat diet anyway. Furthermore, these negative effects might have been side effects of the old generation of cholesterol-lowering drugs (Jacobs 1993). Second, fat-rich diets are also thought to contribute to some forms of cancer. Third, and perhaps most importantly, fat-rich diets are one of the major risk factors for overweight. Persuading people to lower the fat content of their diets might therefore help them to control their weight without needing to restrict their calories. Thus, public health campaigns directed at healthy eating might help to reduce the negative health consequences of both overweight and calorie-restrictive diets.

Salt intake and hypertension

Hypertension (i.e. high blood pressure) is a major risk factor for strokes and coronary heart disease. There may be many causes of hypertension but the one that has most frequently been cited is intake of salt. Thus, the World Health Organization Expert Committee on Prevention of Coronary Heart Disease felt sufficiently confident of the link to advocate a general reduction in the consumption of salt (WHO 1982). These recommendations have been reiterated by other expert panels. For example, the Committee on Diet and Health of the National Research Council in the USA recommended that the total daily intake of salt be limited to six grams or less (Committee on Diet and Health 1989). The same recommendation has been given in the manual of nutrition of the British Ministry of Agriculture, Fisheries and Food (MAFF 1995).

Although a heated debate between proponents and opponents of salt reduction is still ongoing, there is reason to believe that this recommendation may be overstating the case. As Taubes (1998a) recently commented, two conspicuous trends have characterized the salt dispute over the past five years: 'On the one hand, the data are becoming increasingly consistent – suggesting at most a small benefit from salt reduction – while on the other, the interpretations of the data, and the field itself, have remained polarized' (p. 906). The anti-salt lobby continues to maintain its recommendation of a general reduction in daily salt intake.

As observers of these 'salt skirmishes' have noted, the results from the advocates of strict salt restriction and those from authors with more liberal views are fairly similar: salt reduction would decrease blood pressure among normotensive persons by approximately 2 mm Hg, and in the hypertensive patients about 5 mm Hg (e.g. Luft 1997). These findings support researchers who have argued that salt restriction is only beneficial for *some* individuals, namely those who are particularly salt-sensitive, because of a decreased capacity of the kidney to excrete sodium (e.g. Haddy 1991). Thus, the benefits of a reduction in dietary salt intake are likely to be clinically meaningless to individuals with normal blood pressure, even though there may be a public health impact on the population level. In contrast, individuals who suffer from mild hypertension may benefit from a moderate reduction in daily salt intake. It is essentially without side effects, and even if drug therapy is finally required to lower blood pressure, dietary sodium restriction may reduce the effective dose of the drug and thereby also reduce potential side effects (Haddy 1991). However, at the same time, other dietary changes should be recommended which may even be more effective in lowering blood pressure. Thus, a recent randomized controlled study has indicated a diet rich in fruits, vegetables, and low-fat dairy foods and reduced in saturated fats and total fat content lowered systolic blood pressure in both hypertensive (11.4 mm HG) and normotensive (3.5 mm HG) participants, even though it had the same salt content as the control diet (Svetkey *et al.* 1999). This diet has the additional advantage that it is likely to reduce cholesterol levels and thus another factor contributing to high blood pressure in the long term.

EXERCISE

If one were to conduct a survey of beliefs about what people should do to improve their health, regular exercise would probably be mentioned by most respondents. However, such beliefs do not always translate into action. Even in the United States, where health consciousness appears to be much higher than in Europe, only 15 per cent of the adult population exercise regularly and intensively enough in their leisure time to meet current guidelines for fitness (three times a week for at least 20 minutes) and this percentage has changed very little during the last decade (USDHHS 1996b). The percentage is much higher for adolescents but declines strikingly as age or grade in school increases (USDHHS 1996b).

There is strong evidence that regular vigorous dynamic exercise decreases the risk of hypertension, cardiovascular disease, colon cancer, non-insulin dependent diabetes mellitus, and mortality from all causes (USDHHS 1996b). Regular physical activity also appears to relieve symptoms of depression and anxiety and improve mood (USDHHS 1996b). Such *aerobic* or *endurance* exercises, intended to increase oxygen consumption, include jogging, bicycling and swimming. All these are marked by their high intensity, long duration, and need for high endurance. The regimen most effective in developing and maintaining cardiorespiratory fitness is to exercise three to five days a week for 15 to 60 minutes per session at more than 60 per cent of maximum heart rate (American College of Sports Medicine 1979). *Strength* or resistance training (e.g. weight lifting) increases the size and strength of muscles without improving endurance. The importance of resistance training is increasingly being recognized as a means to preserve and enhance muscular strength and to prevent falls and improve mobility in the elderly (USDHHS 1996). However, because most research has been conducted on the health consequences of aerobic exercise, our discussion of exercise in this section will focus nearly exclusively on this type of exercise.

Exercise and physical health

Physical activity is difficult to measure directly. Three types of indirect measures of physical activity have been used: the early studies often relied on occupation to classify people according to the level of physical activity required by their work. More recent studies have used self-report measures of levels of physical activity. A more objectively measured indicator of physical activity is cardiorespiratory fitness, which is measured by aerobic power.

Occupational activity

Some of the pioneering research on the health benefits of vigorous physical activity was conducted by Morris and his colleagues in Great Britain,
who related both vocational and leisure-time physical activity to a reduction in CHD risk (e.g. Morris *et al.* 1953; Morris *et al.* 1980). Paffenbarger
and his colleagues at Stanford continued the work of Morris on the impact
of occupational activity on health (Paffenbarger and Hale 1975; Brand
et al. 1979). In their study, a group of 3975 longshoremen (i.e. wharf
labourers who load and unload cargo) aged 35 to 75 years were followed
for a 22-year period from 1951 to 1973. Their work activity involved a
wide range of energy expenditure which was evaluated by physical measurements taken in actual on-the-job situations and then converted into
energy-output values (kcal/week).

It was found that 11 per cent (395) of the longshoremen died of coronary heart disease during the 22-year period. Men who expended 8500 or
more kcal/week at work (heavy work) had significantly less risk of fatal
heart disease at any age than men whose jobs required less energy. The
relative risk of individuals engaged in moderate and light physical activity
was nearly twice that of workers doing the heavy jobs. There was practically no difference in risk between individuals engaged in moderate or
light physical activity. The negative relationship between physical activity
and coronary mortality remained when other known factors that contribute to coronary heart disease, such as heavy cigarette smoking and high
systolic blood pressure, were controlled for. Similar findings were reported
in other studies relating work activity to mortality from coronary heart
disease (for a review, see Powell *et al.* 1987). While most of these studies
used all-male samples, some studies have replicated these findings for
both sexes (e.g. Brunner *et al.* 1974; Salonen *et al.* 1982).

As the researchers themselves are the first to admit, 'a leap of faith is
required in any non-experimental study when one attempts to draw causal
interpretations from statistical associations' (Brand *et al.* 1979: 60). One
weakness of these kinds of correlational studies is that it is nearly impossible to control for the possibility that symptoms of clinical illness several
years earlier may have led to switches from higher to lower energy output
jobs. Thus workers who became ill while in a high-activity job may have
been switched to one involving lower activity level before their death.
However, this interpretation is rendered less plausible by the fact that
Brand and his colleagues (1979) were able to rule out the possibility that
job changes less than 4.5 years prior to death accounted for the relationship between work activity and coronary health.

Leisure-time activity

It would be very difficult for people who work in sedentary jobs to
achieve, in their leisure time, such a high level of energy expenditure as
the longshoremen in the study described above. Fortunately, much lower
levels of leisure-time energy expenditure appear to be sufficient to achieve a
marked decrease in the risk of coronary heart disease. This was first demonstrated by Morris and his colleagues, who reported that middle-aged male

office workers who kept fit and engaged in vigorous sports during an initial survey in 1968 to 1970 had an incidence of coronary heart disease in the next eight and a half years that was somewhat less than half that of their colleagues who engaged in no vigorous exercise (Morris *et al.* 1980).

These findings were replicated in the USA with a large sample of male graduates of Harvard University (Paffenbarger *et al.* 1978; Paffenbarger *et al.* 1986). In this study 16,936 male alumni who had entered Harvard between 1916 and 1950 returned a questionnaire concerning their physical activities (e.g. walking, stair climbing, sports) either in 1962 or in 1966. A second questionnaire in 1972 identified the non-fatal heart attacks that had occurred in the meantime. Records of fatal heart attacks were obtained for a period of 12 to 16 years.

During the first six to ten years there were 572 first heart attacks. Age-specific rates of coronary heart disease declined consistently with increasing energy expended per week on exercise. Energy expenditure was again aggregated into a composite index of physical activity and expressed in terms of kilocalories per week. Men with an index below 2000 kcal/week were at 64 per cent higher risk than peers with a higher index. Heart attack risk was clearly related to present-day activity rather than activity during student days. Thus, the fact that an alumnus had engaged in competitive sports as student was unrelated to heart attack risk in later life. Furthermore, as Figure 5.1 indicates, the inverse relationship between activity and heart attack risk could be demonstrated even when other risk factors were controlled for. This is very important since risk factors such as body weight or smoking are strongly and negatively related to exercise adherence.

Of the alumni who returned the questionnaire, 1413 died during the 12 to 16 years of follow-up. Exercise was negatively related to mortality. Death rates from coronary heart disease and from all causes declined steadily as energy expenditure increased from less than 500 to 3500 kcal/week. Beyond this point there was only a slight increase in rates. Men who expended less than 2000 kcal/week were at a 31 per cent higher risk of death than more active men.

Physical fitness

In most of the studies reviewed here, some screening was used to exclude individuals who were already suffering from some diagnosed illness. However, the most extensive clinical screening was probably done in a study by Blair *et al.* (1989), in which male and female participants received a preventive medical examination at a clinic at the outset of the study. All individuals who had a personal history of heart attack, hypertension, stroke or diabetes were excluded, as were respondents who had abnormal responses to a resting or exercise electrocardiograph.

Physical fitness, which can be considered an objective indicator of habitual physical exercise, was measured directly by a treadmill exercise test assessing treadmill test endurance. The average follow-up of the participants (10,224 men and 3120 women) was slightly more than eight years. Fitness was negatively related to mortality. This inverse relationship was significant for mortality from all causes and for mortality from coronary heart disease. It remained significant even after statistical adjustment for

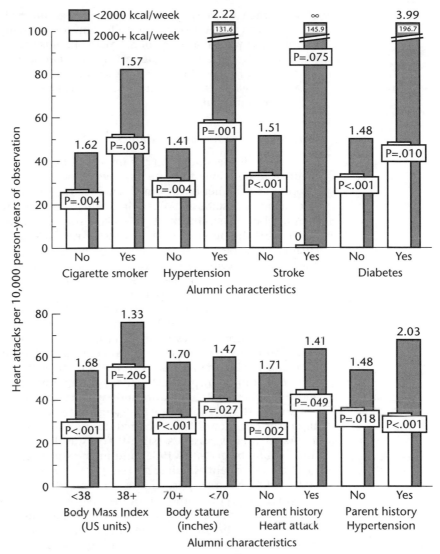

Figure 5.1 Physical activity and first heart attack.
Note: Given here are paired combinations of the physical activity index and other characteristics of Harvard male alumni.
Relative risk is calculated as follows:

$$\frac{\text{rates for alumni with low physical activity index}}{\text{rates for alumni with high physical activity indx}}$$

Source: Paffenbarger *et al.* (1978).

age, smoking habits, cholesterol level, systolic blood pressure, fasting glucose level and parental history of coronary heart disease.

Extended follow-up of this sample provided the opportunity to evaluate the relationship of changes in physical fitness with mortality in a cohort of 9777 men (Blair *et al.* 1995). The average interval between the two examinations was 4.9 years and follow-up for mortality after the second examination was an average of 5.1 years. Results indicated that improvements in fitness were associated with a substantial reductions in mortality risk. Thus, men who were unfit at their initial examination but who became fit by the time of their subsequent examination had a 44 per cent reduction in mortality.

Control of confounding variables

Since none of the studies on the impact of exercise used random assignment of respondents to levels of physical activity, the issue of temporal priority (i.e. whether the assumed cause really preceded the assumed effect) is difficult to establish. When individuals are free to determine their own level of physical activity, it is likely that they choose to become less active with the onset of some disease process. Health screening of participants at the beginning of a study enables exclusion of individuals who already suffer from coronary heart disease or some other serious illness. However, with medical diagnoses being less than perfectly reliable, even careful medical screening could not rule out the possibility that the lowering of activity levels was due to some undiagnosed illness. However, as Powell and associates (1987) argued, if self-selection by illness were an important factor, studies with medical screening before the observation period should show smaller and less consistent associations between activity and health than those without prior screening. In their extensive review of studies on physical activity and coronary heart disease, Powell and colleagues (1987) failed to find evidence for such a difference.

A second strategy to safeguard against self-selection by illness is to omit all deaths or illnesses that occurred during the first two or three years of follow-up after exercise assessment. This was done in the Harvard alumni study (Paffenbarger *et al.* 1986) and in the study relating physical fitness to all-cause mortality (Blair *et al.* 1989). A strong negative relationship still pertained between exercise and death from cardiovascular diseases. Since one would expect the strength of the inverse relationship to weaken considerably over time if individuals with subclinical heart disease were overrepresented in the inactive group, the persistence of a strong relationship makes an interpretation in terms of this type of self-selection less plausible.

There is a second type of self-selection, however, that cannot be controlled by these procedures, namely, self-selection by risk factors. There is evidence that people who are older, of lower socio-economic status, overweight, or smokers are more likely to drop out of voluntary exercise programmes than younger, middle- or upper-class, normal weight, nonsmoking individuals (for a review, see p. 179 below). Since all these variables are also related to increased risk of morbidity and mortality, this type of selection could account for the health difference. However, in many of the studies reported earlier (e.g. Paffenbarger *et al.* 1978, 1986; Blair *et al.* 1989), the health benefit of exercise could be demonstrated even when these risk factors were statistically controlled.

In conclusion, the evidence from these and other studies on the health impact of physical exercise is quite consistent in demonstrating an inverse relationship between physical activity and coronary heart disease. In a meta-analysis of the findings of 27 cohort studies, Berlin and Colditz (1990) found the relative risk of death from coronary heart disease of 1.9 for sedentary occupations as compared with active occupations and of 1.8 for sedentary as compared to strenuous activity in the better quality studies. Similarly, a more recent review in the report of the Surgeon General concluded that the 'numerous estimated measures of association for cardiovascular outcomes presented in this chapter generally fall within the range of 1.5 to 2.0-fold increase in risk of adverse health outcomes associated with inactivity' (USDHHS 1996b: 144).

Even though a controlled intervention study is still needed in this area, the studies described earlier have been very thorough in controlling for all suspected confounding variables. Studies of leisure-time activity suggested that a weekly energy expenditure in excess of 1500 to 2000 kcal is sufficient to reduce the risk of mortality from heart disease. It is left to the reader to judge whether one can, as most writers in this area appear to do, consider a vigorous daily half-hour run or daily walk of an hour to be a moderate level of physical activity that is attainable by most adults. Fortunately for those who are satisfied with less than maximal health benefits, the relationship between activity level and health appears to be monotonic, at least for leisure-time activity. In other words, there is a consistent association between exercise and health benefits: every increase in exercise will benefit our health.

Mediating processes

A number of biological mechanisms have been proposed to explain how physical activity might prevent the development of coronary heart disease (Powell *et al.* 1987). It has been suggested that muscular activity may directly protect the cardiovascular system by stimulating the development of collateral vessels that support the heart muscle. There is evidence from animal studies that physical activity increases the diameter of epicardial coronary arteries (e.g. Kramsch *et al.* 1981) and enhances coronary collateral development (Neil and Oxendine 1979). However, there is no evidence from humans to support this hypothesis (Powell *et al.* 1987).

Exercise could also prevent sudden cardiac death by enhancing myocardial electrical stability. This could be responsible for the lower rate of sudden deaths reported for the more active participants in several studies. There is some evidence that physical training increases cardiac parasympathetic tone in humans (Kenney 1985). Parasympathetic stimulation reduces ventricular fibrillation that can be caused by insufficient blood supply to the heart muscle (Kent *et al.* 1973). There is also evidence from animal studies of a heightened resistance to ventricular fibrillation after exercise training (e.g. Billman *et al.* 1984).

Finally, physical exercise may have beneficial effects on factors that contribute to the development of coronary heart disease, such as overweight, high blood pressure and atherosclerosis. Evidence has shown that exercise has positive effects on weight control (p. 148) and reduces the risk of hypertension. Several randomized controlled trials conducted to determine the effect of exercise on blood pressure indicated that regular exercise lowers both systolic and diastolic blood pressure by 6mm HG (for a review, see USDHHS 1996b). However, since the positive effects of exercise on health have been demonstrated in studies that controlled for weight and hypertension (e.g. Paffenbarger *et al.* 1978), these factors are unlikely to be the major mediators of the exercise–health relationship. Regular exercise may also lower the risk of atherosclerosis. There is evidence that exercise training is associated with an increase in high-density lipoproteins (USDHHS 1996b).

How much exercise is needed for physical health?

The majority of prospective studies which have examined the relationship between physical activity or physical fitness and all-cause mortality or CHD reported strong inverse relationships (Powell *et al.* 1987; Berlin and Colditz 1990). However, because there is no standardized measure of physical activity, it is difficult to derive recommendations from these studies with regard to what type of exercise and how much of it a person should do for maximum health benefit. The nearest approximation to a standardized measure of physical activity are the estimates of average caloric expenditure for the various activity categories studied (e.g. Paffenbarger *et al.* 1978, 1986). Based on studies which reported estimates of 'average daily kilocalories expended', the Report of the Surgeon General (USDHHS 1996b) concludes that 'activities leading to an increase in daily expenditure of approximately 150 kilocalories/day (equivalent to about 1000 kilocalories/ week) is associated with substantial health benefits and that the activity does not need to be vigorous to achieve benefit' (p. 146).

As we saw in Table 4.7 (p. 150), the average adult weighing 70 kg has to walk at a moderate pace for 37 minutes or jog for 18 minutes in order to expend 150 kilocalories. The activity does not have to be vigorous to confer health benefits. For example, there is some evidence to suggest that older adults who walk four hours a week have a significantly lower risk of cardiovascular disease than men and women who walk less than one hour each week (LaCroix *et al.* 1996). Although the relationship between level of physical activity and health benefits appears to be monotonic, indicating that any further increases in activity above the moderate level recommended in the Surgeon General's Report will confer further health benefits, there is some evidence to suggest that health benefits increase more steeply with increasing activity at the low rather than the high end of the activity scale. In other words, increasing from no, or very little, physical activity to light or moderate amounts results in greater health benefits than the same difference between moderate and high activity levels (Dunn and Blair 1997).

Exercise and psychological health

It is widely believed that aerobic exercise has a beneficial effect on mental health. Aerobic fitness programmes such as jogging, dancing or swimming have come to be frequent prescriptions for treating depression. There is indeed empirical evidence from correlational and intervention studies that physical activity relieves symptoms of depression and anxiety and improves mood (McDonald and Hodgdon 1991; USDHHS 1996b; Martinsen and Morgan 1997).

The impact on mood

Mood is usually defined as an individual's feeling at a specific moment and thus reflects a temporary state rather than an enduring trait. From a meta-analytic review of 26 correlational and experimental studies that have been conducted on the impact of exercise on mood, McDonald and Hodgdon (1991) concluded that aerobic fitness training produces positive changes in mood states. However, findings from an experimental study by King *et al.* (1989) which was not included in the meta-analysis suggest that, at least in healthy populations, the immediate impact of regular exercise may be limited to those psychological variables which are closely associated with exercise-induced physical changes, such as satisfaction with shape, appearance and fitness. It is possible, however, that the changes in satisfaction with these aspects may in turn have a significant impact on other psychological variables.

Exercise and depression

Evidence from community studies among men and women indicates that physical activity is associated with substantially reduced symptoms of depression and reduced occurrence of clinical depression (USDHHS 1996b). For example, data from a telephone survey conducted in the state of Illinois indicated that adults who spent more time participating in regular exercise, sports, or other physical activities had fewer symptoms of depression than people reporting no physical activity (Ross and Hayes 1988). Similar results were reported in a community study conducted in the German state of Bavaria (Weyerer 1992). However, this kind of correlational evidence is ambiguous with regard to causality. Although participants may be depressed *because* they are unfit and inactive, other explanations are equally consistent with the evidence. Thus, respondents may also be inactive because they are depressed. There could also be a third factor (e.g. some physical illness) that is responsible for both reduced activity and depression.

Support for the hypothesis that physical activity reduces depressive symptomatology and clinical depression comes from experimental and quasi-experimental intervention studies (for a review, see Martinsen and Morgan 1997). Findings from studies by McCann and Holmes (1984), Martinsen *et al.* (1985) and Doyne *et al.* (1987) illustrate the beneficial effect of aerobic exercise on depressive symptomatology. Participants in the McCann and Holmes study were 43 female students who had scored above the cut-off point for mild depression on the Beck Depression Inventory (BDI), a frequently used self-report measure of depressive symptomatology. These individuals were randomly assigned to either an aerobic exercise treatment condition in which they participated in vigorous exercise for

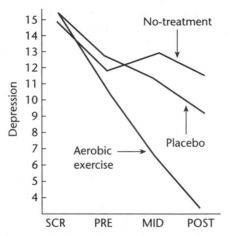

Figure 5.2 Depression and exercise.
Note: Given here are mean screening (SCR), pre-treatment (PRE), mid-treatment (MID) and post-treatment (POST) depression scores for subjects in aerobic exercise, placebo and no-treatment conditions.
Source: McCann and Holmes (1984).

one hour twice a week for 10 weeks, a placebo treatment condition in which they practised relaxation training, or a no-treatment condition. Depressive symptomatology was assessed with a self-report measure (BDI) before, during and after the intervention period. Results indicated that participants in the exercise condition showed a greater decrease in depressive symptomatology than did those in the other two conditions (see Figure 5.2).

The studies of Martinsen and colleagues (1985) and Doyne and colleagues (1987) are interesting because they demonstrate that exercise also helps to reduce depression in individuals who are clinically depressed. Participants in the study of Martinsen and colleagues were male in-patients diagnosed with major depression according to the DSM-III criteria. They were randomly assigned to either aerobic exercise or control groups. The aerobic exercise group engaged in jogging or brisk walking for one hour three times a week for six to nine weeks. The control group took part in occupational therapy without any physical exercise. Patients in both groups also received some psychotherapy. The exercise group experienced a significantly greater decrease in depression (measured with the BDI) than the control group.

These findings were replicated by Doyne *et al.* (1987) in a study of 40 women, who had been screened for major or minor depressive disorder. These women were randomly assigned to an eight-week running, weight lifting or waiting control condition. Participants were also assessed before, during and after the treatment by various self-rating scales of depression, which included the BDI. Results indicated statistically and clinically significant decreases in depression in both the exercise groups relative to the waiting list control group. These improvements were remarkably consistent across the different measures and were reasonably well maintained through the one-year follow-up.

Finally, there is suggestive evidence that exercise may even protect individuals against developing depression. A prospective study of 10,201 Harvard male alumni found an inverse relationship between the level of physical activity assessed in 1961 or 1966 and the incidence of depression during the following 23 to 27 years (Paffenbarger 1994). Respondents were asked in 1988 whether any health problems had ever been diagnosed by a physician and to indicate the year of onset. They were given a list which included depression among other health problems (e.g. CHD, emphysema). Incidence of depression was determined by an attack first experienced during the follow-up period. Results indicated an inverse relationship between physical activity reported at intake and the incidence of depression during the follow-up period. The relative risk of depression was 27 per cent lower for men who had reported playing three or more hours of sports each week than for men who had reported playing no sports.

Thus there is consistent evidence that physical exercise reduces depressive symptoms in individuals who suffer from clinical depression. There is less agreement regarding the influence of vigorous exercise on depression in non-clinical groups. Vigorous exercise appears to be helpful for individuals who have elevated depression scores on standardized scales such as the BDI (e.g. McCann and Holmes 1984), but antidepressant effects have rarely been demonstrated in individuals whose scores are within the normal range on depression (Martinsen and Morgan 1997). Finally, there is some indication that engaging in regular exercise may even protect individuals against developing depression.

Mediating processes

A number of physiological and psychosocial mechanisms have been suggested to account for the impact of exercise on depression (for a review, see Morgan 1997). It has been suggested that aerobic exercise may facilitate the production of brain norepinephrine. Low norepinephrine levels in the central nervous system have been suspected as a cause of some depressions. Another hypothesis is that improved mood states following exercise are stimulated by the release of endorphins, which are opium-like substances produced by the body.

At the more psychological level it has been argued that exercise may reduce anxiety and depression because it distracts individuals and prevents them from focusing on their problems (Bahrke and Morgan 1978). Although this could account for some immediate effects of exercise on anxiety and mood, it is difficult to see how it could explain long-term effects.

A better explanation of such long-term effects is the assumption that exercise may increase individual feelings of self-efficacy. The fact that one is regularly exercising or participating in an exercise group may increase one's feeling of being disciplined, effective and competent. Some of the positive effects of exercise may also stem from factors associated with exercise, such as social activity and a feeling of involvement with others.

Thus, for example, bicycling with friends, swimming with a companion, or running with others may improve mood because of the companionship provided.

Exercise and healthy aging

Exercise can play an important role in slowing down the decline in physical fitness associated with advancing age, in preventing disability and in helping the elderly to preserve their independence (for reviews, see Buchner et al. 1992; Wagner et al. 1992). Aging is characterized by a diffuse loss of physiologic capacity and reserve. The older we become, the less physically fit we become. This decline in physical fitness with advancing age does not develop suddenly at age 65, but begins at middle age and progresses steadily thereafter. Data from cross-sectional studies suggest that between the ages of 30 and 80, we lose approximately 50 per cent of aerobic capacity (i.e. the ability of the body to produce energy by using oxygen) and between 30 and 40 per cent in the strength of back, leg and arm muscles (Buchner et al. 1992). For many years, it was generally accepted that such decline was genetically programmed and, as a result, inevitable.

Replicating a development which took place in the study of aging and intelligence more than a decade earlier (e.g. Baltes and Schaie 1976), researchers have recently noted that the effect of age on physical fitness appears to differ widely between individuals. Whereas some older individuals show substantial physical decline, for others the decline with age is minimal. This suggests that the steep mean decline in physical fitness which appeared to be 'normal' or 'usual' consequences of aging may not be inevitable. Rowe and Kahn (1987, 1997) coined the term 'successful aging' to refer to this type of preservation of function. Successful aging is characterized by three components, namely low probability of disease and disease-related disability, high cognitive and physical functional capacity, and active engagement with life. Successful aging is thus more than the absence of disease, and more than the maintenance of functional capacities. It is their combination with active engagement with life that reflects successful aging most fully.

Evidence from epidemiological studies strongly supports a role of regular physical activity in successful aging by preserving muscle performance, promoting mobility, and reducing fall risk. Several large-scale longitudinal studies observed that for men and women (aged 65 and older) who were functionally intact (e.g. were able to climb stairs and walk half a mile) at baselines measurement, inactivity was associated with a markedly increased risk of losing mobility during the following few years (Wagner et al. 1992). Intervention studies have also demonstrated that aerobic and strength exercise can improve aerobic capacity and muscle strength in older adults (Buchner et al. 1992). Although somewhat less conclusive, the evidence is also supportive of the effectiveness of exercise regimens in improving gait and balance, which are both risk factors for injurious falls in the elderly (Buchner et al. 1992).

The preservation of physical fitness alone would not enable elderly individuals to 'actively engage with life', unless their cognitive functional capacity was also maintained at a high level. There is evidence from non-intervention studies that physically active seniors have better cognitive functions than inactive ones (Wagner *et al.* 1992). Further support comes from a longitudinal study conducted by the MacArthur Foundation Research Network on Successful Aging (Albert *et al.* 1995). This study, which followed a sample of more than a thousand high-functioning elderly (70 to 79) for a two-year period, identified 'strenuous activity in and around the house' as one of four predictors of maintenance of cognitive functions over a two-year interval. In contrast, the evidence from intervention studies, which would be less ambiguous with regard to causal interpretations, is inconsistent. But most of these programmes have been of short duration, and small sample sizes have limited their statistical power (Buchner *et al.* 1992; Wagner *et al.* 1992). Furthermore, there are other ways to slow down or even reverse the age-related decline in cognitive functions. Evidence is accumulating for the effectiveness of cognitive training in enhancing cognitive abilities in old age (e.g. Schaie and Willis 1986).

The determinants of regular exercise

Who are the people who keep fit, and how can we persuade those who do not do so to engage in regular exercise? Unfortunately, from a perspective of health education, many of the variables which have been found to be related to exercise participation and adherence, such as age, education, smoking and proximity to the exercise facility are difficult or impossible to influence (Dishman 1982; Sonstroem 1988). Even self-motivation, which has been found to be significantly related to adherence in several studies (Dishman and Gettman 1980; Dishman *et al.* 1980; Dishman and Ickes 1981; Olson and Zanna 1982), appears to be a fairly stable personality disposition. Self-motivation is conceptualized as a behavioural tendency to persevere independent of situational reinforcements and is measured by a paper-and-pencil test.

Among the *physical variables*, body fat and body weight appear to be major determinants of adherence to exercise programmes. Thus, in one prospective study, Dishman and Gettman (1980) found that body fat, body weight, and self-motivation (which were determined at the beginning of the study) predicted 45 per cent of the variance in adherence in a sample that consisted of 21 male cardiac patients and 45 healthy male individuals. More than half of this variance (24 per cent) was accounted for by percentage of body fat.

Research on the *attitudes* which characterize participants in exercise programmes has often relied on rather global measures of attitudes towards physical activity and sports such as the Physical Estimation and Attraction Scales (Sonstroem 1978; Sonstroem and Kampper 1980). These global measures have been only moderately successful as predictors of recruitment into exercise programmes (for reviews, see Dishman 1982; Sonstroem 1988). This is not surprising, because global attitudes are notoriously poor predictors of specific behaviour (see Chapter 2).

According to the compatibility principle discussed earlier (p. 16), the best predictor of the performance of specific exercises should be the individual's attitude and intention towards performing this exercise. Riddle (1980) collected data on attitudes and behavioural intentions towards regular jogging from several hundred joggers and non-exercisers using a mail questionnaire that was based on the theory of reasoned action (Fishbein and Ajzen 1975). In support of this model, the intention to jog was successfully predicted from the attitudinal and normative components of the model, and the correlation between intention and behaviour was high. Riddle (1980) also found a number of meaningful differences between the beliefs of joggers and non-exercisers. Non-exercisers thought jogging would require too much discipline, take too much time, and make them too tired. Joggers were more likely than non-exercisers to believe that regular jogging would have positive effects, and they also evaluated being in good physical and mental condition more positively. Non-exercisers also indicated that it was unlikely that important reference persons (particularly their physicians) thought that they should jog regularly.

That intention to exercise is in turn closely related to the position an individual holds on the stages of change continuum (Prochaska *et al.* 1992) has been demonstrated with a sample of elderly individuals. These respondents completed to a questionnaire which assessed not only the components of the model of planned behaviour but also the position of these individuals on the continuum of stages of readiness ranging from precontemplation through contemplation, preparation, action to maintenance (Courneya 1995). Analyses showed a close association between the particular stage of a given individual and his or her attitude ($r = .56$), subjective norm ($r = .47$), perceived behavioural control ($r = .55$), and intention to exercise ($r = .75$). Overall, the components of the model of planned behaviour accounted for 63 per cent of the variance in stages of change.

The theories of reasoned action and planned behaviour are also quite successful in predicting actual *exercise behaviour*. In a prospective study of exercise behaviour, Kimiecik (1992) analysed the data of 332 male and female corporate employees who had responded to two questionnaires sent one month apart. The first questionnaire assessed the theoretical predictors (attitudes, subjective norms, perceived control, intention formulated with regard to physical exercise) and the second measured exercise behaviour. When attitude and subjective norm were entered into the regression in a first step to predict intention, only attitude made a significant contribution ($R^2 = .59$). Consistent with the theory of planned behaviour, the addition of perceived control significantly improved the prediction of intentions from .59 to .66.

Exercise intention accounted for 46 per cent of the variance in (self-reported) exercise behaviour. The addition of perceived control to intention increased the variance in behaviour accounted for by a further 3 per cent, to 49 per cent. The addition of the interaction between intention and perceived control raised the variance to 54 per cent. Thus more than half of the variance in exercise behaviour one month after the assessment of the predictors could be accounted for on the basis of the individuals' intentions to engage in physical exercise and their perception of control over their exercise behaviour. The significant intention–control interaction indicates that the association between intention and behaviour is stronger when individuals perceive their control over the behaviour to be high rather than low.

According to the theories of reasoned action and planned behaviour, *continued participation* in exercise programmes (i.e. adherence) should be predicted from attitudes toward continued participation in a programme of physical activity, rather than from attitudes toward the specific physical activity. Since only individuals with positive attitudes towards physical activity are likely to be recruited into the group of exercisers, programme adherence should only be weakly related to general attitudes towards physical exercise. In line with this argument, global measures of attitudes towards physical activity have typically been unsuccessful in predicting adherence, even in cases where they were reasonable predictors of recruitment into the exercise programme (e.g. Sonstroem and Kampper 1980).

In contrast, studies that assessed attitudes and behavioural intentions towards continued programme participation have been fairly successful in predicting programme adherence (e.g. Jonas *et al.* 1993; Theodorakis 1994). For example, in a prospective study of a sample of more than 100 men and women who had registered for university fitness courses at the University of Tübingen (Germany) for a four-month exercise programme, Jonas and colleagues predicted intention to participate ($R^2 = .45$) during the second half of the semester on the basis of attitudes towards participation and perceived control (but not subjective norm). Whereas intention accounted for 25 per cent of the variance of actual participation, perceived control did not make a significant contribution to the prediction of behaviour.

Similar findings were reported by Theodorakis (1994) in a prospective study with a sample of 395 females who participated in physical fitness programmes in fitness clubs in a large city in Northern Greece. Attitude and perceived control accounted for 35 per cent of the variance in intention. Both intention and perceived control made a significant contribution to the prediction of behaviour ($R^2 = .37$). Thus, the model of reasoned action and its extension, the model planned behaviour, do quite well in accounting for both exercise behaviour in general and regular attendance in exercise programmes.

What conclusions can we draw about how to persuade people to exercise and how to increase adherence to exercise programmes? Researchers in this area seem to agree that people join exercise programmes to obtain some health-related benefits (e.g. improvement in cardiovascular fitness, weight loss), but that they stay because the programme is convenient and enjoyable, which suggests a two-step procedure. Since convenience is likely to be a predictor of involvement as well as adherence, mass media campaigns should not only emphasize the health-related benefits of specific exercise, but should also point out that it takes less effort to stay healthy than most people might anticipate. Furthermore, whereas it is difficult to persuade people to join a health club or even to take a daily half-hour walk, it may be much easier to persuade them to rearrange their daily lives and become more physically active.

That individuals can be persuaded to change minor routines has been demonstrated by Brownell *et al.* (1980). These authors observed that only 6 per cent of the people in shopping malls, railway stations and bus stations tended to use stairs rather than elevators. When a simple sign pointing out the benefits of exercise was placed at the bottom of the stairs and escalators, stair use was nearly tripled. Similarly, one might be able to persuade people to walk to work instead of driving or, at least, to park their cars further away from the place of work. Who knows? People who enjoy these small activities and who have become more physically fit as a result may even decide to take up jogging or join an exercise class.

Research on interventions to promote physical activity

Interventions designed to promote physical activity have not been very effective. Thus, the review of studies of the impact of individual-level interventions in the Surgeon General's Report concluded that 'behavioural management approaches have been employed with mixed results. Where an effect has been demonstrated, it has often been small. Evidence of the effectiveness of techniques like self-monitoring, frequent follow-up telephone calls, and incentives appear to be generally positive over the short run, but not over long intervals. Evidence on the relative effectiveness of interventions on adherence to moderate or vigorous activity is limited and unclear' (USDHHS 1996b: 226).

Community-wide interventions have been similarly unsuccessful. Of the three community interventions which included a component that promoted physical exercise, the Minnesota Heart Health Program (Luepker et al. 1994), the Pawtucket Heart Health Program (Carleton et al. 1995) and the Stanford Five-City Project (Farquhar et al. 1990), only one, namely the Minnesota Heart Health Program (MHHP), had a significant, albeit small, effect on levels of physical activity. The MHHP advocated regular physical activity as part of its effort to reduce risk factors for coronary heart disease. Three intervention communities received a five- to six-year programme designed to reduce smoking, influence diet and increase physical activity levels. Mass media were used to educate the public about the relationship between regular physical exercise and reduced risk for CHD, and health professionals promoted physical activity through their local organizations. Three other communities which received no intervention served as comparison sites. Leisure-time physical activity was assessed as the percentage of participants who described themselves as regularly active. Cross-sectional comparisons between intervention and control communities indicated small but significant increases in levels of physical activity in the intervention communities during the first three years. This effect was no longer significant after the third year when activity levels increased also in the control communities. The Surgeon General's Report therefore rightly concludes that the 'result of community-based interventions to increase physical activity have been generally disappointing' (USDHHS 1996b).

School-based interventions have been somewhat more effective. This is important because schools offer an almost population-wide setting for promoting physical activity to young people, primarily through classroom curricula for physical education and health education. One of the most extensive controlled school-based interventions has been the Child and

Adolescent Trial for Cardiovascular Health (CATCH), a controlled intervention trial in elementary schools described earlier (Luepker *et al.* 1996). Outcomes were assessed at pre-test before randomization (fall 1991) and at follow-up (spring 1994). A major component of CATCH was an innovative health-related physical education intervention. For two and a half years, the intervention schools received a standardized physical education intervention, including new curriculum and staff development training. In these intervention schools, daily moderate-to-vigorous activity during physical education classes in which students reported breathing hard was significantly higher in the intervention (58.6 minutes) than the comparison schools (46.5 minutes). However, total minutes of reported physical activity did not differ significantly between intervention and control schools. The unique aspect of this study is that the findings based on self-report measures were backed up by observational data collected by trained observers during physical education.

Significant intervention effects were also reported by the Class of 1989 Study, which was part of the MHHP community study (Kelder *et al.* 1993). The first physical activity intervention took place in the schools of the intervention communities in 8th grade. It consisted of a peer-led physical activity programme. It took place in classes other than physical education and encouraged regular aerobic physical activity though a four-week community-wide competition. Students in intervention communities were challenged to make a special effort to exercise outside school. A second physical activity intervention was implemented in 10th grade. The programme's assessment included annual measurements in intervention and comparison communities collected from a large number of students (baseline 2376 students) for seven years, beginning in sixth grade (1983). The measures of physical activity included self-reported hours of exercise per week out of class and a physical activity score. The physical activity score was created out of two variables which assessed the frequency and intensity of regular physical activity. Physical activity rates throughout the follow-up period were substantially higher in the intervention than the control communities. In the 12th grade, females reported 48 minutes more exercise in the intervention than the comparison communities. For males, a similar intervention trend was observed, even though the differences did not reach acceptable levels of significance. The fact that males and females maintained higher levels of activity throughout most of the follow-up period may lead to higher levels of activity as adults.

As this review has shown, the effects of the individual, community-based or school-based interventions to increase physical activity levels have not been impressive. Although it is difficult to infer from the brief descriptions of the interventions given in many of these reports, one of the reasons for their moderate impact could have been their reliance on health education and health appeals. If one wants to persuade people to change health-impairing behaviour patterns and to adopt healthy behaviour, one has to analyse the belief structure underlying each of these lifestyles. The a priori assumption implicit in the design of many health promotion campaigns that people engage in health-impairing behaviour patterns out of ignorance of negative health consequences is often wrong. Although some people may engage in health-impairing behaviour patterns out of ignorance, more often there are other reasons. In order for a campaign to be effective, these other reasons need to be identified and persuasive arguments developed to focus on these reasons.

THE PRIMARY PREVENTION OF AIDS

By June 1995 more than a million cases of AIDS (Acquired Immune Deficiency Syndrome) had been reported to the World Health Organization (WHO). This is only the tip of the iceberg. According to an estimate by WHO, 18.5 million adults and 1.5 million children were infected with the virus which causes AIDS in 1995 (Adler *et al.* 1997). There is presently neither a vaccine nor a cure. Even though the new combination retroviral therapy is effective in suppressing the infection and delaying the development of the illness (Kelly *et al.* 1998), the only means by which people can escape the infection is by avoiding behaviours that are essential to the transmission of the AIDS virus. Thus, programmes aimed at changing behaviour are still the only strategy to stop the AIDS epidemic.

The cause of AIDS

AIDS is caused by a human immunodeficiency virus (HIV) which attacks the immune system. The immune system reacts with the formation of antibodies. Although these antibodies do not play a protective role as they do in more familiar virus infections, they can be used as indicators of the presence of the virus. These antibodies can be detected in the blood serum by simple tests, two weeks to three months after the infection. Individuals who have developed antibodies are said to be seropositive. But even before the development of antibodies, the individual can be infectious to others through sexual intercourse or blood donations. More recently, it has been discovered that a second human immunodeficiency virus exists (HIV-2) which is mainly restricted to parts of West Africa (Adler *et al.* 1997). Although this virus has also been known to induce AIDS in some cases, it appears to do so more slowly than the original virus (HIV-1). When referring to HIV in this book, I will be referring to the HIV-1 virus, which accounts for most of the HIV infections worldwide.

The period between contracting the virus and developing symptoms of AIDS was highly variable even before the introduction of the new drug treatments. Some individuals develop the symptoms within one to two years while others remain free of symptoms some 15 years later. Approximately 50 per cent of infected individuals develop AIDS by 12 years after the infection (Adler *et al.* 1997). There is evidence to suggest the recent generation of combination anti-retroviral drugs will considerably extend the time between HIV infection and the onset of AIDS (Kelly *et al.* 1998).

Infection with HIV damages the immune system by infecting and killing one type of white blood cell, the T-helper cell. The T-helper cells serve an important function in the regulation of the immune system. They stimulate other cells to mount an attack on invading germs. By infecting and ultimately killing the T-helper cells, the HIV stops the process of responding to invading germs at the beginning and thus severely reduces a person's ability to fight other diseases. Without a functioning immune system to ward off other germs, the individual is vulnerable to becoming infected by germs (bacteria, protozoa, fungi, other viruses) and malignancies, which would ordinarily not have been able to gain a foothold. Usually AIDS is diagnosed through the presence of unusual opportunistic infections (i.e. infections that use the opportunity of lowered resistance) or unusual forms of cancer (e.g. Kaposi's sarcoma, a cancer of the skin and connective tissues). The AIDS virus also appears to attack the nervous system, causing damage to the brain.

Modes of transmission

The virus is transmitted by the exchange of cell-containing bodily fluids. For transmission to occur, these bodily fluids must contain a sufficient concentration of the virus. Only three bodily fluids pose an infection risk, namely blood, semen and vaginal secretions. Other bodily fluids such as saliva, urine and faeces (in the absence of blood) do not contain sufficient concentrations of the virus to pose a risk of infection (Kalichman 1998).

One common route of HIV transmission is sexual intercourse. Anal intercourse is a high-risk activity for both partners, but the risk of infection is greater for the receptive than the insertive partner. The risk of HIV infection through vaginal intercourse is lower than through anal intercourse, because there is less likelihood of lesions. As with anal intercourse, both partners run the risk of infection but the risk is two to four times higher for the receptive (female) partner (Kalichman 1998). Although oral–genital sex is also a biologically plausible route of transmission, the amounts of virus in the saliva are so small that there appears to be little risk of infection. However, there may be some risk in involved in oral–penile sex when ejaculation occurs into the mouth. Exposure of semen to the oral cavity has been reported to be the sole risk factor in a number of cases (Kalichman 1998).

Among injection drug users, the risk of infection is not caused by the drug use *per se*, but by the sharing of injection equipment. The HIV is carried in contaminated blood left in the needle or syringe and the virus is injected into the new victim when dirty syringes or needles are reused. In general, the risk of contracting AIDS through contact with infected blood is very high. Thus, blood transfusions from infected donors carry an extremely high risk of infection (Friedland and Klein 1987).

There is no evidence that HIV can be transmitted through casual contact. It does not seem to enter the body across skin that is intact, and thus is not transmitted by touching, hand shaking, sharing eating utensils, sneezing or living in the same household (Curran *et al.* 1988). Thus, in studies of households where one person was HIV infected, none of over 400 family members was infected except for sex partners or children born to infected mothers (Curran *et al.* 1988).

The epidemiology

The first report of AIDS in the United States involved fewer than a dozen men in summer 1981. By mid-1995, the number of cases reported world-wide to WHO had risen to 1,169,811, with the majority coming from Africa. In the WHO European region 218,938 cases of AIDS had been reported by the end of 1998, of whom 131,976 had died (European Centre for the Epidemiological Monitoring of AIDS 1998). In the USA the number of AIDS cases had already accumulated to 441,000 by the end of 1994 and over 270,000 people had died (Holtgrave *et al.* 1996). In 1993, HIV infection had become the leading cause of death for individuals between 25 and 40 in the United States (Holtgrave *et al.* 1996). Due to the long incubation period between infection and the development of symptoms, the num-ber of AIDS cases represents only a small proportion of the individuals infected with HIV.

The degree of risk of infection for a given group of individuals is deter-mined by three factors, namely the frequency of behaviours that allow viral transmission, the risk of infection attached to these behaviours (i.e. the likelihood that a given interaction between individuals differing in serostatus results in infection), and the prevalence of HIV in the popula-tion (or the particular subpopulation with whom the individual engages in the risk behaviour). In the USA sexual intercourse between men has been the most likely source of infection. Thus of the persons with HIV living in the States, 50 per cent are gay and bisexual men, about 25–30 per cent are injection drug users, and about 20 per cent are non-injection drug-using women (Karon *et al.* 1996). This is true for most Northern parts of Europe as well, but there is a North–South differential. Whereas in Northern countries such as Germany, Great Britain or the Netherlands, sex between men is the most likely source of infection, injection drug use is the more important route of transmission in most countries of South-ern Europe. To give an example, in 1998 in Great Britain (population: 51.22 million) 68.4 per cent (10,740 cases) of the cases of AIDS occurred among homosexual men and only 6.5 per cent (1024 cases) among injec-tion drug users. In Italy, a country with a similar population (57.25 mil-lion), the distribution over the two groups is just the reverse: only 13.9 per cent (5962 cases) of the AIDS cases occurred among homosexual men and 61.7 per cent (26,400 cases) involved drug users. In central Africa, HIV transmission is linked to reuse of scarce needles, and lack of infection-control procedures in hospitals and clinics. It is also clearly related to heterosexual rather than homosexual intercourse (Batchelor 1988). Thus, in many African countries the rate of AIDS is roughly equal for both sexes.

Among homosexual men, adolescents are at highest risk because they practise high levels of sexual risk taking (de Wit 1996). For example, in a sample of young homosexual men aged between 18 and 29 years re-cruited into the San Francisco Young Men's Health Study in 1992 to 1993, an HIV prevalence of nearly 18 per cent was found. Twenty-seven per cent of these men had engaged in unprotected anal sex in the year prior to participation (Osmond *et al.* 1994). In a more recent survey of more than 2100 young homosexual men between 15 and 22 in six urban coun-ties across the USA, median HIV prevalence was found to be 7 per cent

(Valleroy *et al.* 1996). Finally, in a cohort study of young men in Amsterdam initiated in 1995, the prevalence of HIV in a sample of 429 young men with an average age of 25 was 5.1 per cent. Of these young men, 38 per cent reported having had unprotected anal sex in the previous six months (van Griensven *et al.* 1999).

However, even in countries where homosexual men constitute the highest risk group, the proportion of women among AIDS cases is rising rapidly. According to a report by Zierler and Krieger (1997), the proportion of AIDS cases in the USA who are women increased from 6 per cent in 1984 to 19 per cent in 1995, with a cumulative number of AIDS cases among women of 71,724. The proportion of AIDS cases in women attributed to heterosexual transmission has also increased steadily, from 15 per cent in 1983 to 38 per cent in 1995. In 1994, HIV infection replaced heart disease as the third leading cause of death in women aged 24–44 in the USA, following cancer and accidents. Similar trends can be observed in Great Britain (Adler *et al.* 1997). There the number of AIDS cases reported for women has also been steadily increasing, even though the absolute number has remained relatively small. More than half the AIDS cases and HIV infections in women were attributed to heterosexual intercourse. Heterosexual transmission of HIV infections also shows a strong proportional increase in many other European countries. It has even become the predominant mode of infection in countries such as France, Sweden and Norway (European Centre for the Epidemiological Monitoring of AIDS 1998).

Prior to the institution of protective measures to make the blood supply secure, haemophiliacs and other blood recipients could contract AIDS through blood transfusions. It has been estimated that 12,000 persons in the USA were infected with HIV through transfusions before screening of donated blood and plasma for antibodies to HIV begun in 1985 (Friedland and Klein 1987). By that time, 70 to 80 per cent of persons with haemophilia had already been infected with HIV (Friedland and Klein 1987).

Methods of safe(r) sex

Abstention from penetrative sex

Sex is considered totally safe only if there is no risk of the partners being exposed to HIV, that is if sex partners do not engage in any activities which result, or can result, in an exchange of blood, semen, or vaginal secretions. Because condoms sometimes fail, penetrative sex cannot be considered totally safe, even when condoms are being used. Only non-penetrative sexual behaviours such as hugging, holding, kissing or massaging qualify as totally safe sex practices (Kalichman 1998). Because individuals often find it difficult to abstain from penetration once they begin a sexual encounter, safe sex is not a very viable goal for prevention interventions. Most interventions therefore aim at persuading individuals to engage in sex which is safer rather than safe. Safer sex is defined by activities which substantially reduce, but do not totally eliminate, the risk of infection (Kalichman 1998).

Condom use

Condom use is the most common way to practise safer sex. The use of latex condoms substantially reduces the risk of HIV infection. This has been demonstrated in research with heterosexual couples in which one partner is HIV infected and the other is not (for a review, see Kalichman 1998). For example, in a prospective study of HIV-seronegative women who were in a stable monogamous relationship with a seropositive man, Saracco and colleagues (1993) found that 2 per cent of the spouses of men who consistently used condoms during sexual intercourse contracted AIDS, as compared to 15 per cent of the partners of men who used condoms inconsistently. Similarly, gay men who used condoms only some of the time were six times more likely to become infected with HIV than those who used condoms all the time (Detels *et al.* 1989).

Condoms can slip or break and this is more likely during anal than vaginal intercourse (Kalichman 1998). In a survey of homosexual men from the Amsterdam Cohort Study who used condoms regularly, condoms were reported to have slid off or become torn during anogenital sex in 3.7 per cent of the cases. However, the magnitude of the failure rate depended on the type of lubricant used by these men. Condoms used with water-based lubricants failed less frequently (1.7 per cent) than condoms used with no lubricants (5.9 per cent) or with oil-based lubricants (10.3 per cent) (de Wit *et al.* 1993).

Not all condoms are made of latex. Some condoms are made of natural membranes, most commonly lambs' intestines. Although these condoms are durable, effective against unwanted pregnancies, and increase the sensation of sexual stimulation during intercourse, they also have larger pores. Because viruses are much smaller than sperms, these condoms offer little protection against HIV (Kalichman 1998). Another option, namely condoms made from polyurethane, appears to offer a safe alternative to latex condoms (Kalichman 1998).

Negotiated safety

If both sexual partners are seronegative, there is no risk of exposure to HIV, even during unprotected penetrative sex. Therefore, unprotected sex within a monogamous relationship where both partners have had their serostatus tested and found that they are seronegative is safe, if the relationship is truly monogamous. The concept of 'negotiated safety' has been suggested by Kippax and colleagues (1993) to refer to agreements between partners to abstain from unprotected sex outside their relationship.

Obviously, the safety of negotiated safety depends on the extent to which both partners keep to their agreements. In the Australian sample of homosexual men studied by Kippax and colleagues (1997), nine of the 181 seronegative men in seroconcordant steady relationships reported unprotected anal intercourse with a casual partner even though they had an agreement with their steady partner not to have unsafe sex outside their relationship. Data collected in the Amsterdam cohort study of homosexual men indicated that of 47 seronegative men with a concordant partner who engaged in unprotected sex within their steady partner, 8 violated a safe sex agreement and engaged in unprotected sex with casual partners (de Vroome *et al.* in press). This type of evidence suggests that negotiated safety substantially reduces but does not totally exclude the infection risk.

Psychosocial determinants of sexual risk behaviour

Because abstention from penetrative sex is a rather unattractive option for most sexually active individuals, research on the factors assumed to influence strategies of AIDS risk reduction has mainly focused on psychosocial determinants of condom use for heterosexual individuals (e.g. Sheeran *et al.* 1999) and homosexual men (e.g. de Wit *et al.* in press).

Condom use among heterosexuals

A recent meta-analysis of factors influencing heterosexual condom use, based on 121 empirical studies, reported strong support for the theories of reasoned action and planned behaviour (Sheeran *et al.* 1999). The three variables specified by the theory of reasoned action, namely attitudes towards condom use, social norms regarding condom use, and intentions to use condoms, were strongly related to condom use in both longitudinal and cross-sectional analyses. The average correlation for perceived behavioural control over condom use approached medium size and thus supported the assumption underlying the model of planned behaviour that the addition of measures of perceived behavioural control is likely to increase substantially the prediction of behaviour which is not totally under the control of an individual. However, in a study of the determinants of condom use intentions among a national sample of 946 young people in England, Sutton and colleagues (1999) failed to find a significant effect of perceived behavioural control while reporting a substantial influence of attitudes and subjective norms. A reason for the lack of impact of perceived behavioural control on intentions to use condoms may have been the fact that, regardless of the extent of their sexual experience, all these individuals believed that they had high control over condom use.

The health belief model fared less well than the theories of reasoned action and planned behaviour in the meta-analysis of Sheeran and colleagues (1999). According to the health belief model, condom use should be determined by the perceived threat of an HIV infection (i.e. severity x vulnerability) and the perceived costs and benefits of condom use. Surprisingly, perceived threat appears to play a rather minor role in motivating precautionary behaviour. Thus, the association between perceived severity of an HIV infection and condom use did not reach acceptable levels of significance. Because AIDS is generally regarded as a deadly disease, this could be a 'ceiling effect'. However, no 'ceiling effect' occurred for the measures of vulnerability. And yet, perceived vulnerability also showed very low correlations with condom use in this meta-analysis. An even weaker and non-significant association between vulnerability and condom use was reported in a meta-analysis of samples of heterosexuals and gay men by Gerrard and colleagues (1996).

I can only suggest two potential explanations for these puzzling findings. One reason for the weak association between measures of perceived susceptibility and protective behaviour could be that most people believe that they are not at risk of HIV infection through sexual contact (Sheeran *et al.* 1999). Although this perception may not be unrealistic for some groups at this point in time, it could also be a reflection of a denial process for others. The latter assumption is supported by the findings of another meta-analysis of sexual risk behaviour. Gerrard and her colleagues (1996) reported that even though perceptions of vulnerability were related to past risk and precautionary behaviours, this association was much stronger for low-than for high-risk groups. A second factor which might have reduced the relationship between perceived vulnerability and precautionary behaviour could be that the threat of HIV has now been known for many years and individuals who were willing and able to adopt precautionary behaviour have already done so.

This latter explanation may also account for the failure of HIV/AIDS knowledge to influence condom use. This failure should not be misinterpreted as an indication that information about this type of health risk is unimportant. Health education has to be continued to maintain this level of knowledge, especially among adolescents who are particularly at risk. But by now very few adult homosexual men are unaware of the health risks involved in unprotected anal intercourse. Thus the people who still engage in this high-risk activity do so knowing that it is dangerous.

Measures of the other determinants of behaviour of the health belief model, namely perceived benefits of, and barriers to, condom use fared marginally better. Perceived benefits such as the efficacy of condom use, the belief that condoms are attractive to use and do not interfere with sexual pleasure, and perceived barriers such as embarrassment when buying condoms were weakly but significantly related to condom use. It is interesting to note that beliefs related to condom attractiveness (e.g. make sex less spontaneous, make sex less enjoyable, reduce partner's sexual pleasure) also showed the highest correlation with the intention to use condoms in the young sample studied by Sutton and colleagues (1999).

Two variables which do not form part of any of these theoretical models have also demonstrated a strong association with condom use (Sheeran *et al.* 1999). This is interesting, because they are likely to be amenable to modification through interventions. One of these variables was 'carrying a condom' or 'condom availability'. The close association of this variable with condom use is hardly surprising since condom availability is one of the preconditions for condom use. Furthermore, carrying a condom is likely to reflect a strong intention to use condoms. Nevertheless, this finding is important in view of the fact that few interventions have focused on this type of preparatory behaviour.

The other variable which showed a strong association with condom use was communication about condom use. Whereas talking about the risk of contracting AIDS had only a small positive association with condom use, discussions with the partner about whether condoms should be used were strongly associated with using a condom during sexual intercourse. This finding is consistent with the results of intervention studies discussed below (p. 193) showing that training in sexual negotiation skills increases safe sex behaviour among homosexual men.

The association between these variables and condom use would probably have been even higher if the joint effect of 'condom availability' and 'discussion of condom use' had been assessed. This is suggested by the finding of Kashim and colleagues (1993) that 71 per cent of the sexually experienced undergraduates who had bought condoms *and* discussed them with their partner actually used condoms in their next sexual encounters, as compared to 0 per cent of those who fulfilled neither of these conditions. In interpreting these findings we have to remember, however, that being prepared is not only a precondition for effective action, but also reflects a strong intention to act.

Condom use among homosexuals

Findings of studies which apply the models of reasoned action and planned behaviour to condom use among homosexual men are less consistent, though still supportive of the models of reasoned action and planned behaviour. Whereas a study by Fisher and colleagues (1995) supported all the specified relations of the model of reasoned action and suggested few differences between their samples of homosexual men and heterosexual men and women, Gallois *et al.* (1994) found substantial differences. They reported that the determinants from the theory of reasoned action were useful in predicting safe and unsafe sexual behaviour in their heterosexual, but not their homosexual, sample. Kelly and Kalichman (1998) reported that the variables of the model of reasoned action accounted for 7 to 12 per cent of the variance in condom use among their sample of self-identified sexually active homosexual men. In this study substantial additional variance was accounted for by a variable not included in the theories of reasoned action and planned behaviour, namely the reported pleasure individuals derived from unprotected anal sex.

The results of a prospective study by de Wit and colleagues (in press) suggest that the differential impact of the variables of the models of reasoned action and planned behaviour observed in the various studies of condom use by homosexual men may be due to differences between samples in the type of relationships in which the sexual behaviour was enacted. De Wit and his colleagues (in press) found that the value of the theories of reasoned action and planned behaviour in predicting safe sex behaviour (i.e. condom use and abstention from anal sex) depended very much on the relationship with the partner. Whereas the intention to engage in safe sex with a steady partner was strongly related to attitudes, subjective norms and perceived behavioural control, only perceived behavioural control emerged as a significant predictor of safe sex intentions with a casual partners (Table 5.1). The same pattern emerged with regard to the prediction of actual behaviour: safe sex with a steady partner was only predicted by intentions, whereas safe sex with a casual partner was only predicted by perceived behavioural control. Finally, the model accounted for 64 per cent of the variance in safe sex behaviour with steady partners, compared to only 21 per cent in safe sex with casual partners. Thus, whether these homosexual men engaged in safe sex with their steady

Table 5.1 Determinants of safe sex intentions and safe sex behaviour of homosexual men by type of relationship

	Casual partners	Steady partners
Intentions		
Attitude	.05	.41*
Subjective norm	−.12	.31*
Perceived behavioural control	.52*	.06
R square	.54*	.79*
Behaviour		
Intention	−.09	.85*
Perceived behavioural control	.52*	−.06
R square	.21*	.64*

Note: Displayed are standardized multiple regression coefficients (ß).
* significant at p < .001.
Source: de Wit et al. (in press).

partner depended to a large extent on their intentions, but their safe sex behaviour with casual partners depended on their assertiveness and their social skills in persuading their casual partner to keep it safe.

Because a substantial proportion of the men in this sample had casual relationships in addition to their steady partner, we wondered whether the quality of their steady relationship would influence whether or not they would also have sex with a casual partner. Bakker and colleagues (1994) had found with a heterosexual sample that the quality of their relationship and their 'relational commitment' was negatively related to the intention of these individuals to engage in extra-relational sex. A prospective study with homosexual men of the impact of the quality of a steady relationship on sexual behaviour outside that relationship revealed an unexpected pattern (de Vroome et al. in press). Whether or not these homosexual men had extra-relational sex was unrelated to the quality of the relationship with their steady partner. However, relationship quality had a strong impact on whether or not they engaged in *safe* sex with a casual partner. The better their relationship with their steady partner, the more likely they were to take protective measures when having sex with a casual partner. It is interesting to note that these relational measures improved the prediction of behaviour even when intention to engage in safe sex and perceived behavioural control were statistically controlled.

Implications for interventions

Three major conclusions can be drawn from these findings with regard to the design of interventions: first, interventions which rely on epidemiological information to emphasize the severity of AIDS and the vulnerability of the target population are likely to fail, because none of these factors appears to be a major determinant of condom use. Instead communications should aim at eroticizing condom use (see e.g. Tanner and Pollack 1988; Kyes 1990 for examples). Second, persuasive communications should not only target the beliefs underlying attitudes, subjective norms and perceived control, but also persuade people to be prepared and to discuss condom use with their prospective partners. Third, persuasive communications aimed at increasing condom use among homosexual men have to differentiate clearly between condom use in steady as compared to casual relationships. Whereas condom use in steady relationships is mainly determined by attitudes and subjective norms, condom use in casual relationships appears to be mainly controlled by perceived behavioural control. Thus, whereas persuasion should be effective in influencing condom use in steady relationships, some kind of skill training would probably be more effective with regard to condom use in casual encounters.

Interventions to reduce risk behaviour: from risk education to skill training

The early interventions were rarely derived from social psychological theories of attitude and behaviour change but based on an 'informal blend of logic and practical experience' (Fisher and Fisher 1992: 463). However, these interventions were probably quite effective despite such shortcomings. Providing individuals with information about the risk of HIV infection and the development of AIDS *and* motivating them to avoid unsafe sexual behaviour was probably sufficient to achieve behaviour change in the early stages of the epidemic. Risk behaviour cohort studies conducted in San Francisco and New York, both epicentres of the AIDS epidemic, reported 60 per cent reductions in unprotected anal intercourse in the late 1980s, with less than 20 per cent of the participants reporting having had unprotected anal intercourse during the previous year. There was also a substantial decline in average number of sexual partners during this period (McKusick *et al.* 1985; Martin 1987; Winkelstein *et al.* 1987; Coates *et al.* 1989). Studies conducted in less affected areas typically reported higher levels of risk behaviour among homosexual men, even though substantial reductions in risk behaviour had occurred even there (e.g. de Wit *et al.* 1992).

With the dangers of HIV widely known today, people who still engage in sexual risk behaviour either believe that they are not at risk or they are unwilling or unable to avoid unsafe sex. Therefore to be effective now, interventions have to do more than provide information and motivate individuals. They also have to incorporate behavioural skill training, teaching individuals the ability to communicate with, and be assertive with, a potential sexual partner. A number of such interventions have been developed and their effectiveness has been tested in several controlled individual- or group-level intervention studies (e.g. Kelly *et al.* 1989; St Lawrence *et al.* 1995a, 1995b, 1997; Kalichman *et al.* 1996; Belcher *et al.* 1998).

Individual- and group-level interventions

The first study to demonstrate the effectiveness of behavioural skill training in reducing sexual risk behaviour was conducted by Kelly and colleagues (1989). Participants in this study were 104 (apparently) healthy gay men

Table 5.2 Frequency of risky and precautionary behaviour for baseline and follow-up assessment among women exposed to either skill training (experimental condition) or risk education (comparison condition)

| | Experimental condition | | | | Comparison condition | | | |
| | Baseline | | 3 month | | Baseline | | 3 month | |
Behaviour[a]	Mean	Standard deviation	Mean	Standard deviation	Mean	Standard deviation	Mean	Standard deviation
Frequency of condom use during vaginal sex	4.4	7.1	13.1	24.2	8.8	21.1	3.6	4.2
Frequency of unprotected vaginal sex	26.1	30.3	8.2	18.5	24.7	36.0	17.2	29.6

[a] Behaviours measured at baseline and 3-month assessment points reference the previous 90-day period. Values refer to group effect.
Source: Adapted from Belcher *et al.* (1998).

with a high behavioural risk for HIV infection. They were randomly divided into an immediate intervention group and a waiting list control group. The members of the intervention group were taught – through modelling, role playing and corrective feedback – how to exercise self-control in relationships and to resist coercive pressure from a sexual partner to engage in unsafe practices. Evaluation at the end of the training programme indicated that the intervention group participants significantly reduced their frequency of unprotected anal intercourse and increased the frequency of condom use. At an eight-month follow-up, frequency of anal intercourse had decreased to near-zero levels and condoms were used in 77 per cent of those few anal intercourse occasions that still took place.

Since then the effectiveness of this type of social skill training has been demonstrated in a series of interventions with other risk groups. For example, in an intervention aimed at adolescent African American males and females, 246 adolescents between 14 and 18 years of age were recruited via brochures distributed in a public health clinic (St Lawrence et al. 1995a). Participants were randomly assigned to either an educational programme or an eight-week behavioural skill training course. The education control condition consisted of a single two-hour session that provided standard AIDS education. The behavioural skill training consisted of eight 90- to 120-minute weekly group meetings and combined education about the HIV risk with training of technical skills (e.g. correct condom use), communication skills (e.g. sexual assertiveness, refusal), and cognitive competency skills (including recognition and avoidance of high-risk situations). The impact of these interventions was assessed immediately and during a 12-month follow-up period. Both male and female participants showed greater benefit from the skill training intervention, but the effects differed between the two sexes. Male adolescents in the behaviour skill training lowered their rates of unprotected vaginal, oral and anal intercourse to a greater extent than male adolescents who received information only. Female participants were at baseline significantly lower on all sexual activities than men, but the extent to which they engaged in unprotected intercourse increased to a lesser extent after receiving behaviour skill training than after participating in the education session. A slightly shortened version of this intervention has also been successfully used with substance-dependent adolescents (St Lawrence et al. 1995b).

That even shorter interventions can also be effective has been demonstrated by Belcher and colleagues (1998) with another high-risk group, namely low-income inner-city community women, nearly all of whom were African American. Following a baseline assessment, the 72 women who had signed up for the project and been found eligible on the basis of screening which identified them as high risk were randomly assigned to a skill training or a risk education control condition. They either received, on a one-to-one basis, a two-hour AIDS education session or a two-hour behaviour skill training session which included a shortened version of the AIDS education. The effectiveness of these interventions was assessed one month and three months later. Again, the skill training proved much more effective than the education session (Table 5.2).

Even though these studies demonstrate the effectiveness of the combination of skill training and risk education over mere risk education, they do not allow one to identify the components of the skill training which are essential for achieving behavioural risk reduction. Kalichman *et al.* (1996) therefore designed a study which factorially manipulated sexual communication skill training (targeting assertiveness, sexual negoti-ation skills, and comfort in discussing sex with a partner) and behavioural self-management skill training (teaching individuals to recognize envir-onmental and cognitive–affective cues that trigger high-risk situations), keeping AIDS risk communication constant in all conditions. Participants in the study were 87 inner-city women, recruited through outreach and flyers distributed through social service agencies, who completed the four-session programme and the three-month follow-up measure. The experi-ment entailed four conditions: Condition 1 consisted only of risk education; Condition 2 combined risk education with sexual communication skill training; Condition 3 combined risk education with behavioural self-management skill training; and Condition 4 combined risk education with both types of skill training. Assessment of the impact of these interven-tions on risk reduction indicated that only Condition 4 resulted in signific-ant risk reduction. That risk education alone was not effective in reducing sexual risk behaviour is consistent with previous findings. What is puzz-ling, however, is that the training in sexual communication skills was insufficient to reduce sexual risk behaviour. One would have expected that once women were motivated to avoid unprotected vaginal sex, teach-ing them skills to negotiate safety measures with their partners should have helped them to act according to their intentions.

Despite such inconsistencies, these studies provide a reasonably clear picture of the components which have to be incorporated into any inter-vention to be effective. Participants have to be informed of HIV transmis-sion routes and of the health consequences, and they have to be motivated to form the intention to take action by being sensitized to their personal risk. Finally, they have to be trained in the technical and social skills necessary to act in line with their intentions. Even though some studies suggest that as little as one session may be sufficient for the delivery of an effective intervention, these sessions do require personal contact between the staff conducting the intervention and the individuals targeted by the intervention. Thus, even though these interventions have good 'efficacy', they have limited 'reach'. Furthermore, the individuals participating in these studies had all chosen to participate on the basis of information about these studies. It can thus be assumed that they were highly motiv-ated to change their sexual behaviour.

Community-level interventions

Fortunately, a number of community-level interventions have been de-veloped which to some extent alleviate both these limitations. For example, Kelly and colleagues (1991) increased the reach of their intervention by training people identified as popular opinion leaders among gays to dis-seminate information to their peers. The study was conducted among men patronizing gay clubs in three small cities in the South of the USA. Baseline risk behaviour in the one intervention city and two comparison cities was assessed before and after the intervention by asking men entering the gay clubs to respond to a questionnaire. Thirty opinion leaders were identified by the club bartenders. These opinion leaders were then trained in four 90-minute group sessions to disseminate messages to friends suggesting change strategies and endorsing the benefits of behaviour change implementation. The surveys conducted three and six months after the intervention indicated that interventions were effective. In the intervention city, the proportion of men who engaged in any unprotected intercourse in a two-month period decreased from 36.9 per cent to 27.5 per cent. There was also a 16 per cent increase in condom use during anal intercourse and a 16 per cent decrease in the proportion of men with more than one sexual partner. Little or no change was observed among men in the comparison cities over the same period of time.

The most ambitious community-level AIDS interventions to date have been the AIDS Community Demonstration Projects, conducted simultaneously in five USA cities, with intervention and control districts within each of these cities (CDC AIDS Community Demonstration Projects Research Group 1999). The projects combine ideas from the theories of reasoned action and planned behaviour and the notion of stages of change of the transtheoretical model. The risk groups targeted in these communities were active injection drug users, female sex partners of injection drug users, female commercial sex workers, and non-gay-identified men who have sex with men. This last group are men who are bisexual, do not consider themselves homosexual, and are not part of any gay network. The intervention had three key components:

1 The mobilization of community members to distribute and verbally reinforce prevention messages among their peers.
2 Creation of small media materials featuring theory-based prevention messages in the form of role model stories.
3 Increased availability of condoms and bleach kits for cleaning needles.

The first phase of the project involved ethnographic research in the five cities to identify the specific subpopulations at risk, the risk behaviour taking place, and specific 'gatekeepers', that is individuals who would provide a link with the specific risk groups. Through the ties with the 'gatekeepers' the project staff were able to interview members of the targeted risk group. These interviews allowed researchers to identify the behavioural, normative and control beliefs which differentiated 'risky' from 'safe' behaviour in a given risk group and the modal position of the members of this risk group on the stages of change continuum. The gatekeepers also helped with the recruitment of community volunteers from each of the risk populations at each of the sites. From July 1991 to June 1994 nearly 1000 volunteers were recruited and trained to distribute materials in the five project communities.

Role model stories were used to convey the information designed to change the relevant beliefs. A role model story is an authentic story about a community member that describes in the person's own words how and why he or she changed risk behaviour, how barriers of change were overcome, and the reinforcing consequences of the change. The stories were conveyed via small media (i.e. community newsletters, brochures, pamphlets) and new stories were distributed each month. The selection of the messages in these role model stories was guided by the data collected from the study population at each site before and during the intervention. For example, if the survey data indicated that at one site most community members were in the precontemplation stage for a particular behaviour, most of the stories dealing with that behaviour would highlight changes from precontemplation to the contemplation stage. Specific factors or beliefs were addressed if data analysis indicated that they were correlated with intention to change or a stage of change. For example, if people who were in the contemplation stage for consistent condom use tended to believe that condom use interferes with intimacy, whereas people who were in the preparation stage did not hold this belief, role model stories would address intimacy issues. Thus, the role model stories were tailored to the specific population in each site and were also changed over time in line with feedback from the various waves of data collection. In addition to role model stories, the small media also contained basic AIDS information, instruction on the use of condoms or bleach, biographies of community members participating in the project, and other community information.

Data collection was based on street interviews in the intervention and control locations. Two waves of baseline data were collected in spring 1991. The intervention began in each city in the summer of 1991 and continued until the summer of 1994. As this intervention continued, two to three waves of data were collected each year.

The main dependent measure was movement along the stages of change continuum for each of the risk behaviours. Differences on this continuum over time between the intervention and control sites were compared for all individuals surveyed and for the sub-group of individuals who reported direct exposure to the intervention. Recent exposure to the intervention increased in the intervention communities from 5 per cent during month two to a peak of 54 per cent during month 27. There were significant movements along the stages-of-change continuum in the intervention but not the control communities for condom use with both the main partner and the other partners. Furthermore, condom carrying increased by 73.4 per cent in the intervention communities, from 17.4 per cent at the beginning to 30.2 per cent at the end of the intervention. It increased only slightly in the control communities. This study demonstrates that community interventions can be effective if they are theory-based, use elicitation research to identify the relevant salient beliefs, and target the communication to specific risk groups in specific communities.

No review of community-level AIDS interventions would be complete without a discussion of school-based programmes. Schools provide an obvious access point for intervening with adolescents, a population which is both at risk and difficult to reach in any other way. The history of the development of school-based programmes has many features in common with interventions implemented outside schools (Kirby and DiClemente 1994; Kalichman 1998). The first generation of sex education curricula focused primarily upon increasing knowledge and emphasizing the risk and consequences of pregnancy. Exposure to these programmes had as little impact on sexual risk behaviour among students as exposure to similar programmes has had on adult populations.

School-based programmes face an additional problem which is less salient in the development of programmes for other settings, namely the degree to which such programmes can address condom use in addition to providing information about sexual abstinence. Abstinence-based programmes focus on the importance of refraining from sexual intercourse until after marriage. These programmes either exclude discussion of contraceptive measures such a condoms or focus on contraceptive failure in preventing pregnancies or infections. These programmes have typically proved to be ineffective (for reviews, see Kirby and DiClemente 1994; Kalichman 1998).

In contrast to abstinence-based interventions, programmes which emphasize that students should avoid *unprotected* intercourse by either abstaining from intercourse or by using condoms have proved to be more effective. Successful programmes include behavioural skill-building activities that enhance self-efficacy for performing risk-reducing and safer sex negotiation strategies. Most of the successful programmes were conducted in groups and combined basic information about the risks of unprotected intercourse with some form of behavioural skills training. It is important to note that none of the programmes accelerated the onset of sexual activity or increased its frequency (Kalichman 1998). These findings are important because concerns about reckless sexual behaviour are the most frequent reason why people oppose programmes that target avoidance of unprotected intercourse rather than promotion of sexual abstinence.

Pharmacological treatment of HIV and AIDS

Although there is still no cure for AIDS, dramatic advances have been made in the treatment of the infection. The combination therapies which have been available since mid-1996 can reduce HIV viral load, improve immune system functioning, and decrease mortality from AIDS (Kelly *et al.* 1998). These therapies combine the medication which has been available since the mid-1980s [nucleoside analogue reverse transcriptase inhibitors (NRTIs)] with newly developed protease inhibitors. Whereas the NRTIs function by interfering with the ability of HIV to produce DNA early in the HIV replication cycle, protease inhibitors block the maturation of viral particles ('virions') released by a mature HIV cell into the bloodstream, an event that occurs late in the replication cycle. Because the presence of therapeutic levels of protease inhibitors prevents immature virions from maturing, they do not become infectious. Patients on combination drug therapies therefore often exhibit marked and relatively rapid reductions in viral load (Kelly *et al.* 1998).

Although there is evidence that the new treatments can extend both the period between infection and the development of AIDS and the time between the development of AIDS and death, these therapies have been developed too recently to allow evaluation of their long-range effectiveness. Thus, we do not yet know how long the clinical health benefits will last, and whether, or how quickly, viral resistance will develop (Kelly *et al.* 1998). It is also not yet known whether the reduction in viral load results in a reduction in infectiousness (Kelly *et al.* 1998). Furthermore, the drug regimen required by these combination therapies is complex, because the three different antiretroviral drugs (one protease inhibitor, two NRTIs) have different dosage interval schedules. Also, some of these drugs have to be taken on an empty stomach, whereas others are taken following certain types of meals. For example, the protease inhibitor Crixivan has to be taken every eight hours, and little should be eaten two hours before and one hour afterwards. If a person decides to take Crixivan at 7.00 am, he or she then has to take two different NRTIs at 11.00 am, and Crixivan again at 15.00 (again with little food before and after). Finally, at 23.00 Crixivan has to be taken with the two NRTIs. Even brief lapses in adherence can result in increased viral load and enhanced HIV replication, permitting the virus to become drug resistant (Kelly *et al.* 1998). Since people often suffer severe side effects from these drugs, they may have to take additional medication to combat the side effects.

The advent of these drug treatments and the premature claims in the popular press that there is a 'cure for AIDS' may have encouraged people to relapse into high-risk behaviour. For example, results of a recent anonymous survey showed that men who practised unprotected anal intercourse as the receptive partner are more likely than men who do not to believe that it is safe to have sex with an HIV-positive man who has an undetectable viral load, and that the new treatments relieve their worries about unsafe sex (Kalichman *et al.* 1998). Thus, benefits of the new treatments in helping those who are infected could easily be counterbalanced by increased sexual risk behaviour of those who wrongly believe that AIDS can be cured.

Summary and conclusions

It is evident that there has been a substantial reduction of behaviours that are known to be involved in the transmission of the HIV. There can be little doubt that the marked behaviour change that has occurred since the advent of the AIDS epidemic has been a reaction to the diffusion of information about AIDS. Although this type of risk education has to be continued in order to maintain the level of knowledge, it also has to be recognized that risk education is not enough. To be effective, any intervention aimed at reducing sexual risk behaviour should complement sexual risk information with some form of training in the skills which people need to engage in safer sex.

INJURY PREVENTION AND CONTROL

One consequence of the dramatic change in causes of death during this century is that injuries have become the major cause of death during the first four decades of a person's life. Whereas previously the greatest threat to the health and welfare of children came from infectious diseases, inadequate nutrition and sanitation, injuries are now the cause of more deaths to children in the United States and most Western countries than the next six most frequent causes combined (Christophersen 1989). Therefore, the loss of potential years of life before age 65 due to injury-caused death is far greater than the loss due to any of the other leading causes (Waller 1987). Thus, a decrease in the death rate due to injuries would save more person-years of life than a decrease in any of the other causes of death.

The epidemiology

In the United States of America, one accidental death occurs every six minutes (National Safety Council 1986). Approximately two-thirds of the injury deaths in the United States in 1986 were due to unintentional injuries, and one-third were due to intentional injuries (suicides, homicides). The most frequent causes of violent death were injuries sustained in motor vehicle collisions, followed by suicide, homicide, falls, and fire or flames (National Centers for Health Statistics 1988).

Unlike deaths, which are reportable, less severe injuries are often not reported. Morbidity due to injury is therefore more difficult to assess than mortality. According to one estimate, one injury is likely to occur every four seconds in the United States, resulting in a weekly total of 173,100 injuries (National Safety Council 1986). At this rate there are 8.7 million injuries per year in the United States (Christophersen 1989).

The control of injury

Injury is usually defined as bodily 'damage resulting from acute exposure to physical and chemical agents' (Haddon and Baker 1981: 109). Injury occurs when these agents impinge on the body at a level which the body cannot resist. There are three public health strategies for injury control: *persuasion, legal requirements*, and *structural change*. While the first two strategies rely on inducing people to change their behaviour, the third approach reduces the risk of injuries by changing the design of equipment, vehicles or the environment.

Strategies of injury protection can be placed on an active–passive continuum, according to the effort they require from the person implementing that strategy. For example, the most *active* strategy to lower the risk that children get scalded by hot tap water would be to prevent children from running hot water. This would involve forbidding them to approach the hot water tap and monitoring them whenever they are near any taps. A less active strategy would involve lowering the setting of the water heater to a level where the water is no longer scaldingly hot. This would require *only one action*, the adjustment of the thermostat. The least active strategy would be a legal requirement for manufacturers of water heaters to fix settings at a level that does not allow water heaters to discharge water that is scaldingly hot (Wilson and Baker 1987). This would make water heaters safe for children without any actions from their caretakers. There is consensus among experts in the area of injury control that protecting people through environmental changes or changes in vehicles or equipment used, whenever possible, is more effective than mass education or the introduction of legal requirements to induce self-protective behaviour.

Persuasion

As with other areas of health behaviour, it is very difficult to persuade people to take actions that protect them against accidental injuries. The use of seat belts provides a good example. In most countries, only 10 to 20 per cent of drivers used their belts before the introduction of laws requiring their use, even though their use requires very little effort and although they reduce mortality risk to wearers involved in accidents by 60 per cent according to some estimates (e.g. Robertson 1986). It should therefore have been easy to persuade people to use their belts.

Despite this, media campaigns persuading drivers to use seat belts have been notoriously ineffective (Robertson 1986, 1987). In one study, radio and television advertisements urging seat belt use were employed extensively in one community, moderately in a second, and not at all in a third. In the five weeks of the study no significant change in seat belt use occurred that could be attributed to the campaign (Fleischer 1972, reported by Robertson 1987). Equally disappointing were the results of a nine-month seat belt use campaign on one cable of a dual-cable television system used for marketing studies. Observation of seat belt use did not show any differences between the households on the experimental cable than in those on the control cable or the community at large, even though the advertisements were shown nearly 1000 times, often during prime time (Robertson *et al.* 1974).

Why are people so resistant to persuasion, even when it is in their own self-interest to take action? One reason is that persuasive strategies usually focus on knowledge and motivation, and thus affect only two of the factors that are involved in self-protection. Obviously, knowledge of both the risk and the protective action is a prerequisite to self-protection. But even if individuals know that a certain action will protect them against some danger, they might forget to implement it at the relevant moment. This is particularly likely to happen when the necessity for the protective behaviour arises infrequently and is also not consistently related to a sequence of action.

But even if people are reminded of the self-protective action, they might not be motivated to engage in that action because it is effortful and/or because the likelihood of an accident seems remote. For example, the reminder systems installed in most USA cars in the early 1970s did little to increase seat belt use (Robertson 1987). In such cases, compliance with protection recommendations can often be increased by linking additional incentives to the behaviour and/or by making the behaviour less effortful. For example, if children's car seats could be made to fasten in more easily, or even be permanently installed from underneath the regular seat such that they could be unfolded when needed, people would probably be more likely to use them every time they have small children as passengers in their cars.

Finally, people might fail to take a self-protective action if they have insufficient control over the behaviour that is required. For example, parents have only limited control over the behaviour of small children. Thus, whenever the safety of small children is involved, structural changes to make the child's environment safer will be particularly effective. Similarly, people convicted of drunken driving are often people with alcohol problems who may be unable to control their drinking (Robertson 1987). In such cases, a withdrawal of their driving licence until they have overcome their alcohol problem would be more effective than education concerning the dangers of drunken driving.

Legal requirements

Legal requirements are effective to the extent that they succeed in linking new incentives to a given behaviour. Thus, seat belt laws introduce a new incentive for seat belt use, namely, the avoidance of paying a fine. There is ample evidence for the success of legal requirements in inducing behaviour change. For example, when the Swedish government made seat belt use compulsory for front seat passengers in private cars, seat belt use increased from 30 to 85 per cent within a few months (Fhanér and Hane 1979). In New York, where use ranged from 10 to 20 per cent prior to the introduction of a seat belt law in 1984, it varied from 45 to 70 per cent after the law went into force in early 1985. The introduction of these laws also resulted in substantial reductions in deaths of vehicle occupants (Robertson 1986).

Laws requiring parents to restrain their infants or toddlers during motor vehicle travel, which have been adopted by all US states, have also been very effective. According to observational surveys at shopping centres in 19 cities, the rate of child restraint use increased from roughly 20 per cent in 1980 to 80 per cent in 1990 (Graham 1993). Recent estimates suggest that the number of infant and toddler fatalities in motor vehicle crashes are 25 to 40 per cent less than they might have been if child restraint laws had not been adopted (Graham 1993). Laws requiring the use of helmets by motorcyclists have been similarly successful (Robertson 1986).

For legal requirements to be effective, the behaviour that is enforced has to be easily monitored. Thus, the law limiting blood alcohol concentration in drivers is difficult to enforce. According to some earlier estimates, only 1 in 2000 drivers illegally impaired by alcohol is actually arrested for the offence (Robertson 1984). However, roadside sobriety checkpoints are increasingly being employed to enhance the probability that drunk drivers will be detected and apprehended. Furthermore, swiftness of punishment has been enhanced by new state legislation that authorizes police to suspend a driver's licence before conviction on the basis of evidence that the driver has exceeded the legal blood alcohol limit (Graham 1993).

Even though laws offer additional incentives to encourage self-protective behaviour, they still have to rely on the motivation of the individuals at risk to be effective. This also limits their usefulness. Thus, they often have least impact on those sub-groups that are at greatest risk, because those likely to be most reckless are least likely to comply with legal requirements. For example, seat belt laws seem to be least observed by the young and the alcohol-impaired (Robertson 1978).

Structural changes

The great advantage of the structural approach to injury control which changes the environment to make it safer is that it protects people without requiring any effort on their part. An example of a successful structural change was the introduction of smaller containers for children's aspirin. The number of children dying after the ingestion of bottles of flavoured aspirin decreased substantially after bottle sizes were reduced to contain only sub-lethal doses, even when all the tablets in a bottle were consumed. This strategy was more effective than the introduction of childproof caps that had to be replaced after every use and that some children were able to circumvent (Wilson and Baker 1987).

In the area of traffic safety, the introduction of federal standards in the USA in 1968 that required new cars to meet performance criteria for crash worthiness and crash avoidance resulted in an estimated reduction of 14,000 traffic deaths per year by 1982 (Robertson 1986). Substantial further reductions in traffic fatalities will be achieved once all cars are equipped with air bags that inflate automatically in the case of severe frontal crashes. It has been estimated that this will reduce traffic fatalities in the USA by 9000 deaths per year (Robertson 1986).

Conclusions

The opinion of experts in the area of injury control that passive strategies are preferable to active strategies is compelling, since any active strategy for controlling injury depends on convincing a large number of people to change their behaviour in a way that protects them against injury, which has proved very difficult to do. Persuasion is particularly liable to fail when the behaviour is effortful, inconvenient, costly, difficult to control and/or when the risk of injury seems rather remote. However, the application of passive strategies is not always possible and even the safest vehicles, agents, etc. can be dangerous in the hands of individuals who behave without regard for their own safety or that of other people. Legal requirements can help in such situations, but again, their application is limited. Thus, there is no substitute for mass education, in addition to the passive strategies outlined above, in the area of injury control.

GENERAL CONCLUSIONS

The second half of the twentieth century witnessed an unprecedented change in health attitudes. It is hard to imagine today that until the early 1960s people believed that they could smoke, eat and drink excessively with nothing worse to fear than a smoker's cough, a degree of overweight and a hangover. This era of happy ignorance ended in 1964 with the first Surgeon General's Report on the dangers of cigarette smoking and the condemnation of food high in cholesterol (USDHEW 1964).

For some time sex appeared be the one behaviour that could be enjoyed with impunity, especially after the invention of the pill. This happy state of affairs was first marred by the genital herpes scare (a sexually transmitted viral infection which received wide publicity in the mid-1980s) and ended with the news of the sexual transmission of the AIDS virus. Exercise had always been considered healthy (like eating an apple a day) but only recently has this belief been supported by scientific evidence.

As the proponents of health promotion like to emphasize, the dissemination of the evidence from epidemiological research on the health impact of various health behaviours to the public resulted in substantial attitude and behaviour change. Gluttony went out of fashion. Perrier-drinking, vegetarian, monogamous non-smokers who jog regularly and never drive without wearing their seat belts have become almost the modal men and women of the postmodern age.

As we have seen, however, there are two ways to evaluate the evidence of the impact of health promotion on health behaviour. We can be elated about the 20 per cent decrease in the number of smokers in the USA in the 20 years after the first report on smoking by the Surgeon General (USDHEW 1964), but we can also be disenchanted by the fact that one-third of the adult population in the USA still smokes cigarettes, in spite of all the research findings establishing smoking as a health hazard.

How can we explain the apparent lack of response to health warnings? Are they suicidal? Does their resistance to persuasion suggest that health promotion is ineffective and should be abandoned? It seems to me that the dramatic changes in health attitudes and behaviours that have occurred over the last 40 years are sufficient evidence that health education can be effective. One has to keep in mind that, even though good health and long life are important goals for most people, they are not the only goals. As Becker (1976) succinctly stated, a person may be a heavy smoker or so committed to work as to omit all exercise, not out of ignorance, but because the lifespan forfeited does not seem worth the cost of giving up smoking or changing his or her diet. And for many others the goal of being healthy may seem difficult to reach because they feel unable give up smoking or change their diet, even if they wanted to.

For those of us who, in our ambition to squeeze the last minute out of our potential lifespan, have had to forfeit many of life's pleasures, it is hard to understand (and to accept) that there are still people around who smoke, drink like fish, and eat greasy food as if there were no tomorrow. It is difficult to resist the temptation to point out to them what damage they are doing to their health. However, in all likelihood they will have heard these arguments before, and hearing them once more will not change their minds or influence their behaviour. If we really want to 'help' them, we have to find out the reasons why they continue to engage in behaviours which they know to be deleterious to their health.

FURTHER READING

CDC AIDS Community Demonstration Projects Research Group (1999) Community level HIV intervention in 5 cities: final outcome data from the CDC AIDS community demonstration. *American Journal of Public Health*, 89: 336–45. This Community AIDS intervention has been designed by a panel of behavioural experts (including M. Fishbein). The study demonstrates that community interventions can work well, if they are designed in line with social psychological theories.

Christophersen, E.R. (1989) Injury control. *American Psychologist*, 44: 237–41. Reviews the research evidence on the effectiveness of major approaches to injury control.

Kalichman, S.C. (1998) *Preventing AIDS: A Sourcebook for Behavior Interventions*. Mahwah, NJ: Erlbaum. Comprehensive and very readable review of the social psychological research on AIDS prevention.

Taubes, G. (1998) The (political) science of salt. *Science*, 281: 898–907. Entertaining discussion of the scientific controversy about the health consequences of salt consumption. Supports the impression that public health research is sometimes motivated by missionary zeal rather than scientific objectivity.

US Department of Health and Human Services (1996) *Physical Activity and Health: A Report of the Surgeon General*. McLean, VA: International Medical Publishing. This is the most comprehensive review of research on the health consequences of physical activity. The chapters are written by experts and provide comprehensive reviews of research findings.

SIX

STRESS AND HEALTH

The present chapter and Chapter 7 focus on stress as a risk factor for ill health and on social and personality variables as moderators of the stress–health relationship. There is ample evidence that stress results in health impairment. Although these health consequences are to some extent mediated by changes in the endocrine, immune and autonomic nervous systems, the experience of stress also causes negative changes in health behaviour that contribute to the stress–illness relationship. The present chapter examines the evidence for the assumption that stress increases the risk of ill health and discusses some of the processes that might mediate the stress–illness relationship. The following chapter considers social and personality variables that moderate the impact of stress on health.

PHYSIOLOGICAL STRESS AND THE BREAKDOWN OF ADAPTATION

The stress concept has been made popular by Selye's seminal work on a pattern of bodily responses that occurs when an organism is exposed to a stressor such as intensive heat or infection. Although much of the theoretical foundation for this work had been prepared by Cannon (1929), Selye's research advanced our understanding of physiological reactions to noxious stimuli and served as a paradigm for later conceptions of stress.

In his highly readable book, *The Stress of Life*, Selye (1976) described how, as a young medical student at the University of Prague, he was impressed by the fact that, apart from the small number of symptoms characteristic of a given illness (and important for the clinical diagnosis of that illness), there appeared to be many signs of bodily distress which were common to most, if not all, diseases (e.g. loss of weight and appetite, diminished muscular strength, and motivational deficits). But it was not until 10 years later, while doing physiological work on animals, that Selye discovered a set of apparently non-specific bodily responses which seemed to occur whenever an organism was exposed to a stressor, whether this stressor was surgical injury, extreme cold, or non-lethal injections of toxic fluids. These bodily reactions consisted of a considerable enlargement of the adrenal cortex, a shrinkage of the thymus and lymph glands, and ulceration of the stomach and duodenum.

The adrenals are two small endocrine glands situated above the kidneys. They consist of two portions: a central part, the medulla, and an outer rind, the cortex. Both synthesize hormones that are involved in mobilizing the organism for action. The thymicolymphatic system, on the other hand, plays an important role in the immune defence of the body. Using these morphological changes as indices of adrenal cortical activity including an involvement of the immune system, Selye suggested that these endocrine responses helped the organism to cope physiologically with the stressor agent. If one assumes that bodily injuries frequently occur in a context in which the animal has to fight or run, physiological responses that mobilize the organism for action are indeed adaptive. Selye defined these non-specific responses as 'stress'.

No organism can stay in a heightened state of arousal indefinitely. Reactions to stressors therefore change over time. Selye argued that with repeated exposure to the stressor, the defence reaction of the organism passes through three identifiable stages. Together these stages represent the General Adaptation Syndrome. First, in the 'alarm' phase, the organism becomes mobilized to meet the threat. In the second stage of 'resistance', the organism seems to have adapted to the stressor and the general activation subsides. However, an extended exposure to the same stressor can 'exhaust' the adaptive energy of the body. Thus, the third stage of 'exhaustion' occurs if the organism fails to overcome the threat and depletes its physiological resources in the process.

There are therefore two ways in which the stressor can harm an organism: it can either cause damage directly if it exceeds the power of adaptation of an organism or indirectly as a result of the processes marshalled in defence against the stressor. Selye termed the diseases in whose development the stress responses of the organism played a major role 'diseases of adaptation'. For example, the ulcers which are typical of the third stage of the general adaptation syndrome would be considered to be a disease of adaptation. Similarly, the various illnesses which seem to be related to the accumulation of stressful life events would also belong in this category. Thus, illness is the price the organism has to pay for the defence against extended exposure to stressor agents.

Over the years Selye's model has been criticized for a number of reasons. One major point of criticism has been that it assigns a very limited role to *psychological* factors. In contrast to Selye, researchers now believe that psychological appraisal is important in the determination of stress (Lazarus and Folkman 1984). It is possible that even with the stressors used by Selye, the stress response was mediated by the emotional disturbance, discomfort and pain rather than being a direct physiological response to the tissue damage caused by these noxious stimuli. Thus Mason (1975) noted that 'conventional laboratory situations designed for the study of physical stressors, such as exercise, heat, cold, etc. very often also elicit an appreciable degree of emotional disturbance, discomfort, and even pain' (p. 24).

If precautions are taken to minimize psychological reactions, there is no activation of the adrenal system. A related criticism concerned Selye's 'non-specificity assumption' that all stressors produce the same bodily response. There is increasing evidence that specific stressors produce distinct endo-crinological responses and that individuals' responses to stress may be influenced by their personalities, perception and biological constitution (Mason 1975; Lazarus and Folkman 1984). These findings challenge Selye's assumption of the uniform response to stress. But this critique should not detract from the fact that Selye's ideas have had a lasting impact on stress research.

PSYCHOSOCIAL STRESS AND HEALTH

A second major impetus in the advancement of stress theory came from psychiatrists, who began to study life events as factors contributing to the development of a variety of psychosomatic and psychiatric illnesses (e.g. Cobb and Lindemann 1943; Holmes and Masuda 1974). Basic to this work is the assumption that psychosocial stress leads to the same bodily changes which Selye observed as a result of tissue damage. This essentially psycho-somatic tradition generated clinical and epidemiological research which tends to support the assumption that the experience of stressful life events increases the risk of morbidity and even mortality.

The assumption that psychosocial stress had a negative impact on health was first studied in the context of major life events. Major life events range from cataclysmic events such as the death of a spouse or being fired from a job to more mundane but still problematic events such as having trouble with one's boss. While some research examined the impact of *specific* life events such as bereavement or unemployment, the majority of studies use self-report lists or interview-based measures of critical life events to investigate the *cumulative* health impact of the number or total severity of stressful life events which subjects reported having experienced during a given period of time. Because the accumulation of minor irritations may also be stressful, attention has also been focused on the cumulative health effects of the more minor stressful events that occur from day to day. Such daily stresses might include having too many meetings or not enough time for one's family. The following section will evaluate the evidence from this research with regard to the health-impairing nature of psycho-social stress.

The health impact of cumulative life stress

Major life events

Although more recently a number of interview-based measures of critical life events have been developed (Wethington *et al.* 1995), early research on the health impact of stressful life events relied nearly exclusively on self-report 'checklists' (Turner and Wheaton 1995) pioneered by Holmes

Table 6.1 The Social Readjustment Rating Scale

Rank	Life event	Mean value
1	Death of spouse	100
2	Divorce	73
3	Marital separation	65
4	Jail term	63
5	Death of close family member	63
6	Personal injury or illness	53
7	Marriage	50
8	Fired at work	47
9	Marital reconciliation	45
10	Retirement	45
11	Change in health of family member	44
12	Pregnancy	40
13	Sex difficulties	39
14	Gain of new family member	39
15	Business readjustment	39
16	Change in financial state	38
17	Death of close friend	37
18	Change to different line of work	36
19	Change in number of arguments with spouse	35
20	Mortgage over US$10,000	31
21	Foreclosure of mortgage or loan	30
22	Change in responsibilities at work	29
23	Son or daughter leaving home	29
24	Trouble with in-laws	29
25	Outstanding personal achievement	28
26	Wife begin or stop work	26
27	Begin or end school	26
28	Change in living conditions	25
29	Revision of personal habits	24
30	Trouble with boss	23
31	Change in work hours or conditions	20
32	Change in residence	20
33	Change in schools	20
34	Change in recreation	19
35	Change in church activities	19
36	Change in social activities	18
37	Mortgage or loan less than US$10,000	17
38	Change in sleeping habits	16
39	Change in number of family get-togethers	15
40	Change in eating habits	15
41	Vacation	13
42	Christmas	12
43	Minor violations of the law	11

Source: Holmes and Rahe (1967).

and Rahe (1967) with their development of the Schedule of Recent Experiences (SRE) and the Social Readjustment Rating Scale (SRRS).

Self-report measures typically consist of lists of life events and require respondents to indicate which of these events they have experienced during a given time period. The checklist developed by Holmes and Rahe (1967) lists 43 items which describe 'life change events'. Life change events were defined as those events that require a certain amount of social readjustment from the individual (Table 6.1). Since it was assumed that any event which forced an individual to deviate from his or her habitual pattern would be stressful, the list included pleasant as well as unpleasant events. The inclusion of positive as well as negative changes is reasonable if, true to the Selye tradition, stress is assumed to be caused by the need to adapt to new situations. However, there is now evidence that only negative events are related to indicators of ill health (e.g. Ross and Mirowsky 1979).

In answering the checklist, respondents are requested to indicate all the life events they have experienced during a given time period. The measure of cumulative life stress can either consist of the number of life events experienced during a given period of time (SRE) or of a weighted score that also takes account of the severity of these events (SSRS). Thus the two scales differ only in the weight assigned to life events. The SSRS provides scale values based on a rating of the magnitude of social readjustment such an event would require (Holmes and Rahe 1967). The unweighted scores (reflecting merely the number of stressful events experienced) or the life change unit scores (reflecting the summed intensity of these events) can then be related to subsequent periods of illness. Surprisingly, weighting scores by the severity of life events rather than using the mere frequency of events does not seem to improve the power of these scales to predict health problems (Turner and Wheaton 1995).

Although the checklist was also used in a great number of studies in which life events were only assessed retrospectively after the onset of some illness (e.g. Rahe and Lind 1971; Rahe and Paasikivi 1971), the ease with which it could be administered made it feasible to screen large numbers of people and thus encouraged investigators to conduct prospective studies (i.e. studies in which life events were assessed before the onset of illness). In one of the most impressive projects of this kind, Rahe (1968) assessed the changes that occurred in the lives of 2500 Navy officers and enlisted men in the six months prior to tours of duty aboard three Navy cruisers. These life change unit scores were then related to shipboard medical records at the end of the six-month tour of duty. Individuals with life change unit scores in the top 30 per cent of the distribution were categorized as a high-risk group, those with the lowest 30 per cent as low-risk group. Rahe found that in the first few months of the tour the high-risk group had nearly 90 per cent more first illnesses than the low-risk group. Furthermore, the high-risk group consistently reported more illnesses each month for the period of the tour than did the low-risk group.

However, other prospective studies were less supportive of the stress–illness relationship. For example, Theorell and colleagues (1975), who studied a sample of over 4000 Swedish construction workers, found no relationship between stressful life events for a given year and mortality, hospitalization, or days off work during the following year. Goldberg and Comstock (1976) were similarly unsuccessful in a prospective study relating life events to death and hospitalization in two American communities. Furthermore, as Rabkin and Struening (1976) pointed out, the correlations between life stress and illness are typically below .30, suggesting that life events account for less than 9 per cent of the variance in illness.

The initial excitement with which the development of these measures had been greeted was soon followed by a period of critical re-evaluation. One line of argument has raised the possibility that the relationship between life stress and health could be due to a reporting bias (e.g. Mechanic 1978). After all, studies that rely on life event scales do not assess the amount of stress and the number of illnesses directly, but relate self-reported life stress to treatment-seeking behaviour. Thus, individuals with low treatment-seeking thresholds, who consult their doctors for even the most minor health problems, may also be more likely to report any upheaval as a major life event. This assumption could account for most of the results of the Navy study of Rahe (1968) described earlier.

Along similar lines, Watson and Pennebaker (1989) argued that self-report measures of both stressful life events and health complaints reflect a pervasive mood disposition of negative affectivity, which represents a stable personality disposition to experience negative mood and is closely related to the dimension of neuroticism. While negative affectivity correlates highly with measures of symptom reporting, it seems to be unrelated to objective health indicators (e.g. blood pressure levels, serum risk factors, immune system functions). Watson and Pennebaker (1989) suggest that individuals who score high on negative affectivity are hypervigilant and are therefore more likely to notice and attend to normal body sensations. Since their scanning is fraught with anxiety and uncertainty, they tend to interpret normal symptoms as painful and pathological.

Negative affectivity could not account for outcomes of studies where life event measures are related to physical health measures. For example, Sibai and colleagues (1989) investigated the association of wartime stress variables and coronary artery disease in the war-torn Lebanon of 1986. Participants were patients undergoing angiography because of clinical evidence of heart disease. Patients filled out a questionnaire before they came to know the results of the arteriogram. In the questionnaire they had to indicate whether they or their nuclear family had recently experienced any of a range of war-time stressors (e.g. injury, kidnapping, assault, serious threats, displacement from home, damage to home). Patients who had more than a 70 per cent narrowing of their arteries were nearly three times as likely than patients whose arteries showed no evidence of atherosclerosis to have experienced exposure to war events. This finding would be difficult to explain in terms of negative affectivity, because it compared two groups of patients. Since report of angina symptoms is one of the reasons why patients have to undergo coronary angiography, one would expect negative affectivity to be higher among the healthy patients for whom no physical basis could be found for those complaints.

That war stress may not only accelerate the development of atherosclerosis but may also induce myocardial infarction has been demonstrated in a study of effects of Iraqi missile attacks on the incidence of myocardial infarction and sudden deaths among Israeli civilians (Meisel *et al.* 1991). This study is also interesting from a methodological point of view, because it relates an objectifiable stressor (the missile attacks) to an objectifiable health measure (myocardial infarction). The authors reported a sharp increase in the incidence of acute myocardial infarctions during the first days of the Gulf war when compared to a number of control periods (e.g. same period one year earlier; the weeks directly before the attacks).

A second line of argument against the use of self-report measures of life events has been that of the contamination of stress and illness measures (e.g. Schroeder and Costa 1984). Life event scales may be confounded with measures of health in at least two ways: first, life event scales frequently include items that may reflect the physical and psychological conditions of the respondent. If items such as 'Personal injury or illness' or 'Pregnancy' are used as measures of stressful life events, then the event score is directly contaminated with concurrent physical health. Second, life event scales often include items that could reflect the result rather than the cause of psychological problems (e.g. troubles with in-laws, fired at work, separation). Consistent with these assumptions, Schroeder and Costa (1984) demonstrated that the correlation obtained between standard measures of life events and physical illness disappeared when 'contaminated items' were eliminated from the life event scale. However, these findings could not be replicated by Maddi *et al.* (1987).

A third line of argument has been that the checklist approach treats all life events of given type as equivalent (Kessler 1997). Death of a spouse, for example, is assigned a Life Change Score of 100, irrespective of the suddenness of the death or any other circumstance surrounding the death which might have made it more stressful. There is evidence from studies of individual events such as bereavement that the strength of the relationship between life events and depression increases substantially when these sorts of distinctions are made (Stroebe and Stroebe 1987).

One strategy to solve this problem has been the 'contextual' approach to using information about the person and his or her life situation to construct an independent judgement of how stressful the event would be for a typical person in such a situation (Wethington *et al.* 1995). This approach, pioneered by Brown and Harris (1978, 1989), involves two stages. The first stage uses a semi-structured interview, the Life Events and Difficulties Schedule (LEDS) (Brown and Harris 1989). This interview consists of a series of questions asking whether certain types of events have occurred over the past 12 months and a set of guidelines for probing positive responses. The aim of the interviewing method is to enable the interviewer to construct a narrative of each event. The LEDS uses strict criteria about what constitutes a stressful life event, and allows a classification of each event on the basis of severity of threat, emotional significance, and domain of life experience in which it occurred. The second stage consists of expert evaluations of the event descriptions developed on the basis of the interviews. These are presented to a panel of raters, blind to the illness status of the respondent, who discuss the appropriate ratings of threat. Thus, the death of a partner would be assigned different scores depending on the circumstances surrounding the death. For example, a sudden loss might be rated as more threatening than a loss following an extended illness. Although this method is in many ways superior to the checklist method, the resulting rating of severity incorporates already some of the psychological assumptions about the severity of an event (i.e. that a sudden loss is more severe than anticipated loss) which the researcher wanted to test in the first place.

Minor life events

Methodological problems increase in severity as one moves from self-report measures of major life events to scales that assess minor events such as 'daily hassles'. Hassles are 'irritating, frustrating, distressing demands that to some degree characterize everyday transactions with the environment' (Kanner *et al.* 1981: 3). Kanner and colleagues (1981) developed a Hassles Scale that consists of a list of 117 potential hassles. Examples of such hassles are 'misplacing or losing things', 'troublesome neighbours', 'thoughts about death', 'concerns about owing money', 'trouble relaxing', 'concerns about job security'. Subjects are asked to mark each hassle that had happened to them during a given period of time and then to indicate how severe each of the hassles had been during this time (somewhat severe, moderately severe, extremely severe). From this information two summary scores can be computed: frequency, reflecting the number of items checked, and intensity, reflecting the mean severity of the items checked. Although developed as a measure of daily stresses, the scale was originally intended for once-a-month administration for several consecutive months.

In one study, the Hassles Scale was given to 100 middle-aged adults for nine consecutive months and related to reported psychological symptoms, including depression and anxiety (Kanner *et al.* 1981). Hassles were found to be a better predictor of concurrent and subsequent psychological symptoms than were more major life events. Furthermore, while major life events had little impact on symptoms independent of the effect of hassles, hassles continued to predict symptoms, even after the impact of major life events had been statistically controlled. That hassles predicted health outcome as well as or better than major life events was also reported by DeLongis *et al.* (1982), Monroe (1983), Zarski (1984) and Weinberger *et al.* (1987).

Research using the Hassles Scale was soon subjected to the same criticism that had been levelled against studies that relied on measures of major life events. Specifically the Dohrenwends and their colleagues raised the issue of contamination (Dohrenwend *et al.* 1984; Dohrenwend and Shrout 1985). They first argued that the Hassles Scale contained many items that may well reflect psychological symptoms (e.g. 'You have had sexual problems other than those resulting from physical problems'; 'You are concerned about your use of alcohol'; 'You have had a fear of rejection'). When Lazarus and colleagues (1985) demonstrated that a hassles sub-scale consisting only of items that were not confounded showed as high a correlation with psychological symptoms as a sub-scale that consisted mainly of confounded items, Dohrenwend and Shrout (1985) changed their argument to suggest that all hassles reflected symptoms, due to the response format of the Hassles Scale. They argued that the fact that the lowest intensity permitted by the response scale is 'somewhat severe' could be interpreted by subjects as implying that an event had to be at least 'somewhat severe' to be reported as a hassle. Thus, only subjects who experienced difficulties in coping with a given hassle would feel that they should report it.

In response to these criticisms, DeLongis and colleagues (1988) modified the Daily Hassles Scale, eliminating contaminated items, changing the response format by having the subject only rate the extent to which an event constituted a hassle, and asking research participants to respond to the scale on a *daily* basis for several consecutive days. This last change made it more plausible that the scale really assessed daily events and was also in line with methodological trends towards the development of measures which assess stressful experiences at the daily level (for a review, see Eckenrode and Bolger 1995). Consistent with the assumption that daily hassles result in health impairment, DeLongis and colleagues (1988) reported a significant relationship between daily stress and the occurrence of both concurrent and subsequent health problems such as flu, sore throats, headaches and backaches. However, this study does not rule out the possibility raised by Watson and Pennebaker (1989) that the association between daily hassles and reported symptomatology is at least partly due to the influence of negative affectivity.

Conclusions

There is evidence that measures of cumulative stress, reflecting both major and minor stressors, are significantly related to psychological and physical health problems. However, with regard to studies based on self-report measures of stress, there is now considerable doubt about how justifiable it is to interpret this relationship in terms of a causal impact of stress on health. There are not only problems of reporting bias and item contamination, but there is also increasing evidence that self-report measures of both stress and health complaints reflect a stable personality disposition of negative affectivity, or neuroticism, that could at least be partly responsible for the relationship observed between these measures. Some of these problems can be addressed by the use of personal interviews, but the costs of administering interviews are high. Because negative affectivity is unrelated to objective health measures, the use of such a measure may constitute a more effective safeguard against this type of criticism.

The health impact of specific life events: the case of partner loss

Most of the ambiguities involved in using cumulative life event measures can be avoided by studying the health consequences of specific stressful life events. The loss of a partner through death combines a number of features which make it particularly suited to the study of the health impact of stressful life events. Partner loss is not only one of the most severely stressful life events, but is also objectifiable (thereby eliminating the risk of reporting biases affecting the measure of stress). Since the loss of a marital partner is also reflected in census and health records, large bodies of data are available which permit the analysis of excess risk in terms of

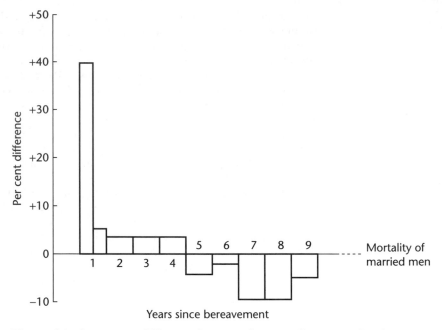

Figure 6.1 Percentage difference between the mortality rates of widowers over age 54 and those of married men of the same age by number of years since bereavement.
Source: Parkes *et al.* (1969).

specific illnesses and even mortality. Finally, with the possible exception of loss due to suicide of the partner (persons might have been driven to it by the illness of their sponse), there can be no doubt that the stressful life event (i.e. the loss) preceded the health problems. Thus, while many of the life events such as 'divorce' or 'separation' typically listed in life event inventories could be consequences rather than the cause of personality problems or depression, this is unlikely in the case of bereavement. A brief overview of the major findings of research on the health consequences of partner loss will therefore be presented.

The loss of a partner through death can indeed adversely affect the health of the surviving partner. This has been shown both in epidemiological surveys comparing marital status groups on various health measures, and in longitudinal cohort studies that examine the health status of bereaved (compared with non-bereaved) persons for a period of time following loss (for reviews, see Stroebe and Stroebe 1987; Stroebe *et al.* 1993; Parkes 1996; Archer 1999).

Consequences can be so direct that the life of the bereaved person is itself threatened. As cross-sectional surveys in many different countries have shown, the widowed have higher mortality rates than their married counterparts. Furthermore, the greatest risk to life appears to be in the first few weeks and months following loss. The classic study by Parkes and colleagues (1969) clearly illustrates this phenomenon. As Figure 6.1. shows, in their longitudinal study of a sample of widowers over the age of 54, there was a 40 per cent increase in mortality during the first half year of bereavement, compared with married controls over an equivalent period. Although there are some variations between studies in patterns of excess mortality rates for the widowed, certain regularities have emerged (for a review, see M. Stroebe and Stroebe 1993). Thus, excesses for widowers are relatively higher than those for widows, as are the excesses for younger as compared with older bereaved spouses. Other studies have confirmed this pattern (Siegel and Kuykendall 1990; Umberson *et al.* 1992).

Despite the excess risk of mortality, expressed in absolute numbers, there are very few bereaved persons who do actually die prematurely. However, for a much larger proportion bereavement is associated not only with intense suffering over an extended period of time, but also with an increased risk of succumbing to a variety of psychological and somatic complaints and illnesses. Thus, depression rates are higher for widowed than non-widowed persons. Visits to physicians are more frequent among the former than the latter, and the physical illness rates of the bereaved are elevated.

Studies are beginning to identify those bereaved individuals who are at particular risk of suffering from the various adverse consequences of loss. There is some evidence (for a review, see Sanders 1993) that health consequences are affected by such factors as the mode of death (more severe consequences after a sudden rather than an expected loss), gender (men suffering more severe consequences) and the extent of social support the individual receives after the loss (more severe consequences for people who do not receive much social support).

While the relationship between bereavement and various mental and physical health debilities has been reasonably well established, this alone is not convincing evidence that it is the stress of bereavement that is the mediating factor. There are a number of alternative explanations. Depression models would tend to look instead to such factors as loneliness consequent upon losing a loved person, or to reactions of helplessness and 'giving up'. Others have argued in terms of artefacts, such as homogamy between spouses (i.e. the similarity of marital partners in sociological, psychological and physical traits), or the fact that partners had joint unfavourable environments (e.g. they breathed the same unhealthy air or both had poor diets).

However, there also seems very little doubt that bereavement is stressful. Longitudinal studies have consistently identified a variety of strains associated with the loss of a spouse, ranging from financial hardships, to social constraints, to problems in the care of bereaved children (Stroebe *et al.* 1993). Systematic analysis of types of stressor encountered by bereaved people has been provided by M. Stroebe and Schut (1999). Criticizing traditional theoretical approaches, these investigators argued that coming to terms with the death of a close person necessitates confrontation with two types of stressor, which they define as *loss-oriented* and *restoration-oriented* coping. Bereaved people have to attend not only to loss of the person him- or herself (going over the events of death, reminiscing, tending the grave, etc.), defined as loss orientation, but also to the changes that come about as a result of loss (taking on the tasks that the deceased had performed; finding new roles and identity, etc.), defined as restoration orientation. A process of oscillation in confronting vs avoiding these two stressors was postulated as critical to successful adaptation.

The results outlined above in relation to risk factors for poor bereavement outcome (low self-esteem, lack of social support, a sudden loss, etc.) can easily be interpreted within a more general stress framework. Thus, traumatic deaths are particularly difficult for survivors to come to terms with, and are associated with high rates of debility (Jacobs 1999). That such circumstances are more stressful for survivors than the peaceful death of an elderly person 'in the fullness of time' seems self-evident. Moreover, such results suggest that it is persons with inadequate coping resources, for example, those people who hold the belief that they have little control over events, who feel particularly unable to cope with the stressful circumstances of bereavement (W. Stroebe and Stroebe 1993).

WHAT MAKES CRITICAL LIFE EVENTS STRESSFUL?

By relating the incidence of illness to specific stressful events, research on the health impact of critical life events evaded the thorny issue of specifying why certain psychological experiences are stressful, how the organism recognizes stressful events and distinguishes them from positive events, and how interindividual differences in reactions to stress can be explained. Thus, while it appears quite plausible that the physical stressors used by Selye, such as extreme cold or the injection of non-lethal amounts of toxic fluids, should challenge the defence systems of an organism, it is less obvious why the death of a partner or the loss of a job should have a similar impact.

These issues have been addressed by psychological approaches to stress which analyse the cognitive processes that mediate between life events and stress. Interactional approaches take the general view that stress is the result of a perceived mismatch between environmental demands and the resources available to the individual in dealing with these demands (e.g. French and Kahn 1962; Lazarus and Folkman 1984). A more specific theory developed by Seligman and his collaborators (Seligman 1975; Abramson *et al.* 1978; Peterson and Seligman 1987) identified perceived lack of control as a key characteristic of stressful situations.

Stress as a person–environment interaction

For several decades, Lazarus (e.g. Lazarus and Folkman 1984) has been the chief proponent of the interactional view of stress. According to Lazarus and Folkman's widely accepted definition, 'Psychological stress is a particular relationship between the person and the environment that is appraised by the individual as taxing or exceeding his or her resources and endangering his or her well-being' (1984: 19). Thus the extent of the stress experienced in a given situation does not depend solely on the demands of the situation or on the resources of the person, but on the relationship between demands and resources as perceived (appraised) by the individual. This is not meant to imply, however, that situations do not differ in the extent to which they are likely to be experienced as stressful.

The two central processes in Lazarus's theory that determine the extent of stress experiences in a given situation are cognitive appraisal and coping. *Cognitive appraisal* is an evaluative process which determines why and to what extent a particular situation is perceived as stressful by a given individual. Lazarus distinguishes three basic forms of appraisal, 'primary appraisal', 'secondary appraisal' and 'reappraisal'. In primary appraisal, individuals categorize a given situation with respect to its significance for their well-being and decide whether the situation is irrelevant, positive or potentially harmful. In secondary appraisal they evaluate the potential threat in terms of their coping resources and also decide on coping options.

Lazarus and Folkman (1984) emphasize that primary and secondary appraisal processes typically occur concurrently. Thus, when confronted with environmental demands individuals evaluate whether the demands pose a potential threat and whether sufficient coping resources are available to cope with them. If they find the environmental demands taxing or threatening, and at the same time view their coping resources as inadequate, they perceive themselves to be under stress, an experience which usually results in negative emotions. Thus, both the evaluation of a situation as stressful, and the intensity of the stress experience depend to some extent on the individual's evaluation of relevant coping resources.

The notion of reappraisal was introduced to emphasize that cognitive appraisal processes are in a permanent state of flux, due to new inputs. Thus the original appraisal of a situation may change as new information about the situation or about the impact of one's own behaviour is received. The realization that what one took to be symptoms of angina pectoris turned out to be only a bad case of heartburn will lead to a reappraisal of the threat signalled by the symptoms.

When a situation has been appraised as stressful, individuals have to do something to master the situation and/or to control their emotional reactions to the situation. These processes of responding to stressful demands have been called *coping processes*. Lazarus and Folkman (1984) distinguish two basic forms of coping: problem-focused coping and emotion-focused coping. Coping is problem-focused when it is directed at managing and altering the problem that is causing distress. For example, a student who is worried about an impending exam will do everything to be well prepared (e.g. attend classes, join a work group). However, the student might also be so anxious that he or she begins to have trouble sleeping or is unable to concentrate. In order to reduce this emotional distress, the student may engage in a range of emotion-focused forms of coping. These could include cognitive operations such as attempts to reappraise the situation as less threatening. But they may also include actions such as taking sleeping pills, smoking or drinking alcohol in order to cope with the emotional distress and calm his or her nerves.

The extent to which the situation is experienced as stressful, as well as the individual's success in mastering it, will depend on his or her *coping resources*. Lazarus and Folkman (1984) distinguish resources that are primarily properties of the person and resources that are primarily environmental.

The person-resources include physical resources such as health and energy, psychological resources such as positive beliefs (e.g. positive self-concept, belief in control) and competencies such as problem-solving and social skills. Examples of environmental resources are material resources (e.g. money) and social support.

It is worth noting that there are important similarities between the cognitive stress model of Lazarus and Folkman (1984) and models of health behaviour such as the health belief model (p. 18) and protection motivation theory (p. 23). This overlap is hardly surprising because both types of theories have been developed to explain how individuals evaluate threats, and how these evaluations determine the way in which people deal with threatening situations. Thus the process of primary appraisal in cognitive stress theory, though much broader (i.e. not restricted to health threats), is structurally similar to the process of threat appraisal as conceptualized for health threats by the health belief model or protection motivation theory discussed earlier. According to models of health behaviour, the probability that an individual engages in a given behaviour to avoid some health threat will depend on the individual's assessment of whether he or she is susceptible to the particular illness and on his or her perception of the severity of the consequences of getting the disease.

The concept of secondary appraisal in cognitive stress theory shares some similarities with the construct of coping appraisal in the revised version of the health protection model (p. 24). Like secondary appraisal, coping appraisal involves both the assessment of whether one has the ability to perform a coping response and of whether the coping response is effective in reducing the threat. However, the inventory of coping strategies incorporated in the cognitive stress model is much broader than the actions assumed by models of health behaviour. Models of health behaviour focus on one coping strategy only, namely problem-oriented coping behaviour designed to reduce or avoid the health threat. Emotion-focused coping, at least if used exclusively, would be considered dysfunctional from the perspective of health behaviour models, because it would not directly contribute to the reduction in health risk. In fact one of the rationales which motivated the development of models of health behaviour was to investigate strategies of persuasion which would motivate problem-oriented coping rather than emotion-focused coping or problem avoidance.

The cognitive stress model developed by Lazarus and his colleagues offers a general framework for the analysis of psychological stress. Although the model identifies many important general principles of stress and coping, its high level of generality can be a disadvantage in research that attempts to use the model to derive testable predictions for specific stressful life events. Therefore a number of more specific stress theories have been developed that either apply the interactive approach to specific life events (e.g. the Deficit Model of Bereavement; Stroebe and Stroebe 1987, or the Person–Environment Fit Model of Work Stress; Caplan 1983) and/or specify more accurately those aspects of a situation that determine the intensity and persistence of the stress experience (e.g. Theory of Learned Helplessness; Seligman 1975). I will focus on the theory of learned helplessness because it has rivalled the model of Lazarus as a major influence on stress research.

Stress as learned helplessness

Although Seligman's (1975; Peterson *et al.* 1993) original interest was in the causes of depression rather than stress ('stress' does not appear as a term in the subject index of his 1975 book), his analysis of the conditions under which life events can result in depression identified perceived lack of control as an essential characteristic of situations that are stressful. The original formulation of the learned helplessness model was derived from escape-avoidance research conducted with animals. These experiments showed that while normal animals, exposed to electric shocks which they can escape, learn to escape after a few shocks, animals that had previously experienced unavoidable shock do not seem to learn the escape response. Later research demonstrated that repeated experiences of uncontrollability had similar effects on humans (e.g. Hiroto 1974; Hiroto and Seligman 1975).

Seligman developed the learned helplessness model as a unified theoretical framework which integrated the data from animal and human research. The basic assumption is that when people or animals experience an event that they cannot control, they develop an expectation of lack of control in similar future situations. This learning results in the helplessness syndrome consisting of motivational, cognitive and emotional deficits: if the persons or animals have learned that the escape from aversive stimulation occurs independent of responses, they will not try very hard to initiate a response that can produce relief; they will also fail to learn new responses that would help them to avoid aversive outcomes and they will react to the traumatic experience first with fear and then depression. On the basis of the similarity of the symptoms of learned helplessness and depression, Seligman proposed that learned helplessness was a major cause of reactive depression.

The extension of the learned helplessness model to depression raised a number of problems. Seligman (1975) had originally emphasized that it was the uncontrollability rather than the aversiveness of outcomes which was responsible for the motivational and emotional deficits. It seemed implausible, however, that people would get depressed because uncontrollable good things tended to happen to them. Furthermore, the view that depressive persons feel helpless is inconsistent with their tendency towards self-blame. If individuals believe that their outcomes are independent of their responses, how could depressed individuals feel responsible for these outcomes? Another inadequacy of the old helplessness model concerned the generality of helplessness across situations and duration over time (Abramson *et al.* 1978). The model does not permit predictions about the conditions under which uncontrollability leads to long-term and broadly generalized helplessness symptoms rather than temporary helplessness that may only concern a very restricted sphere of life (Försterling 1988).

To solve these problems, a cognitive revision of the model was suggested by Abramson and colleagues (1978). According to the revised model, the relation between the experience of uncontrollability and depressive symptoms is mediated by individuals' causal attributions, that is, their interpretations of the reasons for their failure to control a given situation which implies aversive outcomes (Abramson *et al.* 1978). Three attributional dimensions are assumed to be important in producing helplessness: internality, stability and globality. For example, a person who loses his or her job might have reasons to attribute this either internally (e.g. personal incompetence) or externally (bankruptcy of the firm he or she worked for). While he or she might feel depressed in either situation, the attribution to personal incompetence is most likely to result in loss of self-esteem. Personal incompetence would also be a more stable cause than a bankruptcy. While it is relatively unlikely that a future employer would also have to close down, personal incompetence is a stable condition that would also be a problem with the next employer. Globality refers to the extent to which helplessness is confined to specific areas. For example, if an individual merely felt incompetent with regard to a very specific line of work, and that he or she would do much better by changing to another line, helplessness would be much less pervasive than if the individual felt generally incompetent to work in his or her chosen occupation. Finally, the severity and intensity of depressive symptoms will be the greater, the more important and potentially aversive the situation is in which helplessness is experienced.

Thus, according to the attributional theory of learned helplessness, it is not the aversiveness of a negative life event that results in stress and depression, but rather the experience of lack of control induced by negative events that are attributed to internal, stable and global causes. The pre-helplessness phase, in which the individual expends effort to bring the situation under control, is characterized by ongoing stress. During this phase individuals will try to cope with the threat, either by problem-focused coping or by emotion-focused coping. Learned helplessness, when the individual stops trying to cope, is analogous to the phase of exhaustion of resources described by Selye. People often do recover and manage to re-establish control. But the more the individual attributes the helplessness to internal, stable and global causes, the more the stressful experience will result in enduring depressive reactions with the associated cognitive and emotional consequences.

The attributional model further suggested that a characteristic *attributional style* may exist that disposes individuals towards reacting with depression to stressful life events. Seligman and colleagues (e.g. Abramson *et al.* 1978) argued that depression-prone individuals should tend to attribute aversive events to internal, global and stable causes. Two measures of this pessimistic explanatory style were developed: a self-report questionnaire called the Attributional Style Questionnaire (ASQ) and a content analysis procedure called the CAVE (Content Analysis of Verbatim Explanations) technique.

The ASQ presents respondents with six bad events (e.g. you meet a friend who acts hostilely towards you) and six good events (e.g. you did a project which is highly praised). Respondents are asked to imagine themselves in these situations and to provide causal explanations for these events. They are then required to rate each cause in terms of internality, stability and globality. Explanatory style is inferred from the respondents' scores across the three attributional dimensions, computing separate averages for good and bad events. With the CAVE technique, verbatim quotes of causal attributions for good or bad events of the sample of interest are rated by judges in terms of their internality, stability and globality. This technique allows researchers to assess attributional style on the basis of interview material collected for a completely different purpose.

The relationship between attributional style and depression has been observed in numerous studies. A meta-analysis of more than 100 studies found moderate correlations between the predicted attributional pattern and depression (Sweeney et al. 1986). However, critics of the revised theory of learned helplessness doubt the importance of attributions as mediators of depression. In particular, Brewin (1988) argued that some events may have such a major impact on their own account that causal cognitions are relatively unimportant in mediating the emotional response. Thus, there are life events which are so far beyond the range of usual human experience that they would be markedly distressing to almost anyone; examples would be extreme situations as the result of acts of war, collective disasters and accidents, crimes of violence or the violent loss of a loved one. And yet, while powerful events such as the loss of a child or spouse are stressful and saddening for nearly everybody, only a minority of those affected by loss react with enduring depression and health deterioration. It seems plausible that the depressive pattern of attributions is associated with a weakened resistance to, and poorer recovery from, depression. Unfortunately, the theory is somewhat vague about the precise nature of these other factors. Some of these concerns have been addressed in yet another reformulation of the helplessness theory, called the hopelessness theory of depression (Abramson et al. 1989).

In their later research, Seligman and colleagues have begun to relate the pessimistic attributional style to physical illness and even mortality using the CAVE technique to assess attributional style (e.g. Peterson and Seligman 1987; Peterson et al. 1988; for a review, see Peterson et al. 1993). In doing so, Seligman addressed an important claim made in his 1975 book, namely, that learned helplessness would result in an impairment of physical as well as mental health.

In one study the age at death of members of the Baseball Hall of Fame whose playing career occurred between 1900 and 1950 was related to their characteristic attributional style (Peterson and Seligman 1987). Attributional style could be assessed for 24 players on the basis of verbatim quotes reported in sports pages. Peterson and Seligman found a marginally significant correlation ($r = .26$) between the extent to which players offered internal, stable and global explanations for bad events and life expectancy. Players who offered external, unstable and specific explanations for good events also lived shorter lives ($r = .45$).

In another study, attributional style was assessed from interviews completed at the age of 25 years by 99 graduates of Harvard University from the classes of 1942 to 1944, who were mentally and physically fit at the time of the interview. Men who at age 25 explained bad events by referring to their own internal, stable and global negative qualities had significantly poorer health some 20 to 35 years later. Thus, health status assessed by the individual's personal physician at age 45 showed a significant correlation of .37 with pessimistic explanatory style measured at age 25. Health status measured at age 60 correlated .25 with the same attributional style scores. These findings suggest that pessimistic attributional style in early adulthood is a risk factor for poor physical health in middle and late adulthood. However, although Peterson and Seligman (1987) discuss various pathways between explanatory style and physical well-being, there is little empirical evidence concerning the processes which might mediate this relationship.

Conclusions

Both Lazarus and Seligman have developed theories that identify the cognitive processes underlying the stress experience and make predictions with regard to the initiation of coping behaviours. According to the cognitive stress theory of Lazarus, a situation is stressful if it is potentially harmful and if the individual perceives that his or her resources are insufficient to prevent the aversive outcome. While the original theory of learned helplessness conceived of stress as resulting from uncontrollability regardless of whether the event implied harmful or positive outcomes, the stress definition of the revised model is consistent with that of Lazarus and his colleagues in perceiving stress as resulting from the risk of encountering aversive consequences. The revised version of learned helplessness theory further specifies the conditions under which such *aversive* situations are likely to result in persistent feelings of hopelessness and depression. The theory suggests that perceived lack of control over aversive events that is attributed to internal, stable and global causes is likely to result in anxiety and depression. The model further assumes that a characteristic attributional style exists which constitutes a risk factor for depression as well as poor physical health.

With regard to coping, both theories imply that when individuals are exposed to potentially threatening situations, they will initiate coping strategies to contain the threat. These strategies might consist of problem-oriented coping behaviours but they could also involve emotion-oriented coping behaviours. In addition, the learned helplessness model makes the prediction that in chronic stress situations, coping activities will essentially be abandoned if the causes of uncontrollability are perceived as internal, stable and global.

HOW DOES PSYCHOSOCIAL STRESS AFFECT HEALTH?

Stressful life events like the loss of a job or the death of a spouse do not operate on one's bodily system in the same manner as the noxious physical or chemical stimuli studied by Selye. And yet, as we have seen earlier, there can be little doubt that the experience of stressful life events is associated with an increased risk of a wide range of physical and mental disorders. There are two types of mechanisms which mediate the impact of psychosocial stress on health: first, stress can affect health directly through changes in the body's physiology. Second, stress can affect health indirectly through changes in individual behaviour.

Physiological responses to stress

In evolutionary terms, the function of physiological reactions to stress appears to have been to prepare the organism for action. If one assumes that bodily injuries frequently occur in a context in which an animal has to fight or flee, it makes sense that the stress responses consist mainly of catabolic processes, that is, processes involved in the expenditure of energy from reserves stored in the body. It is therefore not surprising that the sympathetic–adrenal–medullary system and the pituitary–adrenocortical system are the two major neuroendocrine systems that are responsible for many of the physiological changes associated with stress. Endocrine refers to the internal secretion of biologically active substances or hormones. Hormones are chemical substances which are released from an endocrine gland (e.g. pituitary) into the bloodstream and act on a distant target site.

Activation of the *sympathetic–adrenal–medullary system* leads to an increase in the secretion of two hormones, norepinephrine and epinephrine. The release of these catecholamines stimulates cardiovascular activity and raises blood pressure. The heart beats faster, increasing the amount of blood pumped with each beat. By constricting peripheral blood vessels and those leading to the gastrointestinal tract, blood pressure is raised. At the same time, the arteries serving muscles (including the coronary arteries of the heart muscle) are dilated, thus increasing their blood supply. Catecholamines also relax air passages. Breathing becomes faster and deeper, the bronchioles of the lungs dilate, and the secretion of mucus in the air passages decreases. Thus more oxygen is available for the metabolism. Catecholamines also cause the liberation of glucose (one of the major sources of usable energy) from the liver, thus availing the muscles of large energy resources. One further effect, which is quite advantageous in the case of physical injury, is that catecholamines increase the tendency of the blood to coagulate.

The activation of the *pituitary–adrenal–cortical system* leads to increases in the secretion and release of corticosteroids from the adrenal cortex. For the physiology of stress reactions, the most interesting corticosteroid is cortisol. Cortisol is important for energy mobilization of the body. It promotes the synthesis of glucose from the liver. Cortisol also mobilizes the fat stores from adipose tissues and increases the level of serum lipids, that is, fat-like substances in the blood such as triglycerides and cholesterol, which also provide energy for skeletal and heart muscles.

The hormones released by sympathetic–adrenal–medullary and the pituitary–adrenal–cortical systems have also been implicated in the modulation of the immune system. Since inflammation of the affected areas (one of the painful side effects of an active immune system) would tend to interfere with fight or flight responses, one could speculate that the prevention of such interference might initially be more important than the destruction of the intruding agent. Suppression of pain is also helped by endogenous opiates, which are morphine-like peptides that are released in the brain in response to stress (O'Leary 1990). Stress-induced opiate activation has been shown to reduce pain reactivity in humans (Bandura *et al.* 1987). There is some evidence that these endogenous opiates also have a suppressive effect on the immune system (O'Leary 1990).

The activation of these physiological stress systems prepares the organism for combat or escape. However, the vigorous physical activity which the stress response prepares us for is rarely an appropriate response to cope with the typical stressful life events encountered today. Instead, in many stressful situations the stress response is likely to hinder rather than help coping and adjustment. Furthermore, while stress responses in the distant past were typically activated by transitory stressors, today many stressors are chronic rather than acute, resulting in more extended elevations of arousal levels. This can impair the functioning of various organ systems, including the immune system, leaving the organism open to infections.

Behavioural responses to stress

The experience of stress motivates individuals to engage in a variety of behavioural strategies which aim to reduce the threat or to cope with the emotions aroused by the potentially aversive experience. For example, an executive who is competing for an important promotion will attempt to enhance chances of success by working longer hours and by generally increasing the quality of his or her performance. When the workload becomes so extreme that people abandon regular meals and just 'grab a quick bite' whenever there is time, when they resort to tranquillizers, cigarettes or alcohol to calm down or go to sleep, coping behaviour can become deleterious to their health.

The assumption that individuals who are under stress are more likely to engage in these kinds of unhealthy behaviour patterns is supported by findings from a survey of a probability sample reported by Cohen and Williamson (1988). In this study, small but statistically significant correlations were observed between perceived stress and shorter periods of sleep, infrequent consumption of breakfast, increased quantity of alcohol consumption, and greater frequency of usage of illicit drugs. Marginally significant relations were also found between stress and (a) smoking and (b) lack of physical exercise.

Similarly, the widows and widowers who participated in the Tübingen Longitudinal Study of Bereavement reported changes in tranquillizer use, smoking and alcohol consumption (Table 6.2). While widows mainly increased their use of tranquillizers and sleeping pills, widowers reported increases in alcohol consumption and smoking. This pattern is consistent with epidemiological data showing that liver cirrhosis is one of the causes of death in which widowers show the greatest excess over married men (M. Stroebe and Stroebe 1993). It is also consistent with reports from relapsed addicts that stress often immediately preceded their return to drug use (e.g. Condiotte and Lichtenstein 1981; Shiffman 1982; Baer and Lichtenstein 1988; Bliss *et al.* 1989). Behavioural factors such as alcohol use and carelessness probably play a role in the relatively high accident rates of people under stress.

Finally, individuals under stress are also likely to draw on their social resources and seek out social support (e.g. Amirkhan 1990). Increased interaction with others results in greater probability of exposure to infectious

Table 6.2 Percentage of men and women interviewed who specified an increase in their use of tranquillizers, sleeping tablets, alcoholic beverages or cigarettes[a]

	Women		Men	
	Married (n = 30)	Widowed (n = 30)	Married (n = 30)	Widowed (n = 30)
Tranquillizers	0.0	24.1	0.0	10.0
Sleeping tablets	3.3	13.3	3.3	6.9
Alcoholic beverages	3.3	6.7	3.3	17.2
Smoking	10.0	17.2	10.0	30.0

[a] Data from the first interviews of the Tübingen Longitudinal Study of Bereavement. Widowed respondents were asked for an increase in use since the death of their partner. Married respondents were asked for increases during the comparable time period.

agents and consequent infection. However, the need to seek out social support under stress is to some extent also influenced by individual differences in affiliative tendencies and the nature of the stressor. Under some conditions, stress could therefore also lead to social withdrawal and decreased risk of exposure to infections.

Stress and disease

The cost of stress is expressed in terms of its effect on health and well-being. Stress has been associated both with impairments in psychological and physical health. With regard to psychological health there is extensive evidence from studies using life stress inventories and assessments of specific life events that chronic stress predicts subsequent depression (for a review, see Kessler 1997). With regard to physical health, the disorders which have attracted most attention are infections, coronary heart disease, alimentary conditions such as dyspepsia and ulcers, and psychopathological problems such as depression. Stress has also been suspected to be important for many other diseases including diabetes mellitus, asthma, and even cancer. However, there is still debate about the causal role of stress in the development of various diseases and the mechanisms that mediate this relationship. I will therefore merely illustrate these stress effects using the role of stress in infections and in coronary heart disease as examples.

Stress, immune functioning, and infectious disease

Infections are caused by some infectious agent, but exposure to such agents does not always cause infection. Whether the individual exposed to an infectious agent actually develops an infection depends on his or her susceptibility to infections, which is primarily mediated by the immune system. There are numerous factors which affect an individual's susceptibility to disease (e.g. prior exposure to the micro-organism and the development of immunity, nutritional status of the host, a wide range of genetic factors). Since Selye's classic work on the effect of stress on the immune system, exposure to stress has to be included among the determinants of individual susceptibility. The three major pathways through which stress influences the immune system are direct innervation of the central nervous system and immune system (nerves ending at immune organs such as the thymus, bone marrow, spleen, and even lymph nodes), the release of hormones (e.g. epinephrine, norepinephrine, cortisol, growth hormones, prolactin), and behaviour (health behaviour).

Research on the impact of stress on susceptibility to immune system-mediated disease such as infections has assessed the effects of stress *either* on indicators of the functioning of the immune system *or* on disease outcome. There are very few studies which have attempted to assess both the impact of stress on disease and the role of immunological changes in mediating this relationship (e.g. Kemeny *et al.* 1989; Cohen *et al.* 1998). I will first discuss studies of the relation between stress and immune functioning, and then go on to consider stress effects on the onset and progression of infectious disease.

Psychoneuroimmunological research on humans has focused on the study of immune processes occurring in circulating peripheral blood which transports the immune components between organs of the immune system and sites of inflammation. The general function of the immune system is to protect the body from damage by invading micro-orgamisms. These foreign substances are called antigens and include bacteria, viruses, tumour cells and toxins. The identification and elimination of antigens is accomplished by several types of lymphocytes (white blood cells). To measure the functioning of the immune system, researchers use either quantitative or functional measures.

Quantitative or *enumerative* tests of the immune system involve counting the number or percentages of different types of immune cells such as T-helper cells, suppressor/cytotoxic T-helper cells and natural killer (NK) cells in the peripheral blood (Cohen and Herbert 1996). Quantifying the number of circulating cells is important for two reasons: first, the body needs a minimum number of each type of immune cell to respond adequately to antigenic response, and second, an optimal response requires a balance of the various cell types. Since these different sub-groups perform specialized functions, it is not possible to use a single measure to determine global immunological competence (Cohen and Williamson 1991; Cohen and Herbert 1996).

Functional measures examine the performance of certain immune cells. The ability of lymphocytes to proliferate rapidly in the face of antigenic challenge is essential to an adequate immune response. Lymphocytic proliferation is a test of cellular immunity that examines how effectively lymphocytes divide when stimulated through incubation with mitogens such as phytohemagglutinin (PHA) or concanavalin A (Con A). Mitogens are substances which are capable of inducing lymphocytes to divide. It is assumed that greater proliferation indicates more effective cell function. The ability of natural killer cells to destroy tumour cells is assessed by incubating natural killer cells with tumour cells. These tests are *in vitro* tests. Cells are removed from the body and their function is studied in the laboratory (Cohen and Herbert 1996; Uchino *et al.* 1996).

There is now ample empirical support for the assumption that psycho-social stress is associated with an impairment of the functioning of the immune system (Kiecolt-Glaser and Glaser 1991; Glaser and Kiecolt-Glaser 1994; Cohen and Herbert 1996). Studies of such diverse groups as bereaved spouses, separated and divorced men and women, psychiatric patients with a major depression, and family care givers of Alzheimer's disease victims have demonstrated that members of such groups are more distressed and show relatively poorer immune functions than well-matched commun-ity counterparts (e.g. Stein *et al.* 1985; Kiecolt-Glaser *et al.* 1987, 1988). Other researchers have observed modest suppression of immune function in medical students during examinations, compared to similar measures taken one month previously when students were less distressed (e.g. Glaser *et al.* 1985). There is also increasing evidence that changes in immune response occur as a function of prolonged and repeated exposure to stress (e.g. Kiecolt-Glaser *et al.* 1987; McKinnon *et al.* 1989). For example, McKinnon and colleagues (1989) found impairment in immune func-tions (relative to a matched control group) in people who lived near the nuclear power station at Three Mile Island and had been exposed to more than six years of stressful uncertainty associated with the accident at this station.

These findings demonstrate the effects of psychological stress on the immune system. It is less clear, however, whether these changes in immune functions really lead to the development of illness (Cohen and Williamson 1991). Although we know that gross alterations in immunity can be asso-ciated with greater morbidity and mortality (e.g. AIDS), little is known about the actual health consequences of these more modest changes in immune functions. It is therefore important to show that psychological stress is related to disease outcome.

The best-controlled studies of the role of stress in increasing suscept-ibility to infection are experimental studies in which volunteers whose exposure to stressful life events has been assessed are exposed to some virus, typically a cold or influenza virus (Cohen *et al.* 1993, 1998). In one of these studies, Cohen *et al.* (1993) exposed 420 male and female volun-teers through a nasal drip to either a cold virus or a saline solution (i.e. placebo group). These volunteers entered quarantine for two days before and the seven days after the viral challenge or saline exposure. Psycho-logical stress was measured by self-reported number of major stressful life events during the previous 12 months, perceptions of current demands exceeding capabilities to cope, and current negative affect. There were two health outcomes in this study, namely infection and clinical disease. Infec-tions result from the multiplication of the invading micro-organism. How-ever, it is possible for a person to be infected without developing clinical symptoms. Whereas none of the individuals in the saline-control group developed an infection, there was a clear association between level of stress and health outcome for those who were exposed to the virus: highly stressed individuals had a significantly higher risk of infection and of developing a cold than persons who were less stressed. Controlling for

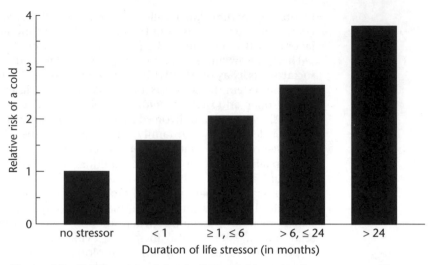

Figure 6.2   Relative risk of developing a cold contrasting persons with stressors of varying duration with those without any stressor.
Source: Cohen *et al.* (1998).

health practices did not reduce the association between stress and susceptibility to illness.

Cohen and his colleagues (1998) recently replicated this study with 276 volunteers who again entered quarantine for six days, one day before being exposed to the virus and five days following the viral challenge. Life stressors were assessed by a standardized semi-structured interview, the Life Events and Difficulties Schedule (LEDS) (Brown and Harris 1989) which allows one to make a reliable classification of stressors in terms of severity and chronicity. Eighty-four per cent of the participants developed an infection but only 40 per cent of the participants actually developed colds. With regard to the influence of stress on susceptibility to disease, an interesting difference emerged between acute and chronic stressors. Whereas there was no association between acute events and susceptibility, the experience of chronic stressors lasting one month or longer was associated with increased risk of infection. Furthermore, the risk of infection increased significantly with the duration of the life stressor (Figure 6.2).

This study is also exemplary in that it assessed the role of a range of potential mediating variables in accounting for the association between stress and risk of infection. To qualify as a potential mediator of the stress–infection–susceptibility relationship, a variable has to be associated with stress and with risk of infection. Thus, one has to demonstrate that the assumed mediator is influenced by stress and that it in turn influences the individual's susceptibility to stress. Finally, it has to be demonstrated that if one statistically controls for this variable in tests of the stress–infection relationship, this reduces or even eliminates this relationship.

Many of the health practices measured (e.g. smoking, exercising, sleep efficiency) were significantly associated with both chronic stress and increased risk of infection. And yet, statistically controlling for these health practices resulted in only minor reductions of the association between chronic stress and susceptibility to infection. Thus, as in their previous study, the authors concluded that the association between stress and susceptibility to colds was not 'primarily mediated by health practices' (Cohen et al. 1998: 222). More puzzling was the finding that chronic stressors in this study were not found to be associated with elevated levels of stress hormones such as epinephrine, norepinephrine, or cortisol. Changes in these stress hormones therefore could not have mediated the relationship between stress and health, even though elevated levels in these hormones were associated with greater risks in colds. Thus, there is now convincing evidence that stress, and particularly chronic stress experiences, are associated with an increased susceptibility to infectious disease. However, despite some support for the assumed impact of stress on endocrine, immune and behavioural variables, there is so far little direct evidence that any of these variables mediate the association between stress and infection.

Stress and coronary heart disease

There are two major forms of coronary heart disease, namely angina pectoris and myocardial infarction. The symptoms of angina pectoris (literally, 'strangling of the chest') are periodic attacks of distinctive chest pain, usually situated behind the sternum and radiating to the chest and left shoulder. Patients suffering from angina pectoris complain of tightening, or pressure, or a 'band' around the chest. Attacks of angina pectoris are typically brought on by physical exercise and emotional exertion and usually disappear within one to two minutes or, at most, five to ten minutes of stopping exertion. They are quickly relieved by rest or medication aimed at dilating blood vessels and reducing blood pressure. The major cause of angina pectoris is an insufficient supply of oxygen to the heart due to atherosclerosis. Attacks of angina pectoris rarely involve permanent damage to the heart muscle.

If plaque grows at a rate exceeding the blood supply available for the nutrition of its cells, it is likely to rupture and form the basis for a thrombosis, which will then completely block an already narrow passage. Such ruptures may also be the result of haemodynamic factors such as high levels of arterial blood pressure (Herd 1978). The formation of blood clots which obstruct the artery and diminish the blood supply to the left ventricle of the heart are the most frequent cause of myocardial infarction, a necrosis (death) of the heart tissue caused by a long-lasting insufficiency of the oxygen supply. Myocardial infarction is one of the major causes of death in most industrialized nations.

Much of the evidence for the relationship between stress and coronary heart disease derives from retrospective studies that use life event scales and are therefore open to methodological criticism (e.g. Rahe and Lind 1971; Rahe and Paasikivi 1971; Theorell and Rahe 1971; Rahe et al. 1974). For example, Rahe and colleagues (1974) gathered life change data on more than 200 survivors of myocardial infarctions and a similar number of cases of abrupt coronary death in Helsinki. Next of kin, most of whom were spouses, provided the life change data for the victims of sudden deaths. Results indicated marked elevation in the magnitude of total life changes during the months prior to infarction compared to the same time period one year earlier. The major problem with this type of study is that the retrospective assessment of life events is likely to be influenced by the respondent's knowledge of the occurrence of an illness. Since the belief that stress is bad for coronary health is part of common culture, respondents inclined to search for explanations for their own or their partner's illness are likely to remember more stressful life events as having occurred just prior to the event.

There are now, however, also many studies on the impact of stress on heart disease which used prospective designs on individuals who were already at high risk (e.g. Byrne *et al.* 1981; Ruberman *et al.* 1984). For example, Byrne and colleagues (1981) examined a cohort of 120 men and women who survived heart attacks. At the first interview, which took place 10 to 14 days following their admission into a coronary care unit, these patients responded to an extensive questionnaire that also contained questions about personal, social and financial worries prior to the heart attack which, in the judgement of the patients, may have contributed to the attack. Of the 102 members of the original sample who could be located eight months later, 20 had a recurrence of the heart disease, and seven had died as a direct consequence of the heart attack. The individuals who had a recurrence of the disease, whether fatal or non-fatal, had reported significantly more worries at the first interview than people who had not suffered a recurrence. Somewhat similar findings were obtained in a large study reported by Ruberman *et al.* (1984). Thus, even though the evidence from retrospective studies of the impact of cumulative life stress on coronary heart disease is somewhat problematic, results from studies of the impact of bereavement and from prospective studies with high-risk groups provide consistent evidence on the relationship between psychosocial stress and heart disease.

These findings from human studies are complemented by results from animal experiments which provide evidence of the importance of experimentally manipulated psychological stress in the development of atherosclerosis. In a series of studies Clarkson *et al.* (1987) subjected cynomolgus monkey colonies to stress by repeatedly reshuffling groups and breaking up stable social structures. Dominant monkeys in unstable and therefore stressful social situations developed increased coronary atherosclerosis in comparison with both subordinates who probably did not struggle very hard to achieve dominance and dominant monkeys in socially stable groups. The administration of beta-blockers reduced the tendency to develop atherosclerosis.

There are several *mechanisms* by which stress can contribute to coronary heart disease. Stress is likely to accelerate the development of atherosclerosis, by increasing the secretion of catecholamines and cortisol (both involved in mobilizing fat stores) and thus increasing the level of serum lipids. An extensive review of research on the impact of stress on the level of serum lipids found that the majority of studies showed significant increases in cholesterol (and especially free fatty acid levels) in response to emotional arousal induced by a variety of stressors (Dimsdale and Herd 1982). Catecholamines also increase the tendency of blood to coagulate, which may contribute to the formation of blood clots and consequent blocking of arteries, especially arteries already narrowed due to the formation of atherosclerotic plaque.

Another line of argument has proposed that an exaggerated *psychophysiological reactivity* to behavioural challenge may be implicated in the development of major cardiovascular disorders such as coronary heart disease and essential hypertension (Manuck and Krantz 1986; Blascovich and Katkin 1995). According to this hypothesis, repeated physiological reactions involving excessive heart rate and/or pressor responses to behavioural stressors promote arterial 'injury' through haemodynamic forces such as turbulence and sheer stress. Cardiovascular reactivity is measured in terms of heart rate, blood pressure or other cardiovascular changes in response to stress, as opposed to measuring only resting levels of these variables.

Evidence for the involvement of physiological reactivity in the development of atherosclerosis comes from animal as well as human studies. Clarkson *et al.* (1986) measured cardiac reactivity in two cohorts of male and female cynomolgus monkeys who were fed a moderately atherogenic diet (i.e. likely to result in atherosclerosis) for approximately two years. These monkeys are particularly suitable for this kind of study because they are known to be highly susceptible to the development of diet-induced atherosclerosis. Heart rate measurements were obtained on each animal under both resting and stressful conditions. 'High' and 'low' heart rate reactors only differed in their responsiveness to the stress situation. They did not differ in average heart rate during baseline measurement. When the coronary arteries of 'high' and 'low' heart-rate reactive animals were investigated at the end of the two-year period, the 'high' heart rate reactors had roughly twice the coronary artery atherosclerosis of the 'low' reactors.

Since physiological reactivity is typically not assessed in epidemiological studies, there is little evidence on the reactivity–CHD relationship in human beings. Probably the only prospective study in which haemodynamic reactivity to stress was assessed and later related to the development of coronary heart disease was reported by Keys *et al.* (1971). These authors reported that the magnitude of participants' diastolic blood pressure response to cold immersion (the cold pressor test) was significantly associated with development of CHD at a 23-year follow up.

In a more recent cross-sectional study reported by Blascovich and Katkin (1995), patients who were referred for coronary angiography underwent psychological stress testing before the medical assessment. Cardiovascular reactivity assessed in terms of changes in blood pressure was a significant predictor of various indicators of the progression of atherosclerosis in these men even when traditional predictors had been controlled for.

In addition to these physiological pathways, there are also behavioural pathways that might mediate the impact of stress on coronary health. As discussed earlier (p. 226), stress is associated with a number of poor health practices which can accelerate the development of atherosclerosis. Individuals under stress are likely to increase their consumption of cigarettes and alcohol, adopt poor eating habits, and engage in very little physical exercise (e.g. Cohen and Williamson 1988).

SUMMARY AND CONCLUSIONS

The stress concept was made popular by Selye's work on the bodily responses of organisms exposed to stressors such as intensive heat or cold, non-lethal injections of toxic substances, and infections. Selye suggested that these bodily reactions to stress were non-specific and helped the organism to cope with the stressor. Diseases of adaptation characteristic of the stage of exhaustion are the price the organism has to pay for the defence against extended exposure to stressor agents.

The psychosocial approach to stress is based on the assumption that psychosocial stress results in the same kind of bodily changes which Selye observed as a consequence of tissue damage. In this tradition, evidence was generated to demonstrate that specific life events or cumulative life stress are associated with an increased risk of morbidity or even mortality.

This research related stressful life events to the incidence of illness, but did not address the question why certain psychological experiences are stressful and how the organism distinguishes stressful from positive events. This issue was later addressed by psychological theories of stress which focus on the cognitive processes that mediate between life events and stress. Two approaches were described, the cognitive stress theory of Lazarus and colleagues and the theory of learned helplessness of Seligman and colleagues. Both theories conceive of stress as resulting whenever events are appraised as potentially harmful and when individuals perceive their resources to be insufficient to prevent the aversive outcome.

The last section of the chapter addressed the question of how stressful events can be detrimental to psychological and physical health. The impact of psychosocial stress is mediated by two pathways, a direct route via the body's physiology and an indirect route, affecting health through the person's behaviour. The joint impact of these reactions to stress contributes to the development of ill health either by interacting with other causes of disease or by affecting the body's ability to resist infection.

FURTHER READING

Blascovich, J. and Katkin, E.S. (eds) (1995) *Cardiovascular Reactivity to Psychological Stress and Disease*. Washington, DC: American Psychological Association. This book evaluates the evidence concerning the cardiovascular reactivity hypothesis. This hypothesis suggests that exaggerated psychophysiological reactivity to stress may be implicated in the development of major cardiovascular disorder.

Cohen, S. and Williamson, G.M. (1991) Stress and infectious disease in humans. *Psychological Bulletin*, 109: 5–24. Comprehensive review of research on the relationship between stress and infectious disease in humans.

Cohen, S., Kessler, R.C. and Gordon, L.U. (eds) (1995) *Measuring Stress*. New York: Oxford University Press. The chapters written by experts review the psychological approaches to stress measurement.

Lazarus, R.S. and Folkman, S. (1984) *Stress, Appraisal, and Coping*. New York, NY: Springer. In this classic monograph the authors review the literature on stress as it related to the cognitive stress theory of Lazarus, Folkman and their colleagues.

Stroebe, M., Stroebe, W. and Hansson, R. (eds) (1993) *Handbook of Bereavement*. New York, NY: Cambridge University Press. This edited volume provides a comprehensive review of scientific knowledge on the psychological and psychobiological consequences of losing a loved person through death.

Watson, D. and Pennebaker, J.W. (1989) Health complaints, stress, and distress. Exploring the central role of negative affectivity. *Psychological Review*, 96: 234–54. Argues that self-report measures of both stressful life events and health complaints reflect a pervasive mood disposition to experience negative mood. While negative affectivity correlates highly with measures of symptom reporting, it seems to be unrelated to objective health indicators.

SEVEN

MODERATORS OF THE STRESS–HEALTH RELATIONSHIP

In interviews with bereaved individuals to assess the health consequences of their loss experience, I have been impressed by the tremendous differences in the way these people coped with the event, differences that were often quite unrelated to situational indicators of the severity of the event (e.g. Stroebe *et al.* 1988). Such differences in adjustment are of course consistent with the interactional concept of stress, according to which individual differences in coping styles and coping resources are as important as variations in situational demands in determining the extent to which stress is experienced. This chapter will present a more detailed discussion of coping processes and of the major coping resources which moderate the relationship between stress and ill health.

STRATEGIES OF COPING

Coping strategies or styles play an important role in an individual's physical and psychological well-being when he or she is confronted with negative or stressful life events (Endler and Parker 1990). Recent research considers coping as 'the person's cognitive and behavioural efforts to manage (reduce, minimize, master, or tolerate) the internal and external demands of the person–environment transaction that is appraised as taxing or exceeding the resources of the person' (Folkman *et al.* 1986: 572). Thus coping encompasses the cognitive and behavioural strategies which individuals use to manage both the stressful situation and the negative emotional reactions elicited by that event.

The most striking feature of this definition of coping is its breadth. Coping processes are not only assumed to include all the decisions and actions taken by an individual faced with a stressful life event but also the attendant negative emotions. The only limiting condition is that to constitute coping, these cognitive and behavioural strategies should have the function of 'managing' the stressful situation. This implies that to constitute coping, strategies should *aim* at lowering the probability of harm resulting from the stressful encounter and/or at reducing negative emotional reactions. Whether or not these strategies are successful in reaching the goal of managing the stressful situation is not part of the definition of coping.

Dimensions of coping

A great deal of research effort has been invested in the identification of basic dimensions of coping. This is not surprising, because analyses of the literature on coping or of self-reports of cognitive or behavioural coping strategies employed by samples of respondents in stressful encounters have suggested an immense variety of coping strategies. In these investigations respondents were presented with lists of coping strategies and asked to indicate which of these they used in coping with a recent stress experience. Responses were then factor-analysed. Factor analysis is a statistical procedure which allows one to identify from the intercorrelations of a set of items a smaller number of basic dimensions assumed to be responsible for these correlations.

Studies which followed such a procedure have uncovered a variety of different basic dimensions (e.g. Folkman and Lazarus 1980; Folkman *et al.* 1986a, 1986b; Amirkhan 1990; Endler and Parker 1990). In a study which resulted in the construction of one of the most widely used coping scales, the Ways of Coping Questionnaire, Folkman, Lazarus and their colleagues (1986a) identified eight distinct coping strategies (see Table 7.1). Endler and Parker (1990), on the other hand, who used a comparable procedure in the development of their Multidimensional Coping Inventory, arrived at three dimensions, namely task-oriented coping, emotion-oriented coping, and avoidance-oriented coping. The factor analytic study of Amirkhan (1990) also led to the identification of three dimensions, but these were somewhat different from those identified by Endler and Parker (1990). Amirkhan (1990) labelled his dimensions problem solving, seeking social support, and avoidance.

There are a number of reasons for these inconsistencies. Far from being an objective procedure, the outcomes of factor analyses are dependent on numerous aspects of a study, such as the composition of the item pool or of the sample of respondents, and the method of factor analysis used. Finally, researchers have great freedom in the labels they attach to their scales, so that even apparent similarities between studies are often more the result of consistencies in labelling than in the items which underlie a dimension.

And yet it is possible to infer some consensus between these studies. There seem to be a number of basic dimensions which emerge in all this research (for a review, see Parker and Endler 1992). Most studies suggest that coping has two major functions, namely to reduce the risk of harmful consequences that might result from a stressful event (i.e. problem-focused coping) and to regulate the distressing emotional reactions to the event (i.e. emotion-focused coping). These two types of coping do not

Table 7.1 The coping strategies identified by Folkman and her colleagues

Scale 1: Confrontive coping
Stood my ground and fought for
  what I wanted
Tried to get the person responsible
  to change his or her mind
I expressed anger to the person(s)
  who caused the problem
I let my feelings out somehow

Scale 2: Distancing
Made light of the situation; refused
  to get too serious about it
Went on as if nothing had
  happened
Didn't let it get to me; refused to
  think about it too much
Tried to forget the whole thing

Scale 3: Self-controlling
I tried to keep my feelings to myself
Kept others from knowing how bad
  things were
I tried to keep my feelings from
  interfering with other things too
  much

Scale 4: Seeking social support
Talked to someone to find out more
  about the situation
Talked to someone who could do
  something concrete about the
  problem
I asked a relative or friend I
  respected for advice
Talked to someone about how I was
  feeling

Scale 5: Accepting responsibility
Criticized or lectured myself
Realized I brought the problem on
  myself
I made a promise to myself that
  things would be different next
  time

Scale 6: Escape–avoidance
Wished that the situation would go
  away or somehow be over with
Hoped a miracle would happen
Had fantasies about how things
  might turn out
Tried to make myself feel better by
  eating, drinking, smoking, using
  drugs or medication, and so forth

Scale 7: Planful problem solving
I knew what had to be done, so I
  doubled my efforts to make things
  work
I made a plan of action and
  followed it
Changed something so things would
  turn out all right
Drew on my past experiences; I was
  in a similar position before

Scale 8: Positive reappraisal
Changed or grew as a person in a
  good way
I came out of the experience better
  than when I went in
Found new faith
Rediscovered what is important in
  life

Source: Adapted from Folkman *et al.* (1986a).

reflect mutually exclusive alternatives but processes that often co-occur. While problem-focused coping is usually reflected by one or two factors, there is often a wide array of emotion-focused factors. Thus, two of the strategies identified by Folkman and colleagues (1986a) appear to be clearly problem-focused (confrontive coping, planful problem solving), five are clearly emotion-focused (distancing, self-controlling, accepting responsibility, positive reappraisal, escape avoidance), and one focuses on both functions (seeking social support).

A second dimension which frequently emerges from this research is approach vs avoidance (Roth and Cohen 1986). Avoidant coping is related to several constructs with a long research history (e.g. repression-sensitization; Byrne 1961 and monitoring vs blunting; Miller 1980). An individual can confront his or her emotions (e.g. by reappraising the situation or confiding in a friend) but he or she can also avoid this confrontation using strategies such as denial, distraction or wishful thinking. Similarly, the individual can confront a health threat by undergoing some extensive diagnostic procedure or a recommended operation, but he or she might also decide that it would be better to avoid seeking a diagnosis or having an operation. The Ways of Coping Questionnaire dimensions of distancing and escape–avoidance reflect avoidance strategies, whereas confrontative coping, seeking social support, accepting responsibility and planful problem solving would seem to involve approach-based coping.

A third dimension which has typically emerged in these studies is the seeking of social support. Individuals might cope with a stressful experience alone or seek social support to help reduce the stress. As a social psychologist I would naturally like to add this social dimension to coping. However, Endler and Parker (1990) were probably right when they argued that social support should be considered a resource for coping strategies rather than a specific coping dimension.

This leaves us with a two-dimensional classification implying four categories of coping, namely problem-focused approach, problem-focused avoidance, emotion-focused approach, and emotion-focused avoidance. However, this type of representation may be somewhat misleading because it suggests that emotion-focused vs problem-focused coping form endpoints on a continuum when in fact they represent two independent dimensions. Stressful situations almost by definition arouse strong emotions which are likely to impair the ability of the individual to proceed through the decision-making and action sequence. Therefore individuals typically have to deal with problems and emotions at the same time. Whether a stress situation elicits predominantly emotion-focused or problem-focused coping will depend on the controllability of the situation. Some stress situations are characterized by the fact that there is very little the individual can do to change the situation, whereas others are controllable and elicit the full choice of coping alternatives. Moreover, it is important to note that controllability, like stress, is a person–environment interaction. Although some stress experiences may be universally uncontrollable, others may be uncontrollable only for individuals who lack some specific ability that is necessary in order to control the situation.

The differential effectiveness of strategies of coping

Given the extensive research devoted to the identification of basic dimensions of coping, it is disappointing how little is known about the differential effectiveness of these coping strategies. Even though numerous studies have related coping strategies to physical and psychological well-being following stressful encounters, few general conclusions can be drawn from this research. There are a number of conceptual and methodological reasons for the failure of this outcome research to produce clear-cut results.

A major problem with much of the early research on coping is that it assessed coping effectiveness in relation to a range of *different* stressful encounters (e.g. Aldwin and Revenson 1986; Folkman *et al.* 1986a; McCrae and Costa 1986). Participants in these studies were asked to indicate the most stressful event they experienced during a specified period. This may have included financial problems, health problems, interpersonal disputes, and difficulties at work. In view of the general consensus in the literature that the effectiveness of a given coping strategy is dependent on the nature of the stressful encounter, the decision to adopt a procedure which aggregates measures of coping effectiveness across different encounters and thus essentially disregards the nature of the stressful encounter is surprising.

This problem has been recognized in more recent studies of coping effectiveness which were explicitly based on the assumption that the degree to which individuals have control over a stress situation moderates the effectiveness of their coping strategies. More specifically, it was predicted that in situations over which the individual has a great deal of control, problem-focused coping strategies should be more effective than emotion-focused strategies, whereas emotion-focused coping strategies should be most effective in stress situations over which the individual has very little control. However, despite the plausibility of this hypothesis, empirical support has been rather mixed (for a review, see Terry and Hynes 1998). One potential reason for these inconsistencies could be psychometric problems with the measures used to assess emotion-focused coping. As Stanton *et al.* (1994) have argued, some of the scales used to assess emotion-focused coping contained items which confound coping strategy with coping outcome. For example, the coping scale developed by Endler and Parker (1990) contains emotion-focused coping items which solely reflect distress (e.g. 'become very tense'). Other items reflect low self-esteem (e.g. 'focus on my inadequacies'). Stanton and her colleagues demonstrated that exclusion of these contaminated items from measures of emotion-focused coping substantially lowered the association between these coping scales and measures of psychological maladjustment.

Even if the assumption that the effectiveness of emotion-focused coping depends on the controllability of the stress situation were empirically well-supported, this would still fail to tell us which of the variety of strategies of emotion-focused coping should be employed in a given stress situation. There is only one general guideline I can offer. Most of the empirical literature suggests that chronic reliance on avoidant coping is associated with poorer adjustment than is emotion-focused coping strategies in which individuals confront their emotions (e.g. Carver *et al.* 1993; Stanton and Snider 1993; Nolen-Hoeksema and Larson 1999). In one study, avoidance was even found to be associated with cancer progression (Epping-Jordan *et al.* 1994).

Evidence that confrontation of one's emotions is associated with better adjustment than avoidance is consistent with research by Pennebaker on the positive health impact of disclosure of previously undisclosed traumatic events. Pennebaker consistently found that subjects who had been instructed to write about past traumatic events (e.g. Pennebaker *et al.* 1988) or recent upsetting experiences (Pennebaker *et al.* 1990) reported fewer health centre visits following the experiment when compared with controls who wrote about trivial events (for a review, see Pennebaker 1989). Originally Pennebaker accounted for these findings in terms of a theory of inhibition, which outlines the processes by which failure to confront traumatic events results in poorer health. The central assumption of this theory is that inhibition of thoughts, feelings and behaviour is an active process requiring physiological work. When individuals inhibit their desire to talk or think about traumatic experiences over long periods of time, cumulative stress is placed on the body resulting in increased vulnerability to stress-related disease. More recently, Pennebaker (e.g. 1997) has changed the focus of his explanation from potential negative effects of suppression to positive effects of disclosure. He now argues that disclosure helps the individual to organize the experience, to clarify psychological states to others, and to translate emotional experiences into the medium of language. Thus Pennebaker's theories point to potential mechanisms that might mediate the health-impairing effect of chronic avoidance.

But even though confrontational varieties of emotion-focused coping appear to be more effective than avoidance coping, this association may be curvilinear. There is evidence to suggest that thinking too much about one's emotions is also associated with poor outcome. Nolen-Hoeksema and her colleagues have identified rumination as an ineffective coping strategy (e.g. Nolen-Hoeksema *et al.* 1997; Nolen-Hoeksema and Larson 1999). Ruminators tend to focus passively on their symptoms of distress and the meaning and consequences of these symptoms, instead of actively working through their emotions. Ruminative response styles may prolong depression by enhancing the effects of negative mood on cognition and by interfering with instrumental behaviour. The difference between good and bad emotion confrontation may be that ruminators engage in wishful thinking and passively reiterating their emotions. In contrast, non-ruminators actively engage in positive reappraisal, trying to reconstruct the meaning of the stress situation in a new and positive way.

There are two further conceptual issues which have so far been neglected in research on coping effectiveness, namely the choice of the criterion used to define effectiveness and the time frame during which effectiveness is assessed. In most of these studies, effectiveness has been defined in terms of the level of distress individuals experienced at some arbitrarily chosen point in time following the stressful encounter. A coping strategy was considered effective if individuals who used this coping strategy experienced less distress, mood disturbance, or depressive symptomatology than individuals who used other coping strategies. It can easily be demonstrated that this choice of criterion is problematic. Although psychological health and physical health are often correlated, there are many instances in which they are not. For example, a man who uses denial to cope with symptoms of an acute coronary illness may have less distress in the short run, but risks serious physical consequences in the long run. Similarly, Pennebaker and his colleagues (1990) found that individuals who expressed their emotions about some undisclosed trauma had increased levels of psychological distress but also fewer health centre visits.

The second conceptual issue concerns the time frame. This refers both to the time elapsed between the stress experiences and the use of a coping strategy, and to the interval between the assessment of the coping strategy and the measurement of outcome. For example, despite the overwhelming support for the superiority of approach over avoidance coping, there is evidence to suggest that avoidant coping strategies such as denial may be quite effective in the initial stages of coping with severely traumatic events. Such strategies can reduce stress and anxiety and allow for a gradual recognition of threat. If one deals oneself with threatening material in a way that prevents it from becoming overwhelming, one is provided with time needed for assimilation of stressful information and for mobilization of efforts to change the environment or provide protection (e.g. Horowitz 1979; Roth and Cohen 1986; Stroebe 1992). Because individuals eventually have to assimilate even the most painful experience, the chronic use of denial is likely to impair the likelihood of adjustment.

A related issue concerns the time between the assessment of a coping strategy and the measurement of outcome. It seems plausible that some coping strategies may have a positive impact in the short run but be counterproductive in the long run. For example, most researchers report that the use of alcohol and drugs in coping with the loss of a loved person is associated with increased distress in the long run (e.g. Nolen-Hoeksema and Larson 1999). And yet, it is quite conceivable that the immediate effect of alcohol and drugs is a positive one.

Conclusions

Much of the early work on effectiveness of coping styles was stimulated by the interactional stress theory of Lazarus, Folkman and their colleagues, a theory which does not make predictions about the choice of coping strategies or effectiveness in coping. As a consequence of the lack of a guiding theory and, at the same time, the ready availability of instruments to measure coping styles, researchers have often adopted the atheoretical research strategy of asking individuals to report (retrospectively) the coping styles they used in stress situations, and then relating these reports to some measure of distress. The methodological weaknesses of this type of research were aggravated by using cross-sectional designs and aggregating findings across different stress situations.

More recently, these problems have been recognized and approaches to coping research have been improved. There are more studies which use a prospective methodology to study individual coping with a specific stress situation. For example, several studies have examined the impact of coping with breast cancer on outcomes assessed at a one-year follow-up. These have showed that avoidant coping was related to higher levels of distress (e.g. Carver et al. 1993; Stanton and Snider 1993) and to poorer disease outcome (Epping-Jordan et al. 1994). More recently, momentary reports of coping have been used to avoid problems related to the retrospective nature of coping reports (Stone et al. 1998). Finally, and probably most importantly, these methodological advances been paralleled by the development of theories which allow one to derive predictions about effective coping (e.g. Carver and Scheier 1990). As a result, the number of studies which use theoretical perspectives to derive predictions about effective or ineffective coping with a particular stressor is increasing. The coming years should bring major advances in our knowledge about the relative effectiveness of different coping styles.

COPING RESOURCES AS MODERATORS OF THE STRESS–HEALTH RELATIONSHIP

According to cognitive stress theories, the impact of stress on health is also dependent on the coping resources which are available to the individual confronted with the stressful life event. In analysing coping resources, researchers distinguish between extrapersonal and intrapersonal resources (e.g. Lazarus and Folkman 1984; Stroebe and Stroebe 1987; Cohen and Edwards 1989). *Extrapersonal coping resources* are resources external to the individual which are potentially helpful in alleviating the stress. Examples of extrapersonal resources likely to help the individual in coping with stressful life experiences are financial resources and social support. *Intrapersonal coping resources* consist of the personality traits, abilities and skills which enable people to cope with the stress experience. Coping resources are sometimes referred to as stress-buffering resources because they are presumed to protect or buffer people against the negative impact of stressful events (e.g. Cohen and Edwards 1989).

Coping resources can moderate the impact of stressful life events by influencing stress appraisal or by affecting the coping process (Cohen and Wills 1985). Most resources intervene at both of these stages. For example, the pessimistic attribution style conceptualized as part of the revised model of learned helplessness is assumed to moderate both appraisal and recovery (e.g. Peterson and Seligman 1987). Similarly, the extent to which individuals perceive that supportive others are available will affect the appraisal as well as the coping process (Cohen and Wills 1985). Much of the empirical research on coping resources investigates whether a person's health status is related to the extent to which he or she possesses a given resource. For example, as will be demonstrated below, there is evidence that individuals who have a great deal of social support suffer a lower risk of mental and physical impairment and even mortality than individuals who have little social support.

EXTRAPERSONAL COPING RESOURCES

Two major extrapersonal coping resources are material resources and social support. Whereas there is an extensive literature on social support as a coping resource (for reviews, see House 1981; Cohen and Wills 1985), economic resources are rarely discussed in this context (Lazarus and Folkman 1984). The role of economic resources will therefore be considered only briefly and most of this section will be devoted to the discussion of the impact of social support on health and well-being.

Material resources

In view of the strong negative relationship which has been observed between social class and illness and between social class and mortality (Adler *et al.* 1994), it is surprising that material resources are so infrequently discussed as a coping resource. It seems plausible that the coping function of economic resources contributes to the negative association between socio-economic status and morbidity or mortality. After all, people with money, especially if they have the skills to use it effectively, should have more coping options in most stressful situations than people without money. Money can provide easier access to legal, medical and other professional assistance.

The problem in using data on the association between socio-economic status and health as evidence in this context is that the relationship itself is not very well understood. However, in addition to the factors discussed earlier (p. 67), namely deficits in knowledge about health risks and poor health habits, differential exposure to stressful life events could also be responsible for the higher morbidity and mortality associated with low socio-economic status. Moderate but significant positive correlations between socio-economic status and life-change scores indicate that stressful life events are over-represented in the lower classes (e.g. Dohrenwend 1973). There is also evidence that exposure to undesirable life events is more likely to evoke mental health problems in low rather than high socio-economic status individuals (e.g. Dohrenwend 1973). The greater vulnerability of lower class individuals seems to some extent to be due to a differential availability of social support (Brown and Harris 1978). However, it is plausible that restricted access to other coping resources due to limited economic means could also contribute to this relationship.

If economic resources form an important coping resource, they should buffer the individual against the deleterious impact of stress. However, at least in bereavement research – the one area in which socio-economic status has been studied as a stress moderator – there does not seem to be any evidence that high socio-economic status buffers individuals against the health-impairing impact of the loss experience. While most studies show that widowed of low socio-economic status are less healthy than those of high socio-economic status, the comparison with non-bereaved control groups indicates that the health differential due to socio-economic status is the same for bereaved and non-bereaved groups (for a review, see Stroebe and Stroebe 1987). However, the fact that economic resources do not appear to buffer the individual against the health impact of bereavement does not preclude the possibility that such resources could not protect against other types of stressful events.

Social support

Over the past few decades, much research effort has been invested in the examination of the beneficial effects of social support on health and well-being. There is now a great deal of evidence that the availability of social support is associated with a reduced risk of mental illness and physical illness, and even mortality (e.g. Cohen and Wills 1985; Cohen 1988; House *et al.* 1988; Schwarzer and Leppin 1989a, b; Pierce *et al.* 1996; Stroebe and Stroebe 1996). Social support has been defined as information from others that one is loved and cared for, esteemed and valued, and part of a network of communication and mutual obligation (Cobb 1976). Such information can come from a spouse, a lover, children, friends, or social and community contacts such as churches or clubs.

Conceptualization and measurement of social support

The measurement of social support has been approached from two perspectives which differ in the way they conceptualize social support: one conceives of social support in terms of the *structure* of the target person's interpersonal relationships or social network, the other in terms of the *functions* that these relationships or networks serve for him or her (for a discussion see Cohen and Wills 1985; House and Kahn 1985; Stroebe and Stroebe 1996).

Structural measures reflect the social integration or embeddedness of the individuals by assessing the existence or quantity of social relationships of the individual. This information is relatively objective, reliable and easy to obtain. It can sometimes be gathered by observation or from behavioural records (e.g. marriage records, organizational memberships). But even if it is based on self-reports, information about whether a person is married, lives alone or belongs to some church is simple to collect, and usually fairly accurate (House and Kahn 1985). A standardized procedure for measuring various social network characteristics (e.g. size, density) has been developed by Stokes (1983) and is known as the Social Network List. There is consistent evidence that low levels of social relationship are associated with an increased risk of mortality (Berkman and Syme 1979; Blazer 1982; House *et al.* 1982).

Functional measures of social support assess whether interpersonal relationships serve particular functions. Various topologies of support functions have been proposed (e.g. House 1981; Cohen and McKay 1984; Stroebe and Stroebe 1987). Most distinguish between emotional, instrumental, informational and appraisal support. *Emotional support* involves providing empathy, care, love and trust. *Instrumental support* consists of behaviours that directly help the person in need; for example, individuals give instrumental support when they help other people to do their work, take care of their children, or help them with transportation. *Informational support* involves providing people with information which they can use in coping with their problems. *Appraisal support* is closely related to informational support. It also involves the transmission of information, but in this case it is information that is relevant for the person's self-evaluation. Thus, by comparing oneself to another person, one may use the other as a source of information in evaluating oneself.

The measurement of social support functions has been based on measures assessing the individual's perception of either the availability of others who provide these functions or the actual receipt of these support functions during a given time period (for a discussion of this distinction, see Dunkel-Schetter and Bennett 1990). Examples of measures of the *perceived availability* of social support are the Interpersonal Support Evaluation List (ISEL) (Cohen *et al.* 1985) and the Social Support Questionnaire (SSQ) (Sarason *et al.* 1983). The ISEL assesses the perceived availability of four types of social support (tangible, appraisal, self-esteem, belonging). For example, respondents have to indicate whether there are people with whom they can talk about intimate personal problems or who would help them with advice. The items of the SSQ consist of two parts, one assessing the number of available others whom individuals feel they can 'count on' for a particular type of support, and another measuring the individual's degree of satisfaction with the perceived support available in that particular situation. The number of available support providers is more similar to structural measures of social network size than to measures of functional support and is only moderately related to the satisfaction with the social support that is available.

A widely used scale to assess *received* social support is the Inventory of Socially Supportive Behaviors (ISSB) (Barrera *et al.* 1981). The items of the ISSB describe specific supportive behaviours that represent emotional, tangible, cognitive–informational, and direct guidance support. Respondents are asked to indicate how often during the past four weeks each supportive behaviour occurred. The individual's score thus represents the average frequency of receipt of these supportive behaviours.

Relationship between measures

It seems plausible that the number of social relationships a person has established is strongly related to the functional support the person perceives as available or actually receives. However, the different types of measures of social support show only weak relationships with each other. For example, Sarason *et al.* (1987) who examined the relationship between the Social Network List and measures of perceived and received social support (SSQ; ISSB) found only modest correlations between network size and satisfaction with perceived or received social support. These findings are reasonable if one considers that adequate functional support might be derived from *one* very good relationship but may not be available from several superficial ones.

The relationship between measures of the perceived availability of social support and received social support is also typically very modest. That low correlations are quite typical can be seen from Dunkel-Schetter and Bennett's (1990) survey of studies of the relationship between these two types of measures. Newcomb (1990), who examined the relationship between these two types of functional measures using structural equation modelling, found strong support for the existence of two latent constructs representing perceived and received social support, as well as evidence for a moderate degree of overlap.

Many researchers have argued that, in view of the modest correlations between these different measures, social support should be regarded as a complex construct consisting of three components, namely social embeddedness or integration, perceived availability of social support and received social support (e.g. Dunkel-Schetter and Bennett 1990). Measures of social integration conceptualize social support in terms of the size and structure of an individual's interpersonal network. They describe the channels through which supportive resources can, but need not, flow and are thus only indirect measures of social support. Perceived availability and the actual receipt of social support conceptualize social support in terms of the support functions served by the individual's interpersonal network. They thus reduce the richness of group interactions in that they reflect only those actions of group members that can be considered positive and helpful. Although from a social psychological perspective the actual exchange of resources would appear to be more central to the concept of social support than their perceived availability, measures of the perceived availability of support have been found to be more closely related to health than measures of received support (e.g. Schwarzer and Leppin 1992). One reason for the weak association of received social support and health outcome is that the supportive behaviour of others is not only a function of who is available but also of the instances in which help might have been needed during the period in question. It is therefore not surprising that, unlike measures of the perceived availability of support, measures of received support have often been found to be positively related to negative life events and symptomatology (Sarason *et al.* 1990).

The impact of social support on health

Much of the impetus for the work on social support and health came from the field of epidemiology. In an impressive early survey, Berkman and Syme (1979) were able to demonstrate a relationship between social support and mortality. These investigators studied social and community ties among a random sample of 6928 women and men whose age varied from 30 to 69 when first interviewed in 1965 in Alameda County, California. Each of the four types of social relationship that was assessed at that time (marriage, contacts with extended family and friends, church membership, membership in other organizations) independently predicted the rate of mortality over the succeeding nine years. Individuals who were low on an overall Social Network Index, which weighted the intimate ties more heavily, had approximately twice the mortality risk of individuals who were high on this index over the nine-year period.

Do these findings really show that the availability of social networks extends one's lifespan? One obvious alternative explanation is that the relationship between networks and mortality could have been due to the fact that isolated people were ill at the time of the survey and unable to maintain their social contacts. However, this appeared not to be the case, because the Social Network Index continued to predict mortality after health status at the time of the baseline survey was statistically controlled.

Berkman and Syme (1979) had to rely on self-reports of physical health, cigarette smoking, alcohol consumption, obesity and level of physical activity. Since self-report health measures are not the most reliable or valid indicator of a person's health status, it was important to replicate these findings with more objective indicators of health status. This was done in a large-scale prospective study which was part of the Tecumseh Community Health Study (House *et al.* 1982). The sample consisted of 2754 men and women who were aged 39 to 69 at the outset of the study in 1967 to

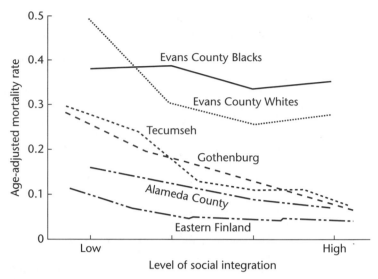

Figure 7.1 Level of social integration and age-adjusted mortality for males in five prospective studies.
Source: Adapted from House *et al.* (1988).

1969. In addition to an assessment of several classes of social relationships and activities, a wide range of health indicators were biomedically measured (e.g. levels of blood pressure, cholesterol, respiratory functions, electrocardiograms). Again, composite indices of these relationship were inversely related to mortality over the 10- to 12-year follow-up period even after adjustment for initial health status. People with low levels of social relationship had approximately twice the mortality risk of those with high levels.

This basic pattern has been replicated in more recent studies in the USA (see Schoenbach *et al.* 1986) and in Sweden (e.g. Welin *et al.* 1985). Of the American studies only the Evans County study (Schoenbach *et al.* 1986) also provided data on blacks. Although the levels of mortality vary greatly across studies, and even though the social support effects are weaker for women than for men, the patterns of prospective association between social integration and mortality are remarkably similar. This can be seen from Figures 7.1 and 7.2, which show the age-adjusted mortality rates for males and females, respectively, from those five studies for which parallel data could be extracted (House *et al.* 1988).

Less dire consequences of the lack of social support have also been established. There is evidence that social support is inversely related to the prevalence and incidence of a number of physical diseases. There is not only empirical evidence that the extent to which individuals experience social support lowers their risk of developing coronary heart disease, but also that social support facilitates recovery from coronary heart disease. The most persuasive evidence for the health-protective effect of social support for patients with established coronary artery disease comes from a prospective study of 1368 symptomatic patients with more than

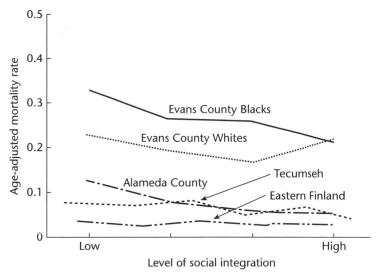

Figure 7.2 Level of social integration and age-adjusted mortality for females in five prospective studies.
Source: Adapted from House *et al.* (1988).

75 per cent closure of at least one major coronary artery (Williams *et al.* 1992). These patients had undergone coronary angiography at the beginning of the study between 1974 and 1980, and at the same time had responded to a measure of perceived social support. Marital status was also recorded as a structural measure of social support. By the end of the study in 1989, 781 patients had undergone surgery, and 237 had died of cardiovascular causes. When survival was assessed over a five-year period, controlling for the extent of cardiac disease at the time of intake, married patients were found to have better survival rates than unmarried patients. There was also a significant interaction between marital status and confidant availability. Unmarried patients without a confidante had a more than threefold increase in the risk of death within five years compared with patients who were either married or had a close confidante.

That social support also aids the recovery from coronary artery bypass surgery (a procedure in which the narrow passage is bypassed by surgically grafted pieces of artery) has been demonstrated in a study in which 155 patients were monitored for a year after their bypass operation (King *et al.* 1993). Social support was measured one day before surgery with the ISEL (Cohen *et al.* 1985). Outcome variables were emotional well-being, function disruption (disruption of usual activities due to illness) and angina symptoms. Controlling for outcome level at baseline, esteem support was found to be significantly related to all three outcome measures at one year after the operation. Instrumental support was related to two of the outcome measures (functional disruption and angina). Belonging support, that is the availability of people one can do things with, was related only to angina symptoms, and appraisal support was unrelated to any of the outcome measures. Thus, the more patients reported before surgery that their spouse

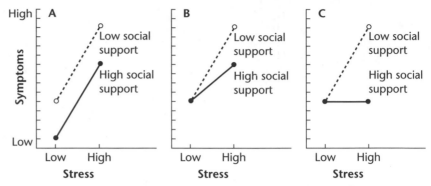

Figure 7.3   An illustration of the two ways in which social support is assumed to benefit health: the direct effect hypothesis (Panel A) proposes that the health benefits of social support occur irrespective of the level of stress; the buffering effect hypothesis proposes that social support protects the individuals to some extent (Panel B) or totally (Panel C) against the negative impact of stress on health.

esteemed them, the higher was their emotional well-being one year later and the less likely they were to experience functional disruption and symptoms of angina pectoris. The recurrence of angina symptoms was also reduced by the personal availability of belonging and instrumental support.

The findings of these studies are not atypical, as can be seen from a meta-analysis of more than 100 studies of relationship between social support and health which appeared between 1976 and 1987 (Schwarzer and Leppin 1989a, b). Schwarzer and Leppin found that social support was significantly related not only to mortality but also to self-report measures of health status, physiological reactivity (e.g. blood pressure, heart rate) and – most strongly – to depression. However, the population effect sizes, which reflect the strength of these relationships, were fairly modest, suggesting that social support on average accounted for between 1 and 4 per cent of the variance in the health measures used in the studies.

Because levels of stress were not assessed in these studies, it is unclear whether these findings merely reflect a generalized beneficial effect of social support, independent of stress, or whether social support buffered individuals against the deleterious impact of stress. Both hypotheses are discussed in the literature. Figure 7.3 illustrates the two ways in which social support can benefit health and well-being.

A *direct effect* of social support on health – independent of the amount of stress individuals experience – could occur because large social networks provide people with regular positive experiences and a set of stable, socially rewarded roles in the community (Cohen and Wills 1985). For example, individuals with high levels of social support may have a greater feeling of being liked and cared for. The positive outlook this provides could be beneficial to health independent of stress experience. A high level of social support may also encourage people to lead a more healthful lifestyle.

According to the *buffering hypothesis*, social support affects health by protecting the individual against the negative impact of high levels of stress (Figure 7.3). This protective effect can best be understood by means of analogy with the effects of an inoculation. Just as a difference in health of individuals who are or are not inoculated should emerge only when they are exposed to the infectious agent, the protective function of social support is only effective when the person encounters a strong stressor. Under low-stress conditions, little or no buffering occurs. Thus, under low-stress conditions, no differences would be expected in the health and well-being of groups enjoying differential levels of social support.

Buffering could operate through two types of processes: first, individuals who experience a high level of social support may *appraise* a stressful event such as a financial crisis or the loss of a job as less stressful than people with little social support, because they know that there are people to whom they can turn for advice or who would even be willing to support them financially. A second way in which social support might buffer the negative impact of stress is by improving people's ability to cope with the stressor. Thus somebody who is experiencing a crisis might be better able to cope if he knows people who can give advice or perhaps even provide a solution to the problem.

To differentiate between the direct effect and the buffering effect of social support, studies have to assess the impact of differential levels of social support under differential levels of stress on health and well-being. The pattern that has emerged from this type of research is less than clear-cut. Some studies reported only main effects while others found interactions between stress and social support. In a review of this literature, Cohen and Wills (1985) examined the hypothesis that these differences in findings are related to the type of measure that was used in a given study. They reasoned that for a buffering effect to occur, the type of social support that is available should be closely linked to the specific coping needs elicited by a stressful event. Since only functional measures assess different types of social support, only studies using functional measures should yield evidence of buffering effects. The use of structural measures of social integration, which assess the existence or number of relationships but not the functions actually provided by those relationships, should only result in main effects. Their review supported this hypothesis.

The role of personality dispositions in research on social support and health

A thorny issue that so far has not been satisfactorily addressed in research on social support and health is the possibility that personality dispositions contribute to the observed relationship between measures of social support and health. There are two different routes by which personality could influence the relationship between social support and health:

1 Personality characteristics could increase an individual's chance of finding social support and at the same time contribute positively to his or her coping ability. For example, it seems plausible that individuals who are socially competent are also more likely to develop strong support

networks and to stay healthy by effectively coping with stressful events or by performing health-enhancing behaviours (Cohen and Wills 1985).

2 Personality characteristics might also bias individual reports of levels of social support and of health symptoms. This issue is particularly problematic where functional measures of social support and self-report measures of stress have been related to self-reports of psychological and physical symptoms. For example, in our Tübingen study of bereavement a significant correlation (−.32) was observed between a scale measuring perceived availability of social support and the neuroticism scale of the Eysenck Personality Inventory. Individuals who have high scores on neuroticism tended to report lower levels of perceived social support. Since, according to Watson and Pennebaker (1989), these individuals are also more likely to report higher levels of stressful life events and higher levels of psychological and somatic symptoms, neuroticism could be partly responsible for relationships observed between measures of perceived social support, perceived stress, and perceived symptomatology.

There are various strategies for dealing with these problems in research on perceived social support and health. One strategy is to reduce the influence of reporting biases by using objectifiable life events (e.g. unemployment, death of a partner) and biomedical health measures. A second safeguard is to use prospective designs which allow one to assess the impact of stress and social support measured at Time 1 on symptomatology at Time 2, while statistically controlling for differences in symptomatology at Time 1. A third strategy involves the inclusion of measures of personality dispositions that are known correlates of social support (e.g. neuroticism, social competence) and using such measures as control variables.

The potential confounding influence of personality dispositions is less problematic in prospective epidemiological studies which relate measures of social integration to mortality. First, personality variables are less likely to influence the simple network measures typically used in these studies (e.g. reports about marriage, membership of organizations) than reports about the perceived availability of social support. Second, mortality is a dependent measure that is uninfluenced by this type of reporting bias. Finally, the alternative possibility that personality influences both the *actual* size of a person's social network (e.g. neurotics may be less likely to find partners or friends) and his or her health can be controlled by using prospective designs that demonstrate the impact of social support on change in health over time.

Mediators of the relationship between social support and health

There are a number of psychological and biological processes through which social support might influence individual health, and many of these could account for main effects of social support as well as stress buffering (for a review, see Stroebe and Stroebe 1996). For example, a person who is integrated into a large social network of family and friends is subject to social controls and peer pressures that influence normative health behaviours. Depending on whether these pressures promote healthy or unhealthy behaviour patterns, social integration could have a positive or negative impact on health. There is some evidence, however, that social support is positively associated with behaviours that are promotive of health (e.g. adherence to medical regimens or traditional health behaviours such as non-smoking, adequate sleep, prudent diet and moderate drinking behaviour). Thus Berkman and Syme (1979) reported a positive relationship between their structural measure of support and various health practices. The possibility that social networks and social support influence health behaviours is also suggested by research on giving up smoking. These studies suggest that success in stopping smoking and the ability to maintain abstinence over a longer period of time has been linked to supportive behaviours from spouses and friends (for a review see Cohen 1988).

Many of the *psychological* processes that link social support to psychological well-being and health may be mediated by self-esteem, that is, the positive or negative beliefs and evaluations that the individual holds towards himself or herself. It is widely accepted among clinical, personality and social psychologists that a positive and stable self-esteem is important for individual well-being. As Tajfel (1978) emphasized, the social groups to which we belong are major determinants of our definition of 'self' and form the basis of social identity. Social identity refers to that part of people's self-concepts which derives from their knowledge of their memberships of various social groups together with the emotional significance attached to these memberships. Thus, embeddedness in a large interpersonal and social network may positively contribute to social identity and self-esteem.

Social relationships may also fulfil a number of support functions which are beneficial for individual self-esteem. There is broad agreement among the helping professions concerning the central role of emotional support for self-esteem and psychological well-being. As Bernard (1968) has described: 'One of the major functions of positive, expressive talk is to raise the status of the other, to give help, to reward; in ordinary human relations it performs the stroking function. As infants need physical caressing or stroking in order to live and grow, and even to survive, so do adults need emotional or psychological stroking or caressing to remain normal' (p. 137).

Group members also serve validational functions which are important for an individual's interpretation of reality. Success or failure in responding to situational demands depends not merely on one's skills but also on whether one is able to assess these abilities and the environmental demands realistically. People often fail because they overestimate their ability or underestimate the difficulty of the task. According to Festinger (1954), the assessment of the validity of one's beliefs about 'reality' and about one's own level of ability frequently depends on social comparison processes, particularly when objective criteria are lacking. Social comparison processes are also important for the evaluation of the appropriateness of one's emotional reactions, particularly in novel, emotion-arousing situations (Schachter 1959). Such processes are therefore likely to play an important role in the perception and evaluation of bodily symptoms.

Ultimately, the impact of social and psychological variables on physical health must be transmitted through *biological* processes. In a recent review of the relationship between social support and physiological processes, Uchino *et al.* (1996) focused particularly on mechanisms underlying the association between social support and physical health. They reported that of the 81 studies which examined social support and physiological processes, 57 focused on aspects of cardiovascular function. The most commonly used cardiovascular measures include heart rate, systolic blood pressure and diastolic blood pressure. In general, the results of correlational studies relating social support to blood pressure are consistent with the assumption that higher social support is associated with better cardiovascular regulation (e.g. lower blood pressure), although the mean effect size (r = .08) was rather modest. Because drawing causal conclusions from correlational findings is always problematic, it is important to note that there is also fairly consistent support from prospective intervention studies on normotensive and hypertensive individuals which suggest a positive effect of social support on cardiovascular regulation (Uchino *et al.* 1996). Finally, there is even evidence from experimental laboratory studies to identify one of the mechanisms by which social support influences cardiovascular regulation: social support reduces cardiovascular reactivity in acute stress situations (effect size: r = .28; Uchino *et al.* 1996). These positive effects may not even require the actual presence of others in acutely stressful situations. Cardiovascular reactivity to stress may even be reduced by the perceived availability of social support (Uchino and Garvey 1997).

Uchino and colleagues (1996) also reviewed the rather small number of studies of the association between social support and endocrine function. An examination of the endocrine function is important because it is associated with both the cardiovascular and the immune system. Whereas a consistent association was found between low social support and higher levels of catecholamines (i.e. epinephrine and norepinephrine), there was little evidence for a relationship between social support and cortisol levels. Finally, Uchino and colleagues (1996) reviewed correlational and prospective studies of the association between social support and indicators of immune functioning. A meta-analysis of nine studies which examined the association between social support and functional immune measures revealed a moderately strong association (r = .21), indicating that higher levels of social support are associated with better immune functioning.

This review revealed relatively strong evidence linking social support to aspects of the functioning of the cardiovascular, endocrine and immune systems. It is interesting to note that the observed association between social support and cardiovascular, endocrine and immune functions did not appear to have been mediated in any substantial way by health behaviour. Thus, despite the impact of social support on health behaviours and of health behaviours on cardiovascular, endocrine and immune functioning, health behaviours did not appear to be the major pathway by which social support influences these physiological functions (Uchino *et al.* 1996).

INTRAPERSONAL COPING RESOURCES

Numerous personality variables have been suggested as moderators of the impact of stress on health, and the list of variables keeps on being extended. Because it would be too ambitious in the context of this chapter to attempt an exhaustive review of this rich but complex body of literature, the discussion will be restricted to two personality variables that have been extensively studied as coping resources which moderate the relationship between stress and health, namely hardiness (e.g. Kobasa *et al.* 1982a) and dispositional optimism (e.g. Scheier and Carver 1987). In a subsequent section, hostility will be discussed as a personality variable which moderates the stress–health relationship without constituting a coping resource (Siegman and Smith 1994; Miller *et al.* 1996).

The hardy personality

Hardiness has been proposed by Kobasa (1979) as a constellation of personality characteristics that protects individuals against the health-impairing impact of stress. There are three components of the hardy personality:

1 Control, which refers to people's belief that they can influence events in their lives.
2 Commitment, which refers to people's sense of purpose and involvement in the events, activities and others in their lives.
3 Challenge, which refers to the expectation that change rather than stability is normal in life and that change in the form of life events can be a positive phenomenon providing an opportunity for growth, rather than a threat to security.

Hardy individuals would score high on all three dimensions and would thus possess a life philosophy which buffers them against the debilitating impact of stressful life events.

The measurement of hardiness

In the course of the development of the concept of hardiness, the scales used to measure it have changed. The most frequently used instrument to measure hardiness in recent research seems to be a composite of five scales. Control is measured by the Powerlessness Scale of the Alienation Test (Maddi *et al.* 1979), and the External Locus of Control Scale (Rotter *et al.* 1962). Commitment is measured by the Alienation from Self Scale and the Alienation from Work Scale of the Alienation Test (Maddi *et al.* 1979). Challenge is measured by the Security Scale of the California Life Goals Evaluation Schedule (Hahn 1966). For each of these scales a high score reflects a relative lack of hardiness.

The practice of combining the various scales used to measure hardiness into one overall score is based on the assumption that individual differences on these measures reflect a common dimension of hardiness. If this assumption were correct, correlations between individual scores on pairs of scales should be high and factor analyses of the five scales should yield a single factor. These assumptions have been questioned (e.g. Funk and Houston 1987; Hull *et al.* 1987; Cohen and Edwards 1989). In fact, Kobasa *et al.* (1981) reported surprisingly low correlations between pairs of scales used to measure hardiness.

Hardiness and health

The concept of hardiness was developed and tested in a study which tried to differentiate people who reacted to stress with illness from those who stayed healthy on the basis of their personality. In a retrospective study, Kobasa (1979) selected from a sample of male executives of a large public utility company who responded to her questionnaires those who reported high levels of stress for the previous three years on the Social Readjustment Rating Scale (Holmes and Rahe 1967). This high-stress group was divided into a high- and a low-illness group on the basis of their responses to a self-report checklist of more than 100 commonly recognized physical and mental illnesses and symptoms. The two groups were then sent a package of personality tests containing five personality scales for each component of the hardiness construct. Statistical analyses identified a number of scales that showed significant differences between the two groups. Kobasa (1979) interpreted these findings as support for her hypothesis that high-stress/low-illness executives indeed showed more hardiness than high-stress/high-illness executives. Although these findings are suggestive, they do not really demonstrate a buffering (i.e. protective) effect of hardiness. They might merely reflect a correlation between the scales used to measure hardiness and the self-report health measure. To rule out this interpretation and demonstrate buffering, Kobasa would have had to show that hardiness was unrelated (or at least substantially less related) to health in a low-stress group.

In two subsequent articles, Kobasa and her colleagues reported a buffering effect for hardiness in a retrospective study that used an adequate design (Kobasa et al. 1982b; Kobasa and Puccetti 1983). Kobasa and her colleagues also conducted a prospective study on executives of the same utility company, in which they collected three sets of data at one-year intervals (Kobasa et al. 1981, 1982a). Using reported illness summed over Years 2 and 3 as the dependent variable, and Year 1 stressful events, hardiness and constitutional predisposition (a measure of parents' illness) as predictors, they found significant main effects for stressful life events, hardiness and constitutional predisposition. Although the pattern of means was consistent with a buffering effect for hardiness, no interactions were significant. However, Kobasa et al. (1982a) reported that an analysis of the same data set controlling for illness at Year 1 and dropping constitutional predisposition from the analysis revealed a significant buffering effect.

Further evidence for a buffering effect of hardiness comes from a retrospective study of a sample of female former students of a small liberal arts college (Rhodewalt and Zone 1989). Life Stress was measured with an adapted form of the Schedule of Recent Life Events. Subjects had to indicate which of the events they had experienced during the last 12 months. They also had to rate whether the event was desirable or undesirable, controllable or uncontrollable, and the amount of adjustment that was necessary for them to cope with the event. Health was assessed with the Beck Depression Inventory (a self-report scale of common symptoms of depression) and the same illness rating scale as the one used by Kobasa (1979). The authors found a buffering effect of hardiness for both depression

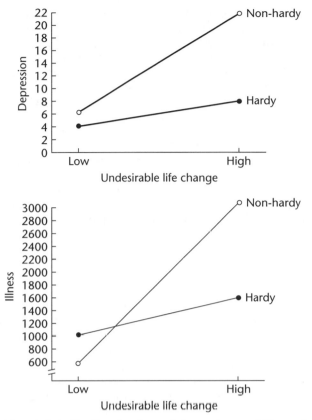

Figure 7.4   Predicted values of depression and illness for the interaction of hardiness with undesirable life change.
Source: Rhodewalt and Zone (1989).

and self-reported physical illness (Figure 7.4). Thus, hardiness seemed to protect these women somewhat against the negative impact of stress on psychological and physical health.

This study is particularly interesting because it also assessed hardiness-related differences in appraisal of stress. Although hardy and non-hardy women did not differ in the absolute number of stressful events reported, non-hardy women reported significantly greater numbers of undesirable life changes. Thus, non-hardy women declared that roughly 40 per cent of their life experiences were undesirable, whereas their hardy counterparts appraised only 27 per cent of their experiences in this manner. In addition to appraising a greater number of events as negative, non-hardy women also reported that the negative events required more adjustment than did hardy women. These findings suggest that the buffering effect of hardiness is at least partly mediated by differences in appraisal processes.

However, there are also several reports of studies which either failed to find any evidence for a buffering effect (e.g. Schmied and Lawler 1986;

Funk and Houston 1987), or only observed buffering effects for one of the components of the Hardiness Scale (e.g. Ganellen and Blaney 1984). Furthermore, there is evidence that hardiness is highly correlated with negative affectivity or neuroticism (Funk and Houston 1987; Hull *et al.* 1987; Allred and Smith 1989). As Watson and Pennebaker (1989) have shown, self-report measures both of stress and of health complaints reflect a pervasive mood disposition of negative affectivity or neuroticism. Thus, it may not be the hardy individuals who are particularly stress-resistant, but the non-hardy individuals who are neurotic and psychologically mal-adjusted and who therefore view their lives as more negative and stress-ful and also report higher levels of health complaints. As the findings of Watson and Pennebaker further suggest, these complaints could be *unrelated* to physical health problems. It would therefore be important in future research to test whether the buffering effect of hardiness can be replicated with objective stress situations using biological or other objective indicators of health status.

Conclusions

There is suggestive evidence that hardiness protects individuals against the impact of stressful life events and that this buffering effect is medi-ated by differences in appraisal processes. Hardy individuals appear to view their lives more positively and as more under their own control. However, the fact that buffering studies have assessed both stress and health with self-report methodology is problematic, particularly in view of the high negative correlation between hardiness and neuroticism. It therefore remains unclear whether the observed interactions between hardiness and stress on health measures should be interpreted in terms of a protective effect of hardiness on health, or in terms of differences in the way neurotic individuals perceive and/or report stress and health symptoms.

Dispositional optimism

Dispositional optimism is a second personality variable which has been suggested as a moderator of the stress–health relationship. It has been proposed that an optimistic nature can motivate people to cope more effectively with stress and consequently reduce the risk of illness (Scheier and Carver 1985, 1987). The crucial factor in optimism, according to Scheier and Carver, is that optimists will be more likely than pessimists to see desired outcomes as within their reach. People who see desired outcomes as attainable should continue to exert effort at reaching these outcomes, even when doing so is difficult. On the other hand, when outcomes are sufficiently unattainable, people will reduce their efforts and eventually abandon the pursuit of a given goal. Since optimists are assumed to see desired outcomes as more attainable than pessimists are, they should also be more likely than pessimists to employ problem-focused coping even in the most stressful situations, when challenged to the limits of their coping resources.

The measurement of optimism

Scheier and Carver (1985) began their research by developing a measure of dispositional optimism, the Life Orientation Test (LOT) which has since been revised (Scheier *et al.* 1994). The LOT has been designed to measure the extent to which individuals hold the general expectation that good things are likely to happen to them. The revised LOT consists of ten items, of which six reflect optimism and four are irrelevant filler items. Three of the optimism items are phrased in a positive way (e.g. 'In uncertain times, I usually expect the best'), and three are phrased in a negative way (e.g. 'If something can go wrong for me, it will'). The irrelevant filler items are included to distract respondents from the purpose of the scale. Respondents answer each item by indicating the extent of their agreement on a five-point scale.

Optimism and health

Evidence for optimism-related differences in coping has been reported in numerous studies (e.g. Scheier *et al.* 1986, 1989; Aspinwall and Taylor 1992; Chang 1998; Segerstom *et al.* 1998). For example, Scheier and colleagues (1986), who administered both the LOT and the Ways of Coping Questionnaire to a sample of undergraduates, found that optimism was associated with more use of problem-focused coping, seeking of social support, and emphasizing the positive aspects of a stressful situation. In contrast, pessimism was associated with denial and distancing, and with focusing on the goal with which the stressor was interfering.

That the impact of optimism on differences in adjustment to life stress is at least partially mediated by differences in coping styles has also been demonstrated in several studies (e.g. Aspinwall and Taylor 1992; Chang 1998; Segerstrom *et al.* 1998). For example, a longitudinal study of college students who were interviewed twice, once shortly after entering college and again three months later, found that optimists made less use of avoidant coping (Aspinwall and Taylor 1992). Avoidant coping in turn predicted less successful adjustment to college life three months later. Greater optimism was also related to greater use of active coping. This in turn predicted better adjustment to college. However, some studies found that the impact of optimism on adjustment was only *partially* mediated by differences in coping strategies (e.g. Chang 1998; Segerstrom 1998). This raises the possibility that differences in coping style are not the only reason why optimists adjust better to stressful situations.

Optimism not only reduces the distress associated with stressful life experiences, but also appears to buffer individuals against the physical effects of life stress. Support for this assumption comes from a prospective study of the impact of what is claimed to be a major stressor, namely the first year of law school at a top American university (Segerstrom *et al.* 1998). Pre-test data were collected during the two weeks preceding law school, and post-test data were collected halfway through the first semester. Optimism was measured with the LOT, supplemented by a situation-specific optimism scale at the pre-test. Dependent measures were mood changes and various measures of the immune system. In support of predictions, dispositional and situational optimism were associated with less mood disturbance and fewer negative effects on the immune system at the post-test taken halfway through the first semester.

This study also examined whether the relationship between optimism and measures of mood and immune functioning was mediated by optimism-related differences in coping styles. As in previous studies, optimism was found to be related to less avoidant coping. Although controlling for difference in coping styles reduced the association between optimism and mood, it did not affect the link between optimism and immune parameters. Since mood disturbances are in turn related to immune measures, the pattern of findings would be consistent with the assumption that coping styles partially mediate the optimism–mood relationship and that the mood disturbances are in turn at the root of the impairment of immune functioning.

That optimists recover more quickly from major surgery has been shown in studies of coronary bypass patients and of women who underwent surgery for breast cancer (Scheier et al. 1989). Optimists recovered faster from the effects of the bypass surgery and there was also a positive relationship between optimism and post-surgical quality of life six months later, with optimists doing substantially better than pessimists. Comparable findings were reported from a longitudinal study of women with early stage breast cancer. These women were interviewed before surgery and several times after surgery. Optimists reported less distress at each point of measurement than pessimists and this effect was mediated by aspects of subjects' coping reactions, particularly the tendency of optimists to make less use of denial and behavioural disengagement.

However, like hardiness research, the research based on the optimism scale has been criticized for its overlap with negative affectivity and neuroticism (Smith et al. 1989). In a replication of the study of Scheier and Carver (1985) on undergraduate stress, Smith and colleagues administered a measure of negative affectivity in addition to the LOT. Their findings for the LOT were comparable to those reported by Scheier and Carver (1985): optimists tended to engage more in problem-focused coping and less in avoidant coping than pessimists and they also reported fewer symptoms at the second assessment. However, these relationships disappeared when level of neuroticism was statistically controlled. In contrast, statistical control of optimism scores did not eliminate the relationship between neuroticism and these same symptoms. As Smith and colleagues (1989) concluded, 'at the very least, these findings suggest that optimism as defined by the LOT is not related to coping and symptom report independently of the influence of neuroticism' (p. 645). Scheier and colleagues (1994) countered this criticism by arguing that since pessimism formed part of the concept of neuroticism, it was to be expected that controlling for neuroticism would reduce the association between optimism and health measures. They further presented data which indicated that control for neuroticism reduced but did not eliminate the association between optimism and depression. Furthermore, since neuroticism is mainly related to symptom reporting but not to actual physical change (Watson and Pennebaker 1989), findings such as the immune changes reported by Segerstrom and colleagues (1998) could not be accounted for in terms of neuroticism.

OTHER MODERATORS OF THE STRESS–HEALTH RELATIONSHIP: THE CASE OF HOSTILITY

Not all personality characteristics which moderate the stress–health relationship are coping resources. There are some personality characteristics which, rather than helping the individual to alleviate the impact of stress experiences, appear to have the opposite effect: they increase vulnerability. This section will discuss hostility as a case in point.

Anger and hostility have long been suspected as risk factors of health impairment, in particular coronary heart disease. However, much of the recent research on the association between hostility and coronary heart disease has been stimulated by attempts to resolve inconsistencies in findings of research on the Type A Behaviour Pattern (Siegman 1994). The Type A 'coronary-prone' behaviour pattern had been identified during the 1950s as a risk factor for the development of coronary heart disease. The Type A individual was described as a person 'who is *aggressively* involved in a *chronic, incessant* struggle to achieve more and more in less and less time, and, if required to do so, against the opposing efforts of other things or other persons' (Friedman and Rosenman 1974: 67).

Although there was quite a bit of positive support for Type A as an independent risk factor in coronary heart disease (e.g. Rosenman *et al.* 1975) there was sufficient negative evidence (e.g. Shekelle *et al.* 1985) to stimulate search for explanations of these inconsistencies. One of the potential causes suggested was the multidimensional nature of the Type A construct (Siegman 1994). The Type A Behaviour Pattern encompasses behaviours reflecting such diverse motives as ambition, hostility, time urgency and aggressiveness, and it seemed likely that not all these factors were associated with coronary heart disease. More specifically, it was suggested that the 'potential for hostility' was the most likely candidate as the 'toxic' component in the Type A Behaviour Pattern (Siegman 1994).

Hostility has been defined as an enduring, negative attitude towards others involving cognitive, affective and behavioural components (Siegman and Smith 1994). The cognitive component reflects negative beliefs about others, including cynicism and mistrust. The affective component consists of a variety of negative emotions, ranging from anger and rage to resentment and contempt. The behavioural component includes aggression and a variety of more subtle form of antagonism. Thus, 'hostility connotes a devaluation of the worth and motives of others, and expectation that others are likely sources of wrong doing, a relational view of being in opposition to others, and a desire to inflict harm or see others harmed' (Smith 1994).

The measurement of hostility

There are a number of different measures of hostility which are based on either the Structured Interview originally developed to assess Type A behaviour, or on self-report questionnaires. The Structured Interview (SI) consists of a series of questions about an individual's characteristic responses to a variety of situations. These interviews are tape recorded and rated for hostile content (e.g. self-reported annoyance), hostile intensity (report or display of intense feelings), hostile style (i.e. behaviour displayed during the interview) and overall potential for hostility (based on clinical judgement). Measures of hostility based on Structured Interviews show the highest association with coronary heart disease (Miller *et al.* 1996).

The most frequently used questionnaire measure of hostility is the Cook–Medley Ho Scale. The Ho scale was originally derived empirically on the basis of those items from the Minnesota Teacher Attitude Inventory that discriminated teachers with good vs poor rapport with students (Cook and Medley 1954). Although the Ho scale is used as an indicator of general hostility, there is evidence that it is multidimensional (e.g. Barefoot *et al.* 1989). The major dimensions measured by this scale are cynicism (negative beliefs about others), hostile affect (negative emotions in relation to others), aggressive responding (a tendency to used aggression as a means of coping with problems), and hostile attribution (reflecting beliefs that others intend to harm the respondent). The popularity of the Ho scale stems from empirical findings that link it to a number of physical health outcomes, including coronary heart disease and premature mortality from all causes, even though the association is less strong and less consistent than that found with the Structured Interview (Miller *et al.* 1996).

Hostility and coronary heart disease

Much of the research on hostility and physical health assessed the association with coronary heart disease. The different endpoints used as indicative of coronary heart disease were angina, myocardial infarction, sudden cardiac death, and the extent of occlusion in coronary arteries. In one of the earliest cross-sectional studies of hostility and coronary heart disease, Williams and colleagues (1980) assessed the association between Ho scores, interview-based ratings of Type A behaviour, and coronary atherosclerosis in a sample of 425 patients undergoing coronary angiography, an intrusive procedure for the diagnosis of the occlusion of coronary arteries. Both Type A Behaviour and hostility scores showed a significant and independent association with the presence of clinically significant coronary artery disease, and hostility turned out to be the stronger predictor. Although other studies using the Ho scale could not replicate this finding, the association between hostility and coronary artery disease has been repeatedly demonstrated in a number of studies using the Structured Interview as well as other self-report measures (for a review, see Helmers *et al.* 1994).

The most persuasive evidence that hostility is a risk factor in the development of coronary heart disease comes from prospective studies of initially healthy individuals. Probably the earliest prospective study was conducted on sub-samples of a larger study of the development of coronary heart disease, namely the Western Collaborative Group Study (Matthews *et al.* 1977). The sub-samples consisted of 62 men who had developed various forms of coronary heart disease over the course of 4.5 years and an age-matched control group of 124 healthy men. The Structured Interviews had been taken prior to the development of symptomatology and were rated blindly on a number of aspects of the Type A coronary-prone behaviour patterns reflecting hostility. The variables providing the best discrimination between men who had developed heart diseases and the healthy controls were ratings of potential of hostility, anger directed outwards, frequent experience of anger, and irritation at waiting in lines. Even more convincing evidence was reported by Barefoot *et al.* (1983) in a 22-year follow-up of a sample of 225 medical students from the University of North Carolina who had filled in the Ho scale when they were students. Subjects who had low hostility scores (below the median) experienced significantly fewer coronary events during the 22-year period than subjects with hostility scores above the median of Cook–Medley scores.

Like the evidence from cross-sectional studies, the evidence from prospective studies has not been totally consistent. But overall it provides strong support for a hostility–heart disease association. Miller and colleagues (1996) concluded from their recent meta-analytic review of the empirical research that 'evidence from both cross-sectional and prospective studies suggests that hostility is a robust risk factor' (p. 344). Although the magnitude of this association varied as a function of the measurement device used, the 'effect sizes for the structure interview measures of hostility are equal or greater in magnitude to those reported for traditional risk factors for CHD-elevated serum cholesterol, blood pressure and cigarette smoking' (Miller *et al.* 1996: 341).

Mechanism linking hostility and health

Having accepted that hostility is a risk factor for coronary heart disease one now has to address the issue of whether it impairs health by contributing to, or more specifically by moderating, the stress–health relationship. To demonstrate that hostility is a (stress-) moderator variable, one has to demonstrate that stressful events have a stronger health impact on individuals who are high rather than low on hostility. A potential link is provided by one of the theoretical explanations offered for the association between hostility and health, namely the explanation in terms of physiological reactivity (Williams *et al.* 1985). Williams and colleagues argued that hostile people are likely to display two psychological responses that are associated with increased physiological arousal: they are prone to experience anger and to engage in vigilant observation of their social environment scanning for signs of hostile behaviour. Anger and vigilance are associated with increases in blood pressure, heart rate and stress-related hormones in response. Given their anger-proneness, hostile people experience anger more frequently and intensely than individuals who are less hostile. More frequent episodes of anger produce elevated levels of cardiovascular and neuroendocrine responses that contribute to coronary heart disease. In support of this model, there is empirical evidence for an association between hostility and cardiovascular reactivity, but the relationship is weak and limited to socially stressful situations (for a review, see Houston 1994). Typical of this pattern are the findings of Suarez and Williams (1989) from male participants who performed an anagram task in which they were either harassed or not harassed. Higher physiological reactivity of high-Ho as compared to low-Ho individuals emerged only under conditions where participants had been harassed.

A second explanation, the psychosocial vulnerability model, suggests that although hostility itself is not a moderator of the stress–health relationship, it is associated with a powerful moderator variable, namely social support. Their mistrust of others and their expectation that others will behave in a hostile manner towards them induces hostile individuals to behave in an antagonistic and aggressive way towards others. This behaviour pattern is likely to reduce the willingness of others to be supportive, and to evoke interpersonal conflict and hostility from others. However, their hostile attitudes towards their social environment not only lower the availability of social support, but also heighten their risk of getting involved in social conflicts and interpersonal stress (Miller *et al.* 1996).

A third explanation suggests that hostile individuals are more likely to engage in health-impairing behaviour patterns and that these behaviours mediate the relationship between hostility and illness (Leiker and Hailey 1988). There is evidence that hostile individuals report more health-impairing behaviours. In a study of undergraduates, Leiker and Hailey (1988) found that high Ho-scores were associated with reports of less physical exercise, less self-care and more alcohol use (including drinking and driving). Similar results were reported by Houston and Vavak (1991). This pattern is also in line with findings from a recent study of a sample of Dutch adolescents in which criminal behaviour was found to be associated with both a tendency to adopt health-impairing behaviour patterns and with ill health (Junger *et al.* 1999). However, Miller and colleagues (1996) found that the association between hostility and coronary disease could even be demonstrated when health behaviour variables were statistically controlled. Similarly, Junger and her colleagues (1999) found that the relationship between criminal behaviour and health remained significant even after controlling for associated differences in health behaviour. Thus, even though the association between hostility and health-impairing behaviour patterns is likely to contribute to the health problems of hostile individuals, the health behaviour model does not provide a complete account of the mechanisms underlying the association between hostility and physical health.

Conclusions

Hostility has been empirically established as a robust risk factor for coronary disease, with effect sizes for the interview-based measure of hostility being equal to or greater than those reported for traditional risk factors. However, the evidence is less clear with regard to mechanisms which mediate the impact of hostility on health. It is therefore still uncertain whether hostility acts as a moderator of the stress–illness relationship or as an independent risk factor.

SUMMARY AND CONCLUSIONS

This chapter has focused on the impact of coping strategies and coping resources as moderators of the impact of stress on health. Research on basic dimensions of coping and on the differential effectiveness of coping strategies in alleviating the health-impairing impact of stress has led to few generalizable findings. The only consistency which emerges is that avoidant coping strategies such as denial, distancing or escape, although sometimes effective in the early stages of coping with some traumatic events, may be a risk factor for adverse responses to stressful events if used chronically.

The discussion of extrapersonal coping resources focused on the beneficial effect of social support on health and the role of social support as a stress-buffering resource. There is consistent evidence from epidemiological studies that individuals with low levels of social support have higher risks of morbidity and mortality. There is also evidence that the perceived availability of social support buffers individuals against the impact of stressful life events. I discussed biological, behavioural and psychological processes which are assumed to mediate the positive impact of social support on health.

The section on intrapersonal coping resources reviewed research on personality characteristics that help to protect individuals from the negative impact of stressful life events. The discussion focused on two personality dimensions which have specifically been developed in the health context, the hardy personality and dispositional optimism. Hardiness consists of three components, namely control, commitment and challenge. It is believed that individuals who are high on these dimensions are better able to withstand the impact of stress and that this relationship is mediated by differences in appraisal processes. Hardy individuals are thought to evaluate stressful events as less stressful and threatening than non-hardy individuals. There is evidence both for the buffering effect of hardiness and for the mediating role of appraisal processes. However, due to the high correlation between hardiness and negative affectivity or neuroticism, it is somewhat unclear whether the buffering effect of hardiness should be interpreted in terms of a protective effect of hardiness on health, or in terms of differences in the way neurotic individuals perceive or report stress and health symptoms.

Dispositional optimism was discussed as a second personality variable which is assumed to moderate the impact of stress on health and wellbeing. It has been assumed that the greater stress resistance of optimists is mediated by differences in coping strategies. In particular, optimists should be more likely to engage in problem-focused coping whereas pessimists should use denial and distancing as preferred ways of coping. Evidence was presented to support this assumption. However, like hardiness, optimism is correlated with neuroticism, and it is not yet clear to what extent neuroticism may be responsible for the relationship between optimism and health and well-being.

Finally, the case of hostility was discussed as an example of a potential moderator of the stress–health relationship which does not constitute a coping resource. There is strong evidence linking hostility to coronary heart disease. It was less clear, however, whether hostility constitutes an independent risk factor or a moderator between stress and health. Explanations which account for the health risk due to hostility in terms of physiological reactivity would suggest a moderator function, even though this may be restricted to interpersonal stressors. The assumption that hostile individuals alienate their friends and thus reduce the availability of social support would also be consistent with a stress-moderating function. In contrast, explanations such as the health behaviour model are more suggestive of an independent effect of hostility on health. The only conclusion one can draw from the evidence to date is that more than one of these mechanisms is likely to contribute to the hostility–health relationship.

The body of research reviewed in this chapter has identified important extrapersonal and interpersonal resources which appear to protect individuals against the deleterious impact of stressful life events, and/or help to reduce exposure to stressful situations. Since the health impact of most of the intrapersonal resources seems to be either mediated by cognitive appraisal or coping processes, this research raises the possibility that one could direct intervention towards the modification of styles of appraisal or coping. Furthermore, since both appraisal and coping are affected by social support, it might also be helpful to provide people with extrapersonal resources such as social support, and thereby improve their capacity to deal with stress.

FURTHER READING

Folkman, S., Lazarus, R.S., Dunkel-Schetter, C., DeLongis, A. and Gruen, R.J. (1986) The dynamics of a stressful encounter. *Journal of Personality and Social Psychology*, 50: 992–1003. This study, in which the authors identified eight distinct coping strategies, resulted in the construction of the Ways of Coping Questionnaire, still one of the most widely used coping scales.

Segerstrom, S.C., Taylor, S.E., Kemeny, M.E. and Fahey, J.L. (1998) Optimism is associated with mood, coping, and immune change in response to stress. *Journal of Personality and Social Psychology*, 74: 1646–65. A prospective study which demonstrated that dispositional optimism to some extent protected individuals undergoing a stressful experience from the negative impact of stress on mood and the immune system.

Siegman, A.W. and Smith, T.W. (eds) (1994) *Anger, Hostility and the Heart.* Hillsdale, NJ: Lawrence Erlbaum. A comprehensive and authoritative review of the relationship between hostility and health.

Stroebe, W. and Stroebe, S. (1996) The social psychology of social support, in T.E. Higgins and A.W. Kruglanski (eds) *Social Psychology: Handbook of Basic Principles*, pp. 597–621. New York, NY: Guilford Press. Reviews the research on the health consequences of social support and provides a social psychological framework for the interpretation of these effects.

EIGHT

THE ROLE OF SOCIAL PSYCHOLOGY IN HEALTH PROMOTION

The epidemiological data presented in this book have identified health-impairing behaviour and psychosocial stress as important factors contributing to ill health. Social psychological knowledge can potentially be used to change health behaviour patterns and to reduce psychosocial stress, thus enabling social psychologists to make a major contribution to the public health effort. In this final chapter I would like to present my personal view on some of the more controversial aspects of the role of social psychology in health promotion.

LIMITS TO PERSUASION

Despite substantial developments in our understanding of the principles that underlie the formation and change of attitudes, the impact of programmes of health education on health behaviour patterns has sometimes been disappointing. Attempts at persuading people to change their lifestyle have been hampered by three factors.

1 It is difficult to convince people that they are vulnerable to a health risk.
2 Even if we do convince them that they are vulnerable, this may not be sufficient to motivate them to change.
3 Even if individuals are persuaded to change health-impairing behaviours, they often find it difficult to act on these intentions.

As discussed in Chapter 3, there is a discrepancy between individual and population perspectives of health risk. While public health policies are guided by the *population attributable risk*, that is, the number of excess cases of disease in a population that can be attributed to a given risk factor, individual decision making is determined by absolute and relative risk. The problem with many health-impairing behaviour patterns is that the *relative risk*, that is, the ratio of chance of the disease for individuals who engage in a risky behaviour vs those who do not, is rather low. For example, even though drinking a bottle of wine every day or having a sedentary lifestyle increases the risk of morbidity and premature mortality, the relative risk is modest. And yet, because these habits are very common in Western societies, the excess burden on the population attributable to these risk factors is quite high.

But even if the *relative* risk attributable to a given behaviour is high, as is the case with smoking, the absolute risk may still be low enough as to make it hardly seem worthwhile for the individual to change. For example, even though a smoker runs a much higher risk of developing lung cancer than does a non-smoker, the ten-year absolute risk of lung cancer for a 35-year old man who is a heavy smoker is only about 0.3 per cent, and the risk of heart disease is only 0.9 per cent (Jeffery 1989). Nevertheless, these small numbers have a great significance from a *population perspective*. In a group of 1,000,000 male smokers aged 35, nearly 10,000 will die unnecessarily before the age of 45 due to their smoking habit. From the *perspective of the individual*, on the other hand, the odds are heavily in favour of individual survival, even in the absence of behaviour change.

Fortunately, from the perspective of public health policy and health promotion, individuals often seem to overestimate the risk attributable to the major behavioural risk factors. And even though they tend to estimate their own risk as considerably lower than that of their fellow citizen, these estimates still surpass by far their (likely) 'true risk'. Finally, there is suggestive evidence that relative risks may be more important than absolute risks in influencing health decisions. In other areas of judgement at least, people tend to under-use prior probabilities derived from base rates and the same may be true for health decisions.

What is difficult to accept for most public health professionals is that convincing people that they are vulnerable may not be sufficient to motivate them to abandon health-impairing in favour of health-enhancing habits. For example, the evidence on determinants of condom use suggests that perceived vulnerability is not a good predictor of condom use. Although methodological factors may be contributing to this particular finding, it may also indicate that vulnerability has been overestimated as a target for health promotion. People often have other important reasons not to adopt safety measures. In the case of condom use, people appear to be more concerned with sexual pleasure than with safety. Thus, as Becker so succinctly put it more than 20 years ago, good health and a long life may be important aims of most people, but they are not the only aim.

Even if health education is effective in persuading people to change, people often fail to act according to their intentions. Thus, the chances of smokers stopping smoking on their first attempt are very low. Most people relapse within the first few months and need repeated attempts before they succeed, if they succeed at all. Some of these individuals can be helped by psychotherapy. But despite recent improvements in therapeutic methods, the painful fact which emerges from a review of the literature is that therapy, like medicine, has to be bitter to be helpful. The most striking demonstration of this fact is provided by the research on the use of anorectic drugs in weight loss: even though a combination of drug and behaviour therapy resulted in much greater weight loss than behaviour therapy alone, behaviour therapy patients were much better able to maintain their weight loss than patients who had undergone the combined treatment (Figure 4.5). It seems to be important that people attribute their weight loss to their ability to control their eating behaviour. This perception of self-efficacy may not develop when weight loss can be attributed to the use of an anorectic drug.

SOME SIDE EFFECTS OF HEALTH EDUCATION

There may also be unpleasant side effects to health education which psychologists have been slow to recognize. By instilling in people the conviction that everybody is responsible for their own health, health education not only increases the motivation of people to improve their own behaviour, but may also motivate them to blame others who fail to live up to these new standards. This point became unpleasantly clear to me a few year ago, when I had to undergo a coronary bypass operation. This is not a pleasant operation and I expected nothing but sympathy from my friends. I was more than a little surprised when I realized that many of them felt that I was myself largely to blame for my illness.

For a social psychologist, this should not have come as a surprise. This reaction could have been predicted from a number of social psychological theories. For example, attribution theory argues that perceptions of causality play an important role in determining affective reactions to an event as well as subsequent behaviour (Weiner et al. 1988). In the case of a serious physical illness, both the patient and the members of his social environment will search for reasons to account for onset of the illness. The outcome of this process of attribution will largely depend on the perceived controllability of the disease in question. If the disease is considered uncontrollable, the patient will be freed of any responsibility for falling ill, and everybody will be full of sympathy and pity. If, however, the disease is considered controllable, then the patient will be seen as responsible and blamed instead of pitied. Research on the perception of persons with AIDS has demonstrated that they are seen as responsible for their own illness and arouse anger rather than pity. These feelings can be changed by changing the attributions, for example, by telling people that the person in question contracted AIDS through a blood transfusion rather than sexual risk behaviour.

Although the contribution of behavioural causes is more substantial in the case of AIDS than it is for coronary heart disease, heart disease was rated in the middle range of controllability in a study conducted by Weiner and colleagues (1988). Furthermore, when participants were given the additional information that the person had been smoking and maintaining a poor diet, perceived controllability increased, and so did the level of blame for the patient.

There are a number of reasons why people may be particularly willing to blame patients for their illness. For example, the perception that a friend who is likely to be similar in many health-relevant characteristics has suddenly fallen ill with a serious illness is highly threatening. After all, if it happened to a friend it could also happen to me. People are therefore highly motivated to find reasons why it should happen to their friend and not to them. Attributing the disease to the friend's lifestyle would offer such a differentiating feature. Another reason why people may be highly motivated to blame others for their illness is that they themselves may have given up some pleasurable but health-impairing behaviour pattern, whilst the other person continued engaging in this behaviour. People who have stopped smoking may be particularly likely to blame others who continue and become sick. After all, by attributing the disease of smokers to their continued smoking, ex-smokers can justify the suffering they have undergone in abandoning the habit.

Unfortunately, this new puritanism may be the price we have to pay for emancipation. We cannot motivate people to change bad health habits and to adopt good ones without placing the responsibility for their health partly on to them. It is only human that, once they have accepted this responsibility, they will turn around and check whether others have also lived up to their responsibilities.

BEYOND PERSUASION: CHANGING THE INCENTIVE STRUCTURE

Many of the problems associated with health education can be avoided by changing the rewards and costs associated with a given behaviour. There is evidence that increases in the price of cigarettes or alcoholic beverages reduce the demand for these goods. Similarly, legal restrictions, like increasing the minimal age at which adolescents are allowed to purchase alcohol, or making seat belt use compulsory, also have a positive impact on behaviour. The advantage of legal and economic strategies is that they are useful for both influencing existing habits and preventing new health-impairing habits from developing.

However, there are also limits to the applicability of these strategies. Thus, economic incentives can only be employed in areas in which substances or goods have to be purchased in order to engage in certain health behaviours. And as the example of drug addiction demonstrates, high prices do not necessarily prevent people from abusive consumption. Similarly, legal sanctions can only be employed in areas where such sanctions are culturally acceptable and also enforceable. For example, a law prescribing that condoms must always be used in sexual intercourse would be neither socially acceptable nor enforceable.

The effectiveness of legal sanctions depends on the acceptance of the law and on individual perception that violation of the law is associated with a high risk of sanction. For example, it is quite likely that the introduction of a law making seat belt use compulsory would not have been as effective as it was if people had not accepted that such a law was in their own best interests. In fact, without the health education campaign that made it widely known that the wearing of seat belts substantially reduces the risk of injuries in traffic accidents, it is unlikely that such a law would have been passed by parliament. Similarly, the significant increases of state taxes for cigarettes in the USA were only possible after extensive health education campaigns changed the public climate regarding smoking. Thus, the war against smoking is an excellent example of the impact of a public health campaign that orchestrates persuasion with economic and legal means of changing health behaviour.

FREEDOM AND CONSTRAINT

The data presented in this book tend to support the argument developed by Gary Becker (1976) that most deaths are to some extent self-inflicted in the sense that they could have been postponed if people had engaged in a healthful lifestyle or abandoned health-impairing behaviour patterns. This has important implications for both individual decision making and public health policy. At the individual level, the implication is that people are free to choose between lifestyles which differ in their impact on their health. For example, it is up to the individual to decide whether he or she wants to smoke and risk premature death or stop the habit and thereby substantially reduce the risk of morbidity and mortality from cancer and heart disease.

The important implication for public health policy is that it has to be ensured that the choices people make are well-informed ones. Individuals must be made to understand the health implications of their chosen lifestyle. But why should governments use legal measures and tax incentives to influence *individual* behaviour and thus infringe on the freedom of their citizens to live according to their chosen lifestyles? After all, the days when suicide was a criminal offence in many countries are over. Accordingly, one could argue that people should be free to choose slow methods of suicide such as chain-smoking cigarettes or drinking too much alcohol.

However, there are reasons for governments to impose some constraint on individual freedom. One reason is that governments tend to discourage individual behaviour which interferes with the health and well-being of others. For example, the laws which forbid people to 'drink and drive' are usually justified with the argument that drunken drivers are a danger to their fellow citizens and actually kill many of them every year. Similarly, passive smoking has now been recognized as a health risk. It has been estimated, for example, that in Great Britain approximately 1000 people die each year from passive smoking. According to one newspaper report, people who believe that their health was damaged in childhood by passive smoking have begun taking legal advice about suing their parents (*Independent on Sunday*, 31 January 1993). This led to the restrictions that have been imposed on smokers in aeroplanes, public buildings and offices.

But is there any justification for constraining people's freedom to choose behaviour patterns that *impair only their own health*, such as imposing legal sanctions for failure to wear seat belts, or increasing taxes on cigarettes to reduce consumption? It has to be recognized that allowing individuals to impair their own health in this way also imposes a burden on their fellow citizens. Health, or more precisely the costs of illness, often constitute public goods. Public goods are goods for which it is not possible for those who supply or produce the good to exclude others who did not contribute from consumption. For example, clean air is a public good in the sense that people who incur costs or suffer discomfort to avoid contributing to pollution (e.g. by using public transport instead of their car) cannot prevent others, who do not incur such costs, from profiting from their actions (i.e. to free ride). Thus, there is a temptation to free ride. Similarly, health costs are a public good in countries in which there is full health insurance coverage, since contributions to insurance are usually independent of lifestyle factors. People who engage in health-impairing behaviour patterns, and as a result incur higher health costs, free ride to some extent on the healthful behaviour of others.

SUMMARY AND IMPLICATIONS

In this book, I have argued for integrated public health interventions that use both health education and fiscal and legal measures to influence a given behaviour. As the war against smoking has demonstrated, the two strategies should be seen as complementary. People are more willing to accept legal and fiscal measures if they know and accept the reasons which persuaded governmental agencies to introduce these measures. Wherever feasible, environmental changes should also be introduced to reduce or eliminate the need for behaviour change. For example, technical appliances should be constructed in ways that minimize the possibility of self-inflicted damage through careless operators.

Finally, I would argue for a change in public health goals from quantity to quality of life. The substantial extension in life expectancy during the twentieth century raised hopes that further improvements in medical treatment and healthy living would enable us to push the limits of mortality further and further. This hope has proved to be misplaced. There are strong indications that the rate at which the average life expectancy increased during the twentieth century declined sharply in the 1980s. The most favoured populations, such as women who have already reached age 65, have a life expectancy today which is exactly the same as it was in 1979 (Fries *et al.* 1989). Furthermore, physicians in the United States, who have modified their own risk behaviours well in advance of the general population and in directions reflecting the most recent knowledge (only 6 per cent of US physicians still smoke cigarettes) hardly live longer than their high-school classmates of the same race (Fries *et al.* 1989). We may have to accept the bitter truth that however far we jog, we will not live to be 140.

Fortunately, there is more to life than the absence of death. Even though healthy living may not substantially extend our lifespan, it is likely to improve the quality of life and to extend *active* life expectancy. The long-held conviction that disease and disability with advancing age results from inevitable, intrinsic aging processes has been replaced by a view that lifestyle factors and the availability of a social support network can modify many of the usual aging characteristics (Hansson and Carpenter 1994; Rowe and Kahn 1997). Thus, by adopting a healthy lifestyle when young, we can substantially increase our chances of successful aging. Furthermore, by significantly reducing the average number of sick days, hospital days or illness symptoms, a healthy lifestyle will not only improve the quality of life for the individual, but it will also result in a significant reduction in population medical expenditure.

GLOSSARY

Absolute risk: the probability that an event will occur, e.g. that an individual will become ill or die within a given period of time.

Acquired immune deficiency syndrome (AIDS): an infectious disease caused by the human immunodeficiency virus (HIV) which attacks the human immune system.

Addiction: the condition of physical and psychological dependence on using a substance (e.g. alcohol, smoking).

Aerobic exercise: energetic and sustained physical exercise intended at increasing the body's capacity to use fuel oxygen; includes jogging, bicycling and swimming.

Alcohol abuse: a maladaptive pattern of alcohol use leading to clinically significant impairment or distress as manifested by one or more of a set of social or legal problems occurring within a 12-month period (e.g. repeated absence from work due to alcohol consumption, driving under the influence of alcohol, recurrent interpersonal problems due to alcohol).

Alcohol dependence: a more serious form of alcoholism than *alcohol abuse*. In addition to the symptoms of alcohol abuse, alcohol-dependent individuals show evidence of tolerance to the effects of alcohol and/or have experienced withdrawal symptoms.

Alcohol myopia: a narrowing of cognitive focus, as a result of a decrease in cognitive capacity due to alcohol consumption. Alcohol myopic individuals are unable to pay attention to any but the most salient features of a situation.

Angina pectoris: a chronic form of *coronary heart disease* marked by periodic attacks of chest pain. It is caused by brief and incomplete blockages of the blood supply to the heart due to *atherosclerosis*.

Anorexia nervosa: an eating disorder which is characterized by self-starvation and refusal to maintain an even minimally normal body weight, combined with an intense fear of becoming fat.

Atherosclerosis: a pathologic process affecting the large muscular and elastic arteries, in which the inner layer of the artery wall is thickened through the deposition of fatty and other materials (*plaque*). Atherosclerosis of the coronary arteries is the major cause of coronary heart disease.

Attitude: the tendency to evaluate a particular entity (e.g. person, group, object) with some degree of favour or disfavour.

Attribution: the process by which people interpret their own and other people's behaviour.

Attributional style: the tendency to make a particular kind of causal inference about behaviour across different situations and across time.

Aversion therapy: therapeutic technique which associates noxious stimuli (e.g. electric shock) with an unwanted behaviour (e.g. drinking alcohol) to arouse aversion to the unwanted behaviour.

Avoidant coping: dealing with a stressful encounter by avoiding confronting the problem or the emotions it arouses. This type of coping relies on strategies such as denial, distraction or wishful thinking.

Behaviour therapy: a set of therapeutic procedures, derived from basic research on human learning, that analyses and targets for modification the stimulus variables that cause and maintain maladaptive behaviour.

Beliefs: the opinions, knowledge and thoughts someone has about some attitude object. Beliefs are perceived links between the attitude object and various attributes which are positively or negatively valued.

Binge eating: refers to consuming, in a discrete period of time, an amount of food which is definitely larger than most individuals would eat under similar circumstances.

Binge eating disorder: a newly described eating disorder characterized by frequent binge eating which is accompanied by emotional distress. These individuals do not engage in the compensatory behaviours (e.g. induced vomiting, use of laxatives) typical for *bulimia*.

Biomedical model: a scientific perspective which assumes that illness is solely the result of physical causes such as infection or injury. Psychological causes are not considered.

Biopsychosocial model: a scientific perspective which assumes that health and illness are the result of an interaction of social, psychological and biological factors.

BMI (Body Mass Index): a height-specific standard for weight obtained by dividing weight in kilograms by height in metres squared [kg/m^2]. This index has a very high correlation with body fat.

Boundary model of eating: a cognitive theory of eating regulation developed to explain differences in the eating behaviour of normal and *restrained eaters*. The model assumes that biological pressures (hunger, satiation) keep food consumption within a certain range for all individuals. Due to their chronic dieting, this range is wider for restrained than unrestrained eaters. Restrained eaters regulate their eating in terms of a self-imposed diet boundary, a cognitive limit which marks their maximum desired consumption. Transgression of this diet boundary induces disinhibitive cognitions ('what the hell' cognitions) and subsequently leads to overeating.

Buffering hypothesis of social support: the hypothesis that social support protects the individual against the negative health impact of high levels of stress.

Bulimia: an eating disorder characterized by binge eating, followed by inappropriate compensatory methods to prevent weight gain (e.g. induced vomiting, use of laxatives).

Cardiovascular reactivity: an exaggerated physiologic responsivity to behavioural challenges (e.g. stress experiences). Cardiovascular reactivity is measured by assessing the changes in heart rate, blood pressure or other cardiovascular variables in response to stress, as opposed to measuring only resting levels of these variables. It is suspected that this kind of reactivity is a factor contributing to the development of *coronary heart disease.*

Cardiovascular system: the system composed of the heart and the blood vessels.

Catecholamines: summary term which subsumes the *hormones epinephrine* and *norepinephrine* (also Dopamine).

Cholesterol: a fat-like substance. Contained in most tissues, it is also the main component of deposits in the lining of arteries. It is carried in the blood mainly by two proteins, namely low-density and high-density *lipoproteins.* Cholesterol is also contained in food (e.g. egg yolk, milk, liver and kidneys).

Cirrhosis of the liver: a disorder of the liver in which healthy liver tissue has been damaged and replaced by fibrous scar tissue. The most common causes of cirrhosis are heavy drinking over years and malnutrition.

Classical conditioning: a kind of learning through which some neutral stimulus initially incapable of eliciting a particular response gradually acquires the ability to do so through repeated association with a stimulus that has already evoked that response.

Cognitive appraisal: the evaluative process which determines why, and to what extent, a particular situation is perceived as stressful.

Cognitive–behavioural therapy: a hybrid form of psychological therapy which emphasizes the importance of cognitive processes and procedures in behaviour change. It places primary importance on cognitive processes and incorporates techniques to change aspects of cognitions as well as of behaviour.

Cognitive response model: the model assumes that attitude change is mediated by the thoughts, or 'cognitive responses', which recipients generate as they receive, and reflect upon, persuasive communications.

Cognitive restructuring: therapeutic technique which help patients to identify and correct self-defeating thought patterns which are frequently associated with emotional upset and *relapse* experiences.

Combination drug therapies for HIV and AIDS: the new, and so far highly effective, therapies which combine the nucleoside analogue reverse transcriptase inhibitors (NRTIs) available since the mid-1980s with the newly developed protease inhibitors.

Compatibility: measures of attitudes and behaviour are compatible to the extent that their target, action, context and time elements are assessed at identical levels of generality.

Confrontative coping: dealing with a stressful situation by trying to solve the problem and/or to confront the emotions it arouses.

Contingency contracting: a therapeutic technique where patients agree with some agency (usually the therapist) on a set of rewards/punishments that will be enacted contingent on their behaviour. For example, smokers who have stopped may forfeit a sum of money if they relapse.

Continuous abstinence: not smoking or drinking since the time of the stop attempt.

Coping: the cognitive and behavioural strategies which individuals use to manage both a stressful situation and the negative emotional reactions elicited by that event.

Coping resources: the extrapersonal (e.g. social support, financial resources) and intrapersonal resources (e.g. optimism, hardiness) available to the individual for *coping* with the demands of a stressful life event.

Coping strategy: the particular mode (or modes) of *coping* chosen by an individual to deal with a stressful situation.

Coping styles: preferred or habitual modes of *coping*.

Coronary angiography: cardiac catheterization to evaluate the extent of *atherosclerosis* or obstruction of the coronary arteries. Blood vessels are made visible to radiography by injecting into them a radio-opaque substance.

Coronary angioplasty: a method of treating blockage or narrowing of arteries in the heart by inserting (and then inflating) a balloon into the narrow passage to widen it. This is used as an alternative to *coronary bypass operations*.

Coronary heart disease (CHD): a disease of the arteries which feed the heart. It is almost always due to *atherosclerosis* causing inadequate blood supply to the heart muscles. There are two major forms of CHD, namely acute myocardial infarction and angina pectoris.

Correlation coefficient: a statistic that reflects the degree and direction of an association between two variables. Ranges from −1.00 (negative association) through 0.00 (no association) to +1.00 (positive association).

Cortisol: a *hormone* secreted by the adrenal cortex which promotes the synthesis and storage of glucose, suppresses inflammation and regulates the distribution of fat in the body.

Cross-sectional study: a research design by which variables are assessed in different groups at the same point in time. For example, the impact of a suspected risk factor on health is assessed by comparing the health of individuals exposed to the risk factor with that of individuals not exposed to the risk factor.

Daily hassles: minor stressors resulting from the irritations and frustrations of daily life.

Defence motivation: the desire to defend and maintain certain beliefs or attitudinal positions which are consistent with existing central attitudes and values.

Detoxification: the process of getting an addicted individual safely through withdrawal after stopping the use of the substance (e.g. drying out of alcoholics).

Disease concept of alcohol abuse: the view that alcoholism is a disease, caused by a psychological predisposition, an allergic reaction to alcohol, or some nutritional deficits. Due to this disease, alcoholics suffer a loss of control when exposed to alcohol, which renders them unable to stop drinking. The only cure is total abstention.

Disulfiram: a drug which induces nausea and vomiting if one drinks alcohol in the days following ingestion of the drug. Administered to deter alcohol abusers from drinking alcohol.

Dual-process theories of persuasion: theories of persuasion (e.g. elaboration likelihood model, heuristic-systematic model) which postulate two modes of information processing that differ in the extent to which individuals engage in content-relevant thoughts. The mode of information processing used by an individual is assumed to depend on processing motivation and ability.

Emotion-focused coping: *Coping* strategies which do not focus on the stressful event but on ameliorating the distressing emotional reactions to the event.

Endocrine system: the system of glands and other structures that produces and secretes *hormones* into the bloodstream.

Epidemiology: the study of the distribution and determinants of health-related states or events in specified populations.

Epinephrine (US term for adrenaline): a *hormone* secreted by the adrenal medulla which stimulates the sympathetic nervous system. It stimulates the heart action and raises the blood pressure, releases glucose and increases its consumption, increases the circulation of the blood in the muscles, relaxes air passages and stimulates breathing. It prepares the body for physical action and at the same time inhibits digestion and excretion.

Expectancy-value models: models which assume that decisions between different courses of action are based on two types of cognitions, namely the subjective probability that a given action will lead to a set of expected outcomes and the valence of these outcomes. Individuals are assumed to choose the course of action which will be most likely to lead to positive consequences or avoid negative consequences.

Experiment: a controlled study where the experimenter deliberately introduces changes in the experimental condition but not the control condition to assess the effects of these changes on some variable of interest (i.e. the dependent variable). The control or comparison condition is comparable to the experimental condition in all respects, except that the changes have not been introduced. In true experiments respondents have to be randomly assigned to conditions.

Externality hypothesis: a cognitive theory of eating regulation which assumes differences in the cues that trigger the eating behaviour of obese and normal weight individuals. Whereas normal weight individuals respond mainly to internal, bodily cues in regulating their eating behaviour, the eating of overweight individuals is strongly influenced by external factors such as the sight and smell of food, social stimuli and habit.

Fear appeals: persuasive communications that attempt to motivate recipients to change behaviour deleterious to their health by inducing fear about the potential health hazards.

Foetal alcohol syndrome: distinct pattern of birth defects as a result of pre-natal exposure to alcohol due to mother's overconsumption of alcohol during pregnancy.

Functional measures of the immune system: measures of the performance of certain immune cells. The ability of lymphocytes to activate other cells to proliferate in the face of antigenic challenge, or to destroy invading cells, is essential to an adequate immune response. Lymphocytic proliferation is a test of cellular immunity that examines how effectively lymphocytes divide when stimulated through incubation with mitogens such as phytohemagglutinin (PHA) or concanavalin A (Con A). The ability of natural killer cells to destroy tumour cells is assessed by incubating natural killer cells with tumour cells.

Functional measures of social support: measures which assess the extent to which interpersonal relationships serve particular support functions (e.g. emotion, instrumental, information and appraisal support).

General adaptation syndrome (GAS): the stages of physiological reaction through which an organism moves when exposed to prolonged and intense stress. The stages consist of alarm, resistance and exhaustion.

Habits: learned sequences of acts which have become automatic responses to specific cues and are functional in obtaining certain goals or end states.

Health: a state of physical, mental and social well-being which changes over time.

Health behaviour: defined either subjectively as behaviour undertaken by individuals to enhance or maintain their health or objectively as behaviours which have been shown to have beneficial health consequences.

Health belief model: the model assumes that people's health behaviour is determined by their perception of the threat of illness or injury and the advantages and disadvantages of taking action.

Health education: the provision of knowledge and/or training of skills which facilitate voluntary adoption of behaviour conducive to health.

Health promotion: any planned combination of educational, economic or environmental measures designed to reduce the vulnerability of individuals, groups or communities to disease in general, or to enhance their health.

Heuristic processing: mode of information processing which assesses the validity of a communication through reliance on heuristics (i.e. simple rules like 'doctors are always right') rather than a critical evaluation of the arguments.

Hopelessness: a state characterized by negative expectations about the occurrence of highly valued outcomes (a negative outcome expectancy) and expectations of helplessness about changing the likelihood of occurrence of these outcomes (a helplessness expectancy).

Hormones: chemical substances which are released from an *endocrine* gland into the bloodstream and act on a distant target site.

Hostility: a personality trait that constitutes a risk factor for coronary heart disease. It reflects a negative attitude towards others involving cognitive (e.g. cynicism, mistrust), affective (e.g. anger) and behavioural components (e.g. aggression).

Human Immunodeficiency Virus (HIV): a virus which attacks and damages the immune system by infecting and killing *T-helper cells*.

Hypertension: high blood pressure.

Ileal bypass: a bypass of the end of the small intestines, used as surgical treatment in cases of extreme obesity.

Incidence: the number of new events, e.g. new cases of a disease in a defined population within a specified period of time.

Learned helplessness: a condition of apathy and depression in reaction to repeated exposure to unavoidable stressors.

Lipoprotein: proteins that transport cholesterol in the blood. Classified into low-density and high-density lipoprotein. High levels of low-density lipoprotein contribute to plaque formation in atherosclerosis. High-density lipoprotein may be involved in transporting surplus cholesterol back to the liver.

Longitudinal study: study in which a cohort of people is followed to allow repeated measurement of variables with the same individuals over time.

Mediating variable or process: a variable or process assumed to account for the cause–effect relationship between two other variables (e.g. differential knowledge about health risks is assumed to be one of the mediators of the relationship between social class and health). The mediating variable is assumed to be (at least partly) responsible for the effect of the cause (i.e. social class) on the outcome variable (i.e. health). To demonstrate that a variable is a mediator, one has to show that it covaries with both changes in the assumed cause and changes in the assumed outcome, and that statistically controlling for the mediator (e.g. through multiple regression) results in a substantial reduction, or even elimination, of the association between the assumed cause and the outcome.

Meta-analysis: a set of statistical techniques for integrating the results of independent studies of a given phenomenon in a common metric (effect size). Use of this common metric permits comparisons across studies and the examination of overall outcomes of findings of all studies combined.

Morbidity: any departure, subjective or objective, from a state of mental or physical well-being.

Mortality: death, usually calculated so that the number of deaths can be expressed as a ratio to number of persons at risk (i.e. still alive) in a specified population.

Myocardial infarction: an acute form of *coronary heart disease* which is commonly called a 'heart attack'. It reflects the death of a heart muscle (myocardium) due to severe and/or prolonged blockage of the blood supply to the tissue.

Negative affectivity: refers to a broad dimension of individual differences (reflected by measures of neuroticism) in the tendency to experience negative distressing emotions. Can affect responses to questionnaire items.

Negotiated safety: refers to agreements between partners to abstain from unprotected sex outside their relationship.

Nicotine regulation model: a theory of smoking which assumes that people smoke to regulate the level of nicotine in the internal milieu. Smoking is stimulated when the nicotine level falls below a certain set point.

Nicotine replacement therapy: nicotine replacement through nicotine chewing gum or nicotine patches helps people who have stopped smoking to overcome withdrawal symptoms.

Norepinephrine (US term for noradrenaline): a hormone released by the adrenal medulla and by the synapses of sympathetic nerves. Whereas epinephrine prepares the body for physical action, norepinephrine deals with the routine jobs such as maintaining an even blood pressure.

Obesity: severe overweight due to excessive body fat. An individual is classified as obese with a body weight which is more than 20 per cent above the ideal weight or a BMI more than 30 kg/m^2.

Operant conditioning: modifies behaviour by manipulating the consequences of such behaviour.

Overweight: a body weight that is between the upper limit of normal and 20 per cent above that limit.

Passive smoking: breathing someone else's smoke in the environment.

Perceived social support: the perception that supportive others are available.

Persuasion: the effects of exposure to relatively complex messages from other persons on the attitudes and beliefs of the recipients.

Placebo control groups: used to check whether the effect of a drug treatment is due to the active ingredient of the drug or some other effects of the treatment. Placebo control groups receive apparently the same drug treatment as the intervention group, except that the administered drug lacks the active ingredient.

Plaque: fatty material that may deposit in arteries. Responsible for narrowing of arteries.

Point prevalence abstinence: not smoking or not drinking around the time when the measurement is being taken.

Population attributable risk: refers to the number of excess cases of disease in a population that can be attributed to a given risk factor.

Prevalence: the number of events (e.g. instances of a given disease) in a given population at a given time.

Primary appraisal: evaluative process by which individuals categorize a given situation with respect to its significance for their well-being and decide whether the situation is irrelevant, positive, or potentially harmful.

Primary prevention: actions undertaken to prevent health problems from occurring.

Problem-focused coping: refers to instrumental behaviour aimed at reducing the risk of harmful consequences that might result from the stressful event.

Prospective study: longitudinal study where the risk factors or variables (e.g. stressful life events) which predict a certain future outcome (e.g. depression or heart disease) are measured first, and the outcome variables are then assessed at some future point in time.

Protection motivation theory: originally an attempt to specify the algebraic relationship between the components of the health belief model. In its most recent version the model assumes that the motivation to protect oneself from danger is a positive linear function of four beliefs: the threat is severe, one is personally vulnerable, one has the ability to perform the coping response, and the coping response is effective in reducing the threat. Two other beliefs have a negative effect on protection motivation: that engaging in the health impairing behaviour is rewarding; and that giving it up is costly.

Psychoneuroimmunology: studies the interaction between psychosocial processes and nervous, endocrine and immune system functioning.

Public health model: a term used here to refer to interventions aimed at changing health behaviour that rely on health promotion and are designed to change the behaviour of large groups.

Quantitative or enumerative tests of the immune system: involve counting the number or percentages of different types of immune cells such as helper T cells, suppressor/cytotoxic T cells, B cells and natural killer (NK) cells in the peripheral blood.

Rapid smoking: a clinical technique which creates aversion to smoking by instructing subjects to smoke continually, inhaling every 6 to 8 seconds, until tolerance is reached.

Received social support: actual social support that has been received over a given period of time.

Relapse: reverting to the full-blown pattern of health impairing or otherwise unwanted behaviour after beginning to change it.

Relative risk: the ratio of the risk of disease or death for individuals who engage in a risky behaviour and those who do not.

Restrained eaters: chronic dieters who try to restrict their food intake and suppress their weight.

Risk factor: any factor (e.g. aspect of personal behaviour, exposure) that increases the probability (determinant), or is associated with an increased probability of occurrence, of a disease (risk marker).

Rumination: an ineffective coping style associated with increased levels of depressive symptomatology. Ruminators tend to focus passively on their symptoms of distress and the meaning and consequences of those symptoms.

Safe sex: sex which involves no risk of the partner being exposed to HIV. Sex is only safe if partners do not engage in any activities which result, or can result, in an exchange of blood, semen, or vaginal secretions.

Safer sex: defined by activities (e.g. condom use) which substantially reduce the risk of infection.

Secondary appraisal: evaluation of the options available to meet the demands of the stressful situation and to avoid the threatened negative consequences.

Secondary prevention: actions undertaken to treat a disease in the early, non-symptomatic stages with the aim of arresting or reversing the condition.

Self-efficacy: refers to beliefs in one's ability to carry out certain actions required to produce a given attainment. For example, the belief that one is capable of giving up smoking or going on a diet.

Self-management procedures: therapeutic procedures where clients are taught to analyse their own behaviour and to manage their own behaviour change.

Set point theory of weight regulation: proposes that each person has a physiologically based weight level (set point) which the body strives to maintain.

Skill training: therapeutic procedure based on the assumption that people engage in health-impairing behaviours because they lack certain skills, such as the skill to cope with stress or with negative emotional states.

Social support: reflects the information from others that one is loved and cared for, esteemed and valued, and part of a network of communication and mutual obligation. Such information can come from a spouse, a lover, children, friends, or social and community contacts such as churches or social clubs.

Stage models of change: theories (e.g. transtheoretical model, precaution adoption process model) which assume that health behaviour change involves progression through a discernible number of stages from ignorance of a health threat to completed preventive action.

Stages of change: the stages through which individuals are assumed to move in their progression from ignorance of a health risk to taking protective action. The different stages are assumed to represent qualitatively different patterns of behaviour, beliefs and experience, and factors which produce transitions between stages vary depending on the specific stage transitions being considered.

Statins: a new generation of cholesterol-lowering drugs which block the endogenous synthesis of cholesterol in the liver.

Stress: the condition which arises when individuals perceive the demands of a situation as challenging or exceeding their resources and endangering their well-being.

Stressful life events: events which represent major changes in an individual's life that range from short-term to enduring and are potentially threatening.

Structural measures of social support: reflect the social integration or social embeddedness of individuals by assessing the existence or quantity of their social relationships.

Subjective norms: (normative) beliefs about how people who are important to us expect us to act weighted by our motivation to comply with their expectations.

Systematic processing: thorough, detailed processing of the information contained in a persuasive communication involving scrutinization of arguments and argument-relevant thinking.

Tailoring: a technique of personalizing persuasive communications on the basis of information about individuals gathered by questionnaire. This technique was originally developed to match persuasive communications to the *stages of change* of the individual, but it can be used to tailor the message to many more individual characteristics.

Tension reduction hypothesis: assumes that alcohol is consumed because it reduces tension. Increased tension constitutes a heightened drive state. By lowering tension and thus reducing this drive state, alcohol consumption has reinforcing properties.

T-helper cells: a class of lymphocytes which serves an important function in the regulation of the immune system by stimulating other cells to attack antigens.

Theory of planned behaviour: the extension of the theory of reasoned action. Besides attitudes and subjective norms, perceived behavioural control is incorporated as the third important predictor of behaviour.

Theory of reasoned action: a theory of the relationship between attitude and behaviour. Assumes that attitudes combine with subjective norms to influence behaviour.

Therapy model: a term used here to refer to interventions aimed at changing health behaviour that rely on methods of psychological therapy. This type of intervention typically involves a one-to-one relationship where 'patients' and therapists are in dyadic interaction, although group treatments and self-therapy programmes are also used.

Very low-calorie diets: supplemented fasts designed to spare the loss of lean body mass through the provision of 70 to 100 grams of protein a day in a total of 300 to 600 calories.

REFERENCES

Abel, E.L. (1980) Fetal Alcohol Syndrome: behavioral teratology. *Psychological Bulletin*, 87: 29–50.

Abraham, C., Sheeran, P., Spears, R. and Abrams, D. (1992) Health beliefs and the promotion of HIV-preventive intentions among teenagers: a Scottish perspective. *Health Psychology*, 11: 369–70.

Abramson, L., Metalsky, G. and Alloy, L. (1989) Hopelessness depression: a theory-based subtype of depression. *Psychological Review*, 96: 358–72.

Abramson, L.Y., Seligman, M.E.P. and Teasdale, J.D. (1978) Learned helplessness in humans: critique and reformulation. *Journal of Abnormal Psychology*, 87: 49–74.

Adler, M., Phillips, A. and Johnson, A. (1997) Communicable diseases: sexually transmitted disease, including AIDS, in J. Charlton and M. Murphy (eds) *The Health of Adult Britain 1941–1994*, Vol. 2, pp. 21–9. London: Government Printing Service.

Adler, N.E., Boyce, T., Chesney, M.A. *et al.* (1994) Socioeconomic status and health: the challenge of the gradient. *American Psychologist*, 49: 15–24.

Ailhaud, G. and Hauner, H. (1998) Development of white adipose tissue, in G.A. Bray, C. Bouchard and W.P.T. James (eds) *Handbook of Obesity*, pp. 359–78. New York, NY: Marcel Dekker.

Ajzen, I. (1988) *Attitudes, Personality and Behavior*. Chicago, IL: Dorsey.

Ajzen, I. (1991) The theory of planned behavior. *Organizational Behavior and Human Decision Processes*, 50: 179–211.

Ajzen, I. (1996) The directive influence of attitudes on behavior, in P.M. Gollwitzer and J.A. Bargh (eds) *The Psychology of Action*, pp. 385–403. New York, NY: Guilford Press.

Ajzen, I. and Fishbein, M. (1977) Attitude–behavior relations: a theoretical analysis and review of empirical research. *Psychological Bulletin*, 84: 888–918.

Ajzen, I. and Madden, T.J. (1986) Prediction of goal-directed behavior: attitudes, intentions, and perceived behavioral control. *Journal of Experimental Social Psychology*, 22: 453–74.

Ajzen, I. and Sexton, J. (1999) Depth of processing, belief congruence, and attitude–behavior correspondence, in S. Chaiken and Y. Trope (eds) *Dual-process theories in social psychology*, pp. 117–38. New York, NY: Guilford Press.

Ajzen, I. and Timko, C. (1986) Correspondence between health attitudes and behavior. *Journal of Basic and Applied Psychology*, 42: 426–35.

Albert, M.S., Savage, C.R., Jones, K. *et al.* (1995) Predictors of cognitive change in older persons: MacArthur studies of successful aging. *Psychology and Aging*, 10: 578–89.

Alcoholics Anonymous (1955) *The Story of How Many Thousands of Men and Women Have Recovered from Alcoholism*. New York, NY: Alcoholics Anonymous Publishing.

Aldwin, C.M. and Revenson, T.A. (1987) Does coping help? A reexamination of the relation between coping and mental health. *Journal of Personality and Social Psychology*, 53: 337–48.

Allred, K.D. and Smith, T.W. (1989) The hardy personality: cognitive and physiological responses to evaluative threat. *Journal of Personality and Social Psychology*, 56: 257–66.

American Cancer Society (1986) *1986: Cancer, Fact and Figures*. New York, NY: American Cancer Society.

American College of Sports Medicine (1979) The recommended quantity and quality of exercise for developing and maintaining fitness in healthy adults. *Medicine and Science in Sports*, 10: 7–9.

Amirkhan, J.H. (1990) A factor analytically derived measure of coping: the coping strategy indicator. *Journal of Personality and Social Psychology*, 59: 1066–74.

Anderson, P. and Scott, E. (1992) The effect of general practitioners' advice to heavy drinking men. *British Journal of Addiction*, 87: 891–900.

Andres, R. (1995) Bodyweight and age, in K.D. Brownell and C.G. Fairburn (eds) *Eating Disorders and Obesity*, pp. 65–70. New York, NY: Guilford Press.

APA (American Psychiatric Association) (1987) *Diagnostic and Statistical Manual of Mental Disorders (DSM-III-R)*. Washington, DC: American Psychiatric Association.

APA (American Psychiatric Association) (1994) *Diagnostic and Statistical Manual of Mental Disorders: Fourth Edition*. Washington, DC: American Psychiatric Association.

Archer, J. (1999) *The Nature of Grief: The Evolution and Psychology of Reactions to Loss*. London: Routledge.

Armitage, C.J. and Conner, M. (1998) Efficacy of the theory of planned behavior: a meta-analytic review. Unpublished manuscript, University of Leeds.

Armitage, C.J. and Conner, M. (1999) Distinguishing perceptions of control from self-efficacy: predicting consumption of a low fat diet using the theory of planned behavior. *Journal of Applied Social Psychology*, 29: 72–90.

Armstrong, G.L., Conn, L.A. and Pinner, R.W. (1999) Trends in infectious disease mortality in the United States during the 20th century. *Journal of the American Medical Association*, 281: 611–67.

Ashley, M.J. and Rankin, J.G. (1988) A public health approach to the prevention of alcohol-related problems. *Annual Review of Public Health*, 9: 233–71.

Aspinwall, L.G. and Taylor, S.E. (1992) Modeling cognitive adaptation: a longitudinal investigation of the impact of individual differences and coping on college adjustment and performance. *Journal of Personality and Social Psychology*, 63: 989–1003.

Autorengruppe Nationales Forschungsprogramm (1984) *Wirksamkeit der Gemeindeorientierten Prävention Kardiovascularer Krankheiten* (Effectiveness of Community-Oriented Prevention of Cardiovascular Diseases). Bern: Hans Huber.

Azrin, N.H. (1976) Improvements in the community-reinforcement approach to alcoholism. *Behaviour, Research and Therapy*, 6: 7–12.

Baer, J.S. and Lichtenstein, E. (1988) Classification and prediction of smoking relapse episodes: an exploration of individual differences. *Journal of Consulting and Clinical Psychology*, 56: 104–10.

Bahrke, M.S. and Morgan, W.P. (1978) Anxiety reduction following exercise and meditation. *Cognitive Therapy and Research*, 2: 323–33.

Bakker, A.B., Buunk, B.P. and Engles, R.C.M.E. (1994) Buitenechetlijke seks en AIDS-preventief gedrag: Een toets van het investeringsmodel, in P.A.M. van Lange, F.W. Siero, B. Verplanken and E.C.M. van Schie (eds) *Sociale psychologie en haar toepassingen*, pp. 40–53. Eburon: Delft.

Baltes, P.B. and Schaie, K.W. (1976) On the plasticity of intelligence in adulthood and old age: where Horn and Donaldson fail. *American Psychologist*, 31: 720–5.

Bandura, A. (1986) *Social Foundations of Thought and Action: A Cognitive Social Theory*. Englewood Cliffs, NJ: Prentice Hall.

Bandura, A. (1997) *Self-efficacy: The Exercise of Control*. New York, NY: Freeman.

Bandura, A., O'Leary, A., Taylor, C.B., Gauthier, J. and Gossard, D. (1987) Perceived self-efficacy and pain control: opioid and non-opioid mechanisms. *Journal of Personality and Social Psychology*, 53: 563–71.

Barefoot, J.C., Dodge, K.A., Peterson, B.L., Dahlstrom, W.G. and Williams Jr, R.B. (1989) The Cook–Medley Hostility Scale: item content and ability to predict surivival. *Psychosomatic Medicine*, 51: 46–57.

Barendregt, J.J., Bonneux, L. and van der Maas, P. (1997) The health costs of smoking. *New England Journal of Medicine*, 337: 1052–7.

Bargh, J.A. (1996) Automacity in social psychology, in E.T. Higgins and A.W. Kruglanski (eds) *Social Psychology: Handbook of Basic Principles*, pp. 169–83. New York, NY: Guilford Press.

Bargh, J. and Barndollar, K. (1996) Automaticity in action: the unconscious as repository of chronic goals and motives, in P.M. Gollwitzer and J.A. Bargh (eds) *The Psychology of Action*, pp. 457–81. New York, NY: Guilford Press.

Baron, R., Inman, M.B., Kao, C.F. and Logan, H. (1992) Emotion and superficial social processing. *Motivation and Emotion*, 16: 323–45.

Baron, R., Logan, H., Lilly, J., Inman, M. and Brennan, M. (1994) Negative emotion and message processing. *Journal of Experimental Social Psychology*, 30: 181–201.

Barrera Jr, M., Sandler, I.N. and Ramsey, T.B. (1981) Preliminary development of a scale of social support: studies on college students. *American Journal of Community Psychology*, 9: 435–47.

Batchelor, W.F. (1988) AIDS 1988: The science and the limits of science. *American Psychologist*, 43: 853–8.

Baucom, D.H. and Aiken, P.A. (1981) Effect of depressed mood on eating among obese and nonobese dieting persons. *Journal of Personality and Social Psychology*, 41: 477–585.

Beck, A.T. (1976) *Cognitive Therapy and the Emotional Disorders*. New York, NY: International Universities Press.

Becker, G.S. (1976) *The Economic Approach to Human Behavior*. Chicago, IL: University of Chicago Press.

Becker, G.S., Grossman, M. and Murphy, K.M. (1994) An empirical analysis of cigarette addiction. *American Economic Review*, 84: 396–418.

Belcher, L., Kalichman, S., Topping, M. *et al.* (1998) A randomized trial of a brief HIV risk reduction counseling intervention for women. *Journal of Consulting and Clinical Psychology*, 66: 856–61.

Bellack, A.S. (1977) Behavioral treatment for obesity: appraisal and recommendations, in M. Hersen, R.M. Eisler and P.M. Miller (eds) *Progress in Behavior Modification*, pp. 1–38. New York, NY: Academic Press.

Belloc, N.B. (1973) Relationship of health practices to mortality. *Preventive Medicine*, 2: 67–81.

Belloc, N.B. and Breslow, L. (1972) Relationship of physical health status and health practices. *Preventive Medicine*, 5: 409–21.

Bem, D.J. (1965) An experimental analysis of self-persuasion. *Journal of Experimental Social Psychology*, 1: 199–218.

Bentler, P.M. and Speckart, G. (1979) Models of attitude–behavior relations. *Psychological Review*, 86: 452–64.

Bentler, P.M. and Speckart, G. (1981) Attitudes 'cause' behaviours: a structural equation analysis. *Journal of Personality and Social Psychology*, 40: 226–38.

Berg, D., LaBerg, J.C., Skutte, A. and Ohman, A. (1981) Instructed versus pharmacological effects of alcohol in alcoholics and social drinkers. *Behavioral Research and Therapy*, 19: 55–66.

Berg, F.M. (1999) Health risks associated with weight loss and obesity treatment programs. *Journal of Social Issues*, 55: 277–97.

Berkman, L.F. and Syme, S.L. (1979) Social networks, host resistance, and mortality: a nine-year follow-up of Alameda County residents. *American Journal of Epidemiology*, 109: 186–204.

Berkowitz, L. and Cottingham, D.R. (1960) The interest value and relevance of fear-arousing communications. *Journal of Abnormal and Social Psychology*, 60: 37–43.

Berlin, J.A. and Colditz, G.A. (1990) A meta-analysis of physical activity in the prevention of coronary heart disease. *American Journal of Epidemiology*, 132: 612–28.

Bernard, J. (1968) *The Sex Game*. Englewood Cliffs, NJ: Prentice Hall.

Best, J.A., Thompson, S.J., Santi, S.M., Smith, E.A. and Brown, K.S. (1988) Preventing cigarette-smoking among schoolchildren. *Annual Review of Public Health*, 9: 161–201.

Bigelow, G., Strickler, D., Liebson, I. and Griffiths, R. (1976) Maintaining disulfiram ingestion among outpatient alcoholics: a security deposit contingency contracting procedure. *Behavior Research and Therapy*, 14: 378–81.

Billings, J.H., Scherwitz, L.W., Sullivan, R., Sparler, S. and Ormish, D. (1996) The lifestyle heart trial: comprehensive treatment and group support therapy, in R. Allan and S. Scheidt (eds) *Heart and Mind*, pp. 233–54. Washington, DC: American Psychological Association.

Billman, G.E., Schwartz, P.J. and Stone, H.L. (1984) The effects of daily exercise on susceptibility to sudden cardiac death. *Circulation*, 69: 1182–9.

Björntorp, P. (1986) Fat cells and obesity, in K.D. Brownell and J.P. Foreyt (eds) *Handbook of Eating Disorders*, pp. 88–98. New York, NY: Basic Books.

Blackburn, G.L., Lynch, M.E. and Wong, S.L. (1986) The very-low-calorie diet: a weight-reduction technique, in K.D. Brownell and J.P. Foreyt (eds) *Handbook of Eating Disorders*, pp. 198–212. New York, NY: Basic Books.

Blackburn, H. (1983) Diet and atherosclerosis: epidemiologic evidence and public health implications. *Preventive Medicine*, 12: 2–10.

Blair, S.N., Kohl, H.W., Paffenbarger Jr, R.S. *et al.* (1989) Physical fitness and all-cause mortality: a prospective study of healthy men and women. *Journal of the American Medical Association*, 3: 2395–401.

Blair, S.N., Kohl, H.W., Barlow, C.E. *et al.* (1995) Changes in physical fitness and all-cause mortality. *Journal of the American Medical Association*, 273: 1093–9.

Blalock, S., DeVellis, R.F., Giorgino, K.B. *et al.* (1996) Osteoporosis prevention in premenopausal women: using a stage model approach to examine the predictors of behaviour. *Health Psychology*, 15: 84–93.

Blane, H.T. and Leonard, K.E. (eds) (1987) *Psychological Theories of Drinking and Alcoholism*. New York, NY: Guilford Press.

Blascovich, J. and Katkin, E.S. (1995) *Cardiovascular Reactivity to Psychological Stress and Disease*. Washington, DC: American Psychological Association.

Blazer, D.G. (1982) Social support and mortality in an elderly community population. *American Journal of Epidemiology*, 115: 684–94.

Bliss, R.E., Garvey, A.J., Heinold, J.W. and Hitchcock, J.L. (1989) The influence of situation and coping on relapse crisis outcomes after smoking cessation. *Journal of Consulting and Clinical Psychology*, 57: 443–9.

Blundell, J.E. and Stubbs, R.J. (1998) Diet composition and control of food intake in humans, in G.A. Bray, C. Bouchard and W.P.T. James (eds) *Handbook of Obesity*, pp. 243–72. New York, NY: Marcel Dekker.

Boer, H. and Seydel, E.R. (1996) Protection motivation theory, in M. Conner and P. Norman. *Predicting Health Behaviour*, pp. 121–62. Buckingham: Open University Press.

Bohman, M., Sigvardsson, S. and Cloninger, C.R. (1981) Maternal inheritance of alcohol abuse. *Archives of General Psychiatry*, 38: 965–9.

Boon, B. (1998) Why dieters overeat: on the cognitive regulation of eating behaviour. Unpublished dissertation, University of Utrecht.

Boon, B., Stroebe, W., Schut, H. and Jansen, A. (1997) Does cognitive distraction lead to overeating in restrained eaters? *Behavioural and Cognitive Psychotherapy*, 25: 319–27.

Boon, B., Stroebe, W., Jansen, A. and Schut, H. (1998a) Food for thought: cognitive regulation of food intake. *British Journal of Health Psychology*, 3: 27–40.

Boon, B., Stroebe, W., Schut, H. and Ijtema, R. (1998b) Reformulating the boundary model: tronic processes in the eating behaviour of restrained eaters. Unpublished manuscript, University of Utrecht.

Borgida, E. and Brekke, N. (1981) The base rate fallacy in attribution and prediction, in J.H. Harvey, W.J. Ickes and R.F. Kidd (eds) *New Directions in Attribution Research*, Vol. 3, pp. 63–95. Hillsdale, NJ: Lawrence Erlbaum.

Borland, R., Owen, N., Hill, D. and Schofield, P. (1991) Predicting attempts at sustained cessation of smoking after the introduction of workplace smoking bans. *Health Psychology*, 10: 336–42.

Boster, F.J. and Mongeau, P. (1984) Fear-arousing persuasive messages, in R.N. Bostrom (ed.), *Communication Yearbook*, Vol. 8, pp. 330–75. Beverly Hills, CA: Sage.

Bouchard, C. and Pérusse, L. (1993) Genetics of obesity. *Annual Review of Nutrition*, 13: 337–54.

Brand, R.J., Paffenbarger, R.S., Sholtz, R.I. and Kampert, J.B. (1979) Work activity and fatal heart attack studied by multiple logistic risk analysis. *American Journal of Epidemiology*, 110: 52–62.

Bray, G.A. (1986) Effects of obesity on health and happiness, in K.D. Brownell and J.P. Foreyt (eds) *Handbook of Eating Disorders*, pp. 3–44. New York, NY: Basic Books.

Breslow, L. (1990) The future of public health: prospects in the United States for the 1990s. *Annual Review of Public Health*, 11: 1–28.

Breslow, L. and Enstrom, J.E. (1980) Persistence of health habits and their relationship to mortality. *Preventive Medicine*, 9: 469–83.

Brewin, C.R. (1988) *Cognitive Foundations of Clinical Psychology*. London: Lawrence Erlbaum.

Brown, G., Zhao, X-Q., Sacco, D. and Albers, J.J. (1993) Lipid lowering and plaque regression. *Circulation*, 87: 1781–91.

Brown, G.W. and Harris, T. (1978) *Social Origins of Depression: A Study of Psychiatric Disorder in Women*. New York, NY: Free Press.

Brown, G.W. and Harris, T.O. (eds) (1989) *Life Events and Illness*. New York, NY: Guilford Press.

Brownell, K.D. (1983) Assessment in the treatment of eating disorders, in D.H. Barlow (ed.) *Behavioral Assessment of Adult Disorders*, pp. 329–404. New York, NY: Guilford Press.

Brownell, K.D. (1995) Exercise in the treatment of obesity, in K.D. Brownell and C.G. Fairburn (eds) *Eating Disorders and Obesity*, pp. 473–8. New York, NY: Guilford Press.

Brownell, K.D. and Rodin, J. (1994) The dieting maelstrom: is it possible and advisable to lose weight? *American Psychologist*, 49: 781–91.

Brownell, K.D., Stunkard, A.J. and Albaum, J.M. (1980) Evaluation and modification of exercise patterns in the natural environment. *American Journal of Psychiatry*, 137: 1540–5.

Brownell, K.D., Marlatt, G.A., Lichtenstein, E. and Wilson, G.T. (1986) Understanding and preventing relapse. *American Psychologist*, 41: 765–82.

Brownson, R.C., Eriksen, M.P., Davis, R.M. and Warner, K.E. (1997) Environmental tobacco smoke: health effects and policies to reduce exposure. *Annual Review of Public Health*, 18: 163–85.

Brug, J., Steenhuis, I. van Assema, P. and de Vries, H. (1996) The impact of a computer-tailored nutrition intervention. *Preventive Medicine*, 25: 236–42.

Brunner, D., Manelis, G., Modan, M. and Levin, S. (1974) Physical activity at work and the incidence of myocardial infarction, angina pectoris and death due to ischemic heart disease. An epidemiological study in Israel collective settlements (kibbutzim). *Journal of Chronic Diseases*, 27: 217–33.

Bruun, K., Edwards, G., Lumio, M. *et al.* (1975) *Alcohol Control Policies and Public Health Perspective*, 25. Helsinki: Finnish Foundation for Alcohol Studies.

Buchner, D.M., Beresford, S.A.A., Larson, E.B., LaCroix, A.Z. and Wagner, E.H. (1992) Effects of physical activity on health status in older adults II: intervention studies. *Annual Review of Public Health*, 13: 469–88.

Budd, R.J. (1986) Predicting cigarette use: the need to incorporate measures of salience in the theory of reasoned action. *Journal of Applied Social Psychology*, 16: 663–85.

Budd, R.J. and Rollnick, S. (1996) The structure of the readiness to change questionnaire: a test of Prochaska and DiClemente's transtheoretical model. *British Journal of Health Psychology*, 1: 365–76.

Byers, T., Mullis, R., Anderson, J. *et al.* (1995) The cost and effects of a nutritional education program following work-site cholesterol screening. *American Journal of Public Health*, 85: 650–5.

Byrne, D. (1961) The repression-sensitization scale: rationale, reliability and validity. *Journal of Personality*, 29: 334–49.

Byrne, D.G., Whyte, H.M. and Butler, K.L. (1981) Illness behaviour and outcome following survived myocardial infarction: a prospective study. *Journal of Psychosomatic Research*, 25: 97–107.

Canning, H. and Mayer, J. (1966) Obesity – its possible effect on college acceptance. *New England Journal of Medicine*, 275: 1172–4.

Cannon, W.B. (1929) *Bodily changes in pain, hunger, fear, and rage*. Boston, MA: C.T. Branford.

Caplan, R.D. (1983) Person–environment fit: past, present and future, in C.L. Cooper (ed.) *Stress Research*, pp. 35–78. New York, NY: Wiley.

Cappell, H. and Greeley, J. (1987) Alcohol and tension reduction: an update on research and theory, in H.T. Blane and K.E. Leonard (eds) *Psychological Theories of Drinking and Alcoholism*, pp. 15–54. New York, NY: Guilford Press.

Carey, M.P., Kalra, D.L., Carey, K.B., Halperin, S. and Richards, C.S. (1993) Stress and unaided smoking cessation: a prospective investigation. *Journal of Consulting and Clinical Psychology*, 61: 831–8.

Carleton, R.A., Lasater, T.M., Assaf, A.R., Feldman, H.A., McKinlay, S. and the Pawtucket Heart Health Program Writing Group (1995) The Pawtucket Heart Health Program: community changes in cardiovascular risk factors and projected disease risk. *American Journal of Public Health*, 85: 777–85.

Caroll, K.M. (1996) Relapse prevention as a psychosocial treatment: a review of controlled clinical trials. *Experimental and Clinical Psychopharmacology*, 4: 46–54.

Carver, C.S. and Scheier, M.F. (1990) Origins and functions of positive and negative affect: a control-process view. *Psychological Review*, 97: 19–35.

Carver, C.S., Pozo, C., Harris, S.D. *et al.* (1993) How coping mediates the effects of optimism on distress: a study of women with early stages breast cancer. *Journal of Personality and Social Psychology*, 65: 375–90.

Cataldo, M.F. and Coates, T.J. (eds) (1986) *Health and Industry: A Behavioral Medicine Perspective*. New York, NY: Wiley.

CDC AIDS Community Demonstration Projects Research Group (1999) Community-level HIV Intervention in 5 cities: final outcome data from the CDC AIDS community demonstration project. *American Journal of Public Health*, 89: 336–45.

Centers for Disease Control (1980) *Risk Factor Update*. Atlanta, GA: US Department of Health and Human Services.

Centers for Disease Control (1994) Cigarette smoking among adults – United States, 1993. *Morbidity and Mortality Weekly Report*, 43: 925–30.

Cepeda-Benito, A. (1993) Meta-analytical review of the efficacy of nicotine chewing gum in smoking treatment programs. *Journal of Consulting and Clinical Psychology*, 61: 822–30.

Chaiken, S. (1980) Heuristic versus systematic information processing and the use of source versus message cues in persuasion. *Journal of Personality and Social Psychology*, 39: 725–66.

Chaiken, S. and Maheswaran, D. (1994) Heuristic processing can bias systematic processing: effects of source credibility, argument ambiguity, and task importance on attitude judgment. *Journal of Personality and Social Psychology*, 66: 460–73.

Chaiken, S., Giner-Sorolla, R. and Chen, S. (1996a) Beyond accuracy: defense and impression motives in heuristic and systematic information processing, in P.M. Gollwitzer and J.A. Bargh (eds) *The Psychology of Action: Linking Motivation and Cognition to Behavior*, pp. 553–78. New York, NY: Guilford Press.

Chaiken, S., Wood, W. and Eagly, A. (1996b) Principles of persuasion, in E.T. Higgins and A.W. Kruglanski (eds) *Social Psychology: Handbook of Basic Principles*, pp. 702–44. New York, NY: Guilford Press.

Chaney, E.F., O'Leary, M.R. and Marlatt, G.A. (1978) Skill training with alcoholics. *Journal of Consulting and Clinical Psychology*, 46: 1092–104.

Chang, E.C. (1998) Dispositional optimism and primary and secondary appraisal of a stressor: controlling for confounding influences and relations to coping and psychological adjustment. *Journal of Personality and Social Psychology*, 74: 1109–20.

Chassin, L., Presson, C.C., Sherman, S.J., Corty, E. and Olshavsky, R. (1984) Prediciting the onset of cigarette smoking in adolescents: a longitudinal study. *Journal of Applied Social Psychology*, 14: 224–43.

Chassin, L., Presson, C.C., Sherman, S.J. and Edwards, D.A. (1990) The natural history of cigarette smoking: predicting young-adult smoking outcomes from adolescent smoking patterns. *Health Psychology*, 9: 701–16.

Cheek, F.E., Franks, C.M., Laucious, J. and Burtle, U. (1971) Behavior modification training for wives of alcoholics. *Quarterly Journal of Studies on Alcohol*, 32: 156–61.

Chick, J., Lloyd, G. and Crombie, E. (1985) Counselling problem drinkers in medical wards: a controlled study. *British Medical Journal*, 290: 965–7.

Christophersen, E.R. (1989) Injury control. *American Psychologist*, 44: 237–41.

Chu, G.C. (1966) Fear arousal, efficacy and imminency. *Journal of Personality and Social Psychology*, 4: 517–23.

Cinciripini, P.M., Lapitsky, L., Seay, S. *et al.* (1995) The effects of smoking schedules on cessation outcome: can we improve on common methods of gradual or abrupt nicotine withdrawal? *Journal of Consulting and Clinical Psychology*, 63: 388–99.

Clark, W.B. and Midanik, L. (1982) Alcohol use and alcohol problems among US adults: results of the 1979 national survey, in *Alcohol Consumption and Related Problems*, pp. 3–52, Alcohol and Health Monograph 1. Washington, DC: National Institute of Alcohol Abuse and Alcoholism (DHHS Publication).

Clarkson, T.B., Kaplan, J.R., Adams, M.R. and Manuck, S.B. (1987) Psychosocial influences on the pathogenesis of atherosclerosis among nonhuman primates. *Circulation*, 76 (Suppl. 1): 29–40.

Clarkson, T.B., Manuck, S.B. and Kaplan, J.R. (1986) Potential role of cardiovascular reactivity in atherogenesis, in K.A. Matthews, S.M. Weiss, T. Detre, T.D. Dembrowksi, B. Falkner, S.B. Manuck and R.B. Williams Jr (eds) *Handbook of Stress, Reactivity and Cardiovascular Disease*, pp. 35–47. New York, NY: Wiley.

Cleary, P.D., Hitchcock, J.L., Semmer, N., Flinchbaugh, L.J. and Pinney, J.M. (1988) *The Milbank Quarterly*, 66: 137–71.

Cloninger, C.R., Bohman, M. and Sigvardsson, S. (1981) Inheritance of alcohol abuse. *Archives of General Psychiatry*, 38: 861–8.

Coates, T., Stall, R., Catania, J., Dolcini, P. and Hoff, C. (1989) Prevention of HIV infection in high risk groups, in P. Volberding and M. Jacobson (eds) *1989 AIDS Clinical Review*. New York, NY: Marcel Dekker.

Cobb, S. (1976) Social support as a moderator of life stress. *Psychosomatic Medicine*, 38: 300–14.

Cobb, S. and Lindemann, E. (1943) Neuropsychiatric observations after the Coconut Grove fire. *Annals of Surgery*, 117: 814–24.

Cohen, S. (1988) Psychosocial models of the role of social support in the etiology of physical disease. *Health Psychology*, 7: 269–97.

Cohen, S. and Edwards, J.R. (1989) Personality characteristics as moderators of the relationship between stress and disorder, in R.W.J. Neufeld (ed.) *Advances in the Investigation of Psychological Stress*, pp. 235–83. New York, NY: Wiley.

Cohen, S. and Herbert, T.B. (1996) Health psychology: psychological factors and physical disease from the perspective of human psychoneuroimmunology. *Annual Review of Psychology*, 47: 113–42.

Cohen, S. and McKay, G. (1984) Social support, stress, and the buffering hypothesis: a theoretical analysis, in A. Baum, J.E. Singer and S.E. Taylor (eds) *Handbook of Psychology and Health*, Vol. 4, pp. 253–67. Hillsdale, NJ: Lawrence Erlbaum.

Cohen, S. and Williamson, G.M. (1988) Perceived stress in a probability sample of the United States, in S. Spacapan and S. Oskamp (eds) *The Social Psychology of Health*, pp. 17–67. Newbury Park, CA: Sage.

Cohen, S. and Williamson, G.M. (1991) Stress and infectious disease in humans. *Psychological Bulletin*, 109: 5–24.

Cohen, S. and Wills, T.A. (1985) Stress, social support, and the buffering hypothesis. *Psychological Bulletin*, 98: 310–57.

Cohen, S., Mermelstein, R., Kamarck, T. and Hoberman, H.N. (1985) Measuring the functional components of social support, in I.G. Sarason and B.R. Sarason (eds) *Social support: Theory, Research, and Applications*, pp. 73–94. Dordrecht: Martinus Nijhoff.

Cohen, S., Lichtenstein, E., Prochaska, J.O. *et al.* (1989) Debunking myths about self-quitting. *American Psychologist*, 44: 1355–65.

Cohen, S., Tyrell, D. and Smith, A. (1993) Negative life events, perceived stress, negative affect, and susceptibility to the common cold. *Journal of Personality and Social Psychology*, 64: 131–40.

Cohen, S., Frank, E., Doyle, W.J. *et al.* (1998) Types of stressors that increase susceptibility to the common cold in healthy adults. *Health Psychology*, 17: 214–23.

Cole, P. and Rodu, B. (1996) Declining cancer mortality in the United States. *Cancer*, 1996: 2045–8.

COMMIT Research Group (1995) Community intervention trial for smoking cessation (COMMIT): I. Cohort results from a four-year community intervention. *American Journal of Public Health*, 85: 183–92.

Committee on Diet and Health (1989) *Diet and Health*. Washington, DC: National Academy Press.

Committee on Trauma Research (1985) *Injury in America: A Continuing Public Health Problem*. Washington, DC: National Academy Press.

Condiotte, M.M. and Lichtenstein, E. (1981) Self-efficacy and relapse in smoking cessation programs. *Journal of Consulting and Clinical Psychology*, 49: 648–58.

Conner, M. (in press) The theory of planned behavior and healthy eating: examining additive and moderating effects of social influence variables. *Psychology and Health*.

Cook, P.J. (1981) The effect of liquor taxes on drinking, cirrhosis, and auto accidents, in M.H. Moore and D.R. Gerstein (eds) *Alcohol and Public Policy:*

Beyond the Shadow of Prohibition, pp. 255–85. Washington, DC: National Academy Press.

Cook, P.J. (1982) Alcohol taxes as a public health measure. *British Journal of Addiction*, 77: 245–50.

Cook, W. and Medley, D. (1954) Proposed hostility for Pharisaic-virtue-skills of the MMPI. *Journal of Applied Psychology*, 38: 414–18.

Cooney, N.L., Zweben, A. and Fleming, M.F. (1995) Screening for alcohol prolems and at-risk drinking in health-care settings, in R.K. Hester and W.R. Miller (eds) *Handbook of Alcoholism Treatment Approaches*, 2nd ed., pp. 54–60. Boston, MA: Allyn and Bacon.

Courneya, K.S. (1995) Understanding readiness for regular physical activity in older individuals: an application of the theory of planned behaviour. *Health Psychology*, 14: 80–7.

Craighead, L.W. (1984) Sequencing of behavior therapy and pharmacotherapy for obesity. *Journal of Consulting and Clinical Psychology*, 52: 190–9.

Craighead, L.W., Stunkard, A.J. and O'Brien, R. (1981) Behavior therapy and pharmacotherapy for obesity. *Archives of General Psychiatry*, 38: 763–8.

Crandall, C.S. (1991) Do heavyweight students have more difficulty in paying for college? *Personality and Social Psychology Bulletin*, 17: 606–11.

Cummings, C., Gordon, J.F. and Marlatt, G.A. (1980) Relapse: prevention and prediction, in W.R. Miller (ed.) *The Addictive Behaviors: Treatment of Alcoholism, Drug Abuse, Smoking, and Obesity*, pp. 291–321. New York, NY: Pergamon.

Curran, J.W., Jaffe, H.W., Hardy, A.M. *et al.* (1988) Epidemiology of HIV infection and AIDS in the United States. *Science*, 239: 610–16.

Curry, S.J., McBride, C., Grothaus, L.C., Louie, D. and Wagner, E.H. (1995) A randomized trial of self-help materials, personalized feedback, and telephone counseling with non-volunteer smokers. *Journal of Consulting and Clinical Psychology*, 63: 1005–14.

Dahlkoetter, J.A., Callahan, E.J. and Linton, J. (1979) Obesity and the unbalanced energy equation: exercise versus eating habit change. *Journal of Consulting and Clinical Psychology*, 47: 898–905.

Dawber, T.R. (1980) *The Framingham Study*. Cambridge, MA: Harvard University Press.

DeJong, W. and Hingson, R. (1998) Strategies to reduce driving under the influence of alcohol. *Annual Review of Public Health*, 19: 359–78.

DeLint, J. (1976) Epidemiological aspects of alcoholism. *International Journal of Mental Health*, 5: 29–51.

DeLongis, A., Coyne, J.C., Dakof, G., Folkman, S. and Lazarus, R.S. (1982) Relationship of daily hassles, uplifts, and major life events to health status. *Health Psychology*, 1: 119–36.

DeLongis, A., Folkman, S. and Lazarus, R.S. (1988) The impact of daily stress on health and mood: psychological and social resources as mediators. *Journal of Personality and Social Psychology*, 54: 486–95.

Detels, R., English, P., Visscher, B.R. *et al.* (1989) Seroconversion, sexual activity and condom use among 2915 HIV seronegative men followed for up to three years. *Journal of Acquired Immune Deficiency Syndromes*, 2: 77–83.

Devor, E.J. and Cloninger, C.R. (1989) Genetics of alcoholism. *Annual Review of Genetics*, 23: 19–36.

De Vries, H., Backbier, E., Kok, G.J. and Dijkstra, A. (1995) The impact of social influences in the context of attitude, self-efficacy, intention and previous behavior as predictors of smoking onset. *Journal of Applied Social Psychology*, 25: 237–57.

De Vroome, E.M.M., Stroebe, W., Sandfort, T.G.M., de Wit, J., van Griensven, G.J.P. (in press) Safe sex in social context: individualistic and relational determinants of AIDS preventive behavior among gay men. *Journal of Applied Social Psychology.*

De Wit, J. (1996) The epidemic of HIV among young homosexual men. *AIDS, 10* (suppl. 3): S21–S25.

De Wit, J.B.F., Kok, G.J., Timmermans, C.A.M. and Wijnsma, P. (1990) Determinanten van veilig vrijen en condoomgebruik bij jongeren. *Gedrag en Gezondheid,* 18: 121–33.

De Wit, J.B.F., de Vroome, E.M.M., Sandfort, T.G.M. *et al.* (1992) Safe sexual practices not reliably maintained by homosexual men. *American Journal of Public Health,* 82: 615–16.

De Wit, J.B.F., Sandfort, T.G.M., de Vroome, E., van Griensven, G.J.P. and Kok, G. (1993) The effectiveness of the use of condoms among homosexual men. *AIDS,* 7: 751–2.

De Wit, J., Stroebe, W., de Vroome, E.M.M., Sandfort, T.G.M. and van Griensven, G.J.P. (in press) Understanding AIDS preventive behavior in homosexual men: the theory of planned behavior and the information–motivation–skills model prospectively compared. *Psychology and Health.*

Dijkstra, A. and de Vries, H. (1999) The development of computer-generated tailored interventions. *Patient Education and Counseling,* 36: 193–203.

Dijkstra, A., de Vries, H., Roijackers, J. and van Breukelen (1996) Voorlichting op maat over stoppen met roken: een veldexperiment. *Gedrag and Gezondheid,* 24: 314–22.

Dijkstra, A., de Vries, H. and Roijackers, J. (1998a) Long-term effectiveness of computer-generated tailored feedback in smoking cessation. *Health Education Research,* 13: 207–14.

Dijkstra, A., de Vries, H., Roijackers, J. and van Breukelen (1998b) Tailored interventions to communicate stage-matched information to smokers in different motivational stages. *Journal of Consulting and Clinical Psychology,* 66: 549–57.

Dijkstra, M., de Vries, H. and Parcel, G. (1992) The linkage approach applied to a school-based smoking prevention program in the Netherlands. *Journal of School Health,* 63: 339–42.

Dimsdale, J.E. and Herd, A.J. (1982) Variability of plasma lipids in response to emotional arousal. *Psychosomatic Medicine,* 44: 413–30.

Dishman, R.K. (1982) Compliance/adherence in health-related exercise. *Health Psychology,* 1: 237–67.

Dishman, R.K. and Gettman, L.R. (1980) Psychobiologic influences on exercise adherence. *Journal of Sport Psychology,* 2: 295–310.

Dishman, R.K. and Ickes, W.J. (1981) Self-motivation and adherence to therapeutic exercise. *Journal of Behavioral Medicine,* 4: 421–38.

Dishman, R.K., Ickes, W.J. and Morgan, W.P. (1980) Self-motivation and adherence to habitual physical activity. *Journal of Applied Social Psychology,* 10: 115–31.

Doherty, K., Militello, F.S., Kinnunen, T. and Garvey, A.J. (1996) Nicotine gum dose and weight gain after smoking cessation. *Journal of Consulting and Clinical Psychology,* 64: 799–807.

Dohrenwend, B.P. (1973) Social status and stressful life events. *Journal of Personality and Social Psychology,* 28: 225–35.

Dohrenwend, B.P. and Shrout, P.E. (1985) 'Hassles' in the conceptualization and measurement of life stress variables. *American Psychologist,* 40: 780–5.

Dohrenwend, B.S., Dohrenwend, B.P., Dodson, M. and Shrout, P.E. (1984) Symptoms, hassles, social supports, and life events: problem of confounded measures. *Journal of Abnormal Psychology*, 93: 222–30.

Douglas, S. and Hariharan, G. (1993) The hazard of starting smoking: estimates from a split population duration model. *Journal of Health Economics*, 13: 213–30.

Doyne, E.J., Ossip-Klein, D.J., Bowman, E.D. *et al.* (1987) Running versus weight lifting in the treatment of depression. *Journal of Clinical and Consulting Psychology*, 55: 748–54.

Dunkel-Schetter, C. and Bennett, T.L. (1990) Differentiating the cognitive and behavioral aspects of social support, in B.R. Sarason, I.G. Sarason and G.R. Pierce (eds) *Social Support: An Interactional View*, pp. 267–96. New York, NY: Wiley.

Dunn, A.L. and Blair, S.N. (1997) Exercise prescription, in W.P. Morgan (ed.) *Physical Activity and Mental Health*, pp. 49–62. Philadelphia, PA: Taylor & Francis.

Eagly, A.H. and Chaiken, S. (1993) *The Psychology of Attitudes*. Fort Worth, TX: Harcourt Brace Jovanovich.

Eckenrode, J. and Bolger, N. (1995) Daily and within-day event measurement, in S. Cohen, R.C. Kessler, L. Underwood Gordon (eds) *Measuring Stress*, pp. 80–101. New York, NY: Oxford University Press.

Egger, G., Fitzgerald, W., Frape, G. *et al.* (1983) Result of large scale media anti-smoking campaign in Australia: North Coast 'Quit For Life' Programme. *British Medical Journal*, 286: 1125–8.

Elkins, R.L. (1980) Covert sensitization treatment for alcoholism: contributions of successful conditioning to subsequent abstinence maintenance. *Addictive Behaviors*, 5: 67–89.

Emrick, C.D. (1975) A review of psychologically oriented treatment of alcoholism: II. The relative effectiveness of different treatment approaches and the relative effectiveness of treatment versus no treatment. *Journal of Studies on Alcohol*, 36: 88–108.

Endler, N.S. and Parker, J.D.A. (1990) Multidimensional assessment of coping: a critical evaluation. *Journal of Personality and Social Psychology*, 58: 844–54.

Engel, G.L. (1977) The need for a new medical model: a challenge for biomedicine. *Science*, 196: 129–36.

Epping-Jordan, J.E., Compas, B.E. and Howell, D.C. (1994) Predictors of cancer progression in young adult men and women: avoidance, intrusive thoughts, and psychological symptoms. *Health Psychology*, 13: 539–47.

Epstein, L.H., Valoski, A., Wing, R.R. and McCurley, J. (1994) Ten-year outcomes of behavioral family-based treatment for childhood obesity. *Health Psychology*, 13: 373–83.

Epstein, S. (1979) The stability of behavior. On predicting most of the people much of the time. *Journal of Personality and Social Psychology*, 37: 1097–126.

Ernsberger, P. and Nelson, D.O. (1988) Effects of fasting and refeeding on blood pressure are determined by nutritional state, not by body weight change. *American Journal of Hypertension*, 1: 153S–7S.

Ernsberger, P. and Koletsky, R.J. (1999) Biomedical rationale for a wellness approach to obesity: an alternative to a focus on weight loss. *Journal of Social Issues*, 55: 221–60.

European Centre for the Epidemiological Monitoring of AIDS (1998) *HIV/AIDS Surveillance in Europe: Quarterly Report No. 60*, 31 December 1998.

Evans, R.I. (1976) Smoking in children: developing a social psychological strategy of deterrence. *Preventive Medicine*, 5: 122–7.

Evans, R.I., Rozelle, R.M., Mittelmark, M.D. *et al.* (1978) Deterring the onset of smoking in children: knowledge of immediate physiological effects and coping with peer pressure, media pressure, and parent modelling. *Journal of Applied Social Psychology*, 8: 126–35.

Ewing, J. (1984) Detecting alcoholism: the CAGE questionnaire. *Journal of the American Medical Association*, 252: 1905–7.

Fairburn, C.G. (1995) Short-term psychological treatments for bulimia nervosa, in K.D. Brownell and C.G. Fairburn (eds) *Eating Disorders and Obesity*, pp. 344–8. New York, NY: Guilford Press.

Fairburn, C.G. and Walsh, B.T. (1995) Atypical eating disorders, in K.D. Brownell and C.G. Fairburn (eds) *Eating Disorders and Obesity*, pp. 135–40. New York, NY: Guilford Press.

Fairburn, C.G., Norman, P.A., Welch, S.L. *et al.* (1995) A prospective study of outcome in bulimia nervosa and the long-term effects of three psychological treatments. *Archives of General Psychiatry*, 52: 304–12.

Farrell, P. and Fuchs, V. (1982) Schooling and health: the cigarette connection. *Journal of Health Economics*, 1: 217–30.

Farquhar, J.W., Maccoby, N., Wood, P.D. *et al.* (1977) Community education for cardiovascular health. *Lancet*, 4 June: 1192–5.

Farquhar, J.W., Fortman, S.P., Flora, J.A. *et al.* (1990) Effects of a community-wide education on cardiovascular disease risk factors: the Stanford Five-City project. *Journal of the American Medical Association*, 264: 359–65.

Fazio, R.H. (1986) How do attitudes guide behavior?, in R.M. Sorrentino and E.T. Higgins (eds) *Handbook of Motivation and Cognition: Foundations of Social Behavior*, pp. 204–43. New York, NY: Guilford Press.

Fazio, R.H. (1990) Multiple processes by which attitudes guide behavior: the MODE model as an integrative framework, in M.P. Zanna (ed.) *Advances in Experimental Social Psychology*, Vol. 23, pp. 75–109. San Diego, CA: Academic Press.

Fazio, R.H. and Towles-Schwen, T. (1999) The MODE model of attitude-behaviour processes, in S. Chaiken and Y. Trope (eds) *Dual-process Theories in Social Psychology*, pp. 97–115. New York, NY: Guilford Press.

Ferruci, L., Izmirlian, G., Leveille, S. *et al.* (1999) Smoking, physical activity, and active life expectancy. *American Journal of Epidemiology*, 149: 645–53.

Festinger, L. (1954) A theory of social comparison processes. *Human Relations*, 7: 117–40.

Festinger, L. (1957) *A Theory of Cognitive Dissonance*. Stanford: Stanford University Press.

Fhanér, G. and Hane, M. (1979) Seat belts: opinion effects of law-induced use. *Journal of Applied Psychology*, 64: 205–12.

Fielding, J.E. (1985) Smoking: health effects and control. *New England Journal of Medicine*, 313: 491–8.

Fielding, J.E. (1986) Evaluations, results and problems of worksite health promotion, in M.F. Cataldo and T.J. Coates (eds) *Health and Industry*, pp. 373–96. New York, NY: Wiley.

Fielding, J.E. (1999) Public health in the twentieth century: advances and challenges. *Annual Review of Public Health*, 20: xii–xxx.

Fielding, J.E. and Piserchia, P.V. (1989) Frequency of worksite health promotion activities. *American Journal of Public Health*, 78: 16–20.

Fiore, M.C., Novotny, T.E., Pierce, J.P. *et al.* (1990) Methods used to quit smoking in the United States: do cessation programs work? *Journal of the American Medical Association*, 263: 2760–5.

Fiore, M.C., Smith, S.S., Jorenby, D.E. and Baker, T.B. (1994) The effectiveness of the nicotine patch for smoking cessation: a meta-analysis. *Journal of the American Medical Association*, 271: 1940–7.

Fishbein, M. and Ajzen, I. (1975) *Belief, Attitude, Intention, and Behavior: An Introduction to Theory and Research*. Reading, MA: Addison-Wesley.

Fishbein, M., Middlestadt, S.E. and Hitchcock, P.J. (1994) Using information to change sexually transmitted disease – related behaviours. An analysis based on the theory of reasoned action, in R. DiClemente and J.L. Peterson (eds) *Preventing Aids: Theories and Methods of Behavioural Interventions*, pp. 61–78. New York, NY: Plenum.

Fisher, J.D. and Fisher, W.A. (1992) Changing Aids-risk behavior. *Psychological Bulletin*, 111: 455–74.

Fisher, K.J., Glasgow, R.E. and Terborg, J.R. (1990) Work site smoking cessation: a meta-analysis of long-term quit rates from controlled studies. *Journal of Occupational Medicine*, 32: 429–39.

Fisher, R.A. (1958) Cancer and smoking (Letter). *Nature*, 182: 596.

Fisher, W.A., Fisher, J.D. and Rye, B.J. (1995) Understanding and promoting AIDS-preventive behavior: insights from the theory of reasoned action. *Health Psychology*, 14: 255–64.

Fleischer, G.A. (1972) An experiment in the use of broadcast media in highway safety. Unpublished paper, University of Southern California, Department of Industrial Systems Engineering, Los Angeles (reported in Robertson 1987).

Folkman, S. and Lazarus, R.S. (1980) An analyis of coping in a middle-aged community sample. *Journal of Health and Social Behavior*, 21: 219–39.

Folkman, S., Lazarus, R.S., Dunkel-Schetter, C., DeLongis, A. and Gruen, R.J. (1986a) The dynamics of a stressful encounter. *Journal of Personality and Social Psychology*, 50: 992–1003.

Folkman, S., Lazarus, R.S., Gruen, R.J. and DeLongis, A. (1986b) Appraisal, coping, health status and psychological symptoms. *Journal of Personality and Social Psychology*, 50: 571–9.

Försterling, F. (1988) *Attribution Theory in Clinical Psychology*. Chichester: Wiley.

Foster, G.D., Wadden, T.A., Kendall, P.C., Stunkard, A.J. and Vogt, R.A. (1996) Psychological effects of weight loss and regain: a prospective study. *Journal of Consulting and Clinical Psychology*, 64: 752–7.

French Jr, J.R.P. and Kahn, R.L. (1962) A problematic approach to studying the industrial environment and mental health. *Journal of Social Issues*, 18: 1–47.

French, S.A. and Jeffery, R.W. (1995) Weight concerns and smoking: a literature review. *Annals of Behavioral Medicine*, 17: 234–44.

French, S.A., Jeffery, R.W., Klesges, L.M. and Forster, J.L. (1995) Weight concerns and change in smoking behavior over two years in a working population. *American Journal of Public Health*, 85: 720–2.

French, S.A., Henrikus, D.J. and Jeffery, R.W. (1996) Smoking status, dietary intake, and physical activity in a sample of working adults. *Health Psychology*, 15: 448–54.

Fried, S.K. and Russell, C.D. (1998) Diverse roles of adipose tissue in the regulation of systemic metabolism and energy balance, in G.A. Bray, C. Bouchard and W.P.T. James (eds) *Handbook of Obesity*, pp. 397–413. New York, NY: Marcel Dekker.

Friedland, G.H. and Klein, R.S. (1987) Transmission of the HIV. *New England Journal of Medicine*, 317: 1125–35.

Friedman, M. and Rosenman, R.H. (1974) *Type A Behavior and Your Heart*. New York, NY: Knopf.

Friedman, M.A. and Brownell, K.D. (1995) Psychological correlates of obesity: moving to the next research generation. *Psychological Bulletin*, 117: 3–20.

Fries, J.F., Green, L.W. and Levine, S. (1989) Health promotion and the compression of morbidity. *Lancet*, I: 481–3.

Fuller, K. (1995) Antidipsotropic medication, in R.K. Hester and W.R. Miller (eds) *Handbook of Alcoholism Treatment Approaches*, 2nd ed., pp. 123–33. Boston, MA: Allyn and Bacon.

Funk, S.C. and Houston, B.K. (1987) A critical analysis of the hardiness scale's validity and utility. *Journal of Personality and Social Psychology*, 53: 572–8.

Furberg, C.D. (1994) Lipid-lowering trials: results and limitations. *American Heart Journal*, 128: 1304–8.

Furst, C.J. (1983) Estimating alcoholic prevalence, in M. Galanter (ed.) *Recent Developments in Alcoholism*, Vol. 1. New York, NY: Plenum.

Gallois, C., Terry, D., Timmins, P., Kashima, Y. and McCamish, M. (1994) Safe sexual intentions and behavior among heterosexual and homosexual men: testing the theory of reasoned action. *Psychology and Health*, 10: 1–16.

Ganellen, R.J. and Blaney, P.H. (1984) Hardiness and social support as moderators of the effects of life stress. *Journal of Personality and Social Psychology*, 47: 156–63.

Gardner, P., Rosenberg, H.M. and Wilson, R.W. (1996) *Leading Causes of Death by Age, Sex, Race, and Hispanic Origin: United States, 1992*. National Center for Health Statistics, Vital and Health Statistics, 20 (29).

George, W.H. and Marlatt, G.A. (1983) Alcoholism: the evolution of a behavioral perspective, in M. Galanter (ed.) *Recent Developments in Alcoholism*, Vol. 1, pp. 105–38. New York, NY: Plenum.

Gerrard, M., Gibbons, F.X. and Bushman, B.J. (1996) Relation between perceived vulnerability to HIV and precautionary sexual behavior. *Psychological Bulletin*, 119: 390–409.

Gibbons, F.X., Eggleston, T.J. and Benthin, A.C. (1997) Cognitive reactions to smoking relapse: the reciprocal relation between dissonance and self-esteem. *Journal of Personality and Social Psychology*, 72: 184–95.

Glaser, R. and Kiecolt-Glaser, J. (eds) (1994) *Handbook of Human Stress and Immunity*. San Diego, CA: Academic Press.

Glaser, R., Kiecolt-Glaser, J.K., Speicher, C.E. and Holliday, J.E. (1985) Stress, loneliness, and changes in herpes virus latency. *Journal of Behavioral Medicine*, 8: 249–60.

Glasgow, R.E. and Lichtenstein, E. (1987) Longterm effects of behavioral smoking cessation interventions. *Behavior Therapy*, 18: 297–324.

Glasgow, R.E., Terborg, J.R., Hollis, J.F., Severson, H.H. and Boles, S.M. (1995) Take Heart: results from the initial phase of a work-site wellness program. *American Journal of Public Health*, 85: 209–16.

Glasgow, R.E., Terborg, J.R., Strycker, L.A., Boles, S.M. and Hollis, J.F. (1997) Take Heart II: replication of a worksite health promotion trial. *Journal of Behavioral Medicine*, 20: 143–61.

Gleicher, F. and Petty, R.E. (1992) Expectations of reassurance influence the nature of fear-stimulated attitude change. *Journal of Experimental Social Psychology*, 28: 86–100.

Godin, G. and Kok, G. (1996) The theory of planned behavior: a review of its applications to health-related behavior. *American Journal of Health Promotion*, 11: 87–97.

Goldberg, E.L. and Comstock, G.W. (1976) Life events and subsequent illness. *American Journal of Epidemiology*, 104: 146–58.

Goldman, L. and Cook, E.F. (1984) The decline in ischaemic heart disease mortality rates: an analysis of the comparative effects of medical interventions and changes in lifestyle. *Annals of Internal Medicine*, 101: 825–36.

Goldman, R., Jaffa, M. and Schachter, S. (1968) Yom Kippur, Air France, dormitory food and the eating behavior of obese and normal persons. *Journal of Personality and Social Psychology*, 10: 117–23.

Gollwitzer, P.M. (1999) Implementation intentions: strong effects of simple plans. *American Psychologist*, 54: 493–503.

Goodrick, G.K., Poston, W.S.C., Kimball, K.T., Reeves, R.S. and Foreyt, J.P. (1998) Nondieting versus dieting treatment of overweight binge-eating women. Journal of Consulting and Clinical Psychology, 66: 363–8.

Goodwin, D.W., Schulsinger, F., Hermansen, L., Guze, S.B. and Winokur, G. (1973) Alcohol problems in adoptees raised apart from alcoholic biological parents. *Archives of General Psychiatry*, 28: 238–43.

Goodwin, D.W., Schulsinger, F., Moller, N. *et al.* (1974) Drinking problems in adopted and nonadopted sons of alcoholics. *Archives of General Psychiatry*, 31: 164–9.

Gortmaker, S.L., Must, A., Perrin, J.M., Sobol, A.M. and Dietz, W.H. (1993) Social and economic consequences of overweight in adolescence and young adulthood. *New England Journal of Medicine*, 329: 1008–12.

Graham, J.D. (1993) Injuries from traffic crashes: meeting the challenge. *Annual Review of Public Health*, 14: 515–43.

Green, L.W. and Kreuter, M.W. (1991) *Health Promotion Planning: An Educational and Environmental Approach*. Mountain View, CA: Mayfield.

Greeno, C.G. and Wing, R.R. (1994) Stress-induced eating. *Psychological Bulletin*, 115: 444–64.

Greenwald, A.G. (1968) Cognitive learning, cognitive response to persuasion, and attitude change, in A.G. Greenwald, T.C. Brock and T.M. Ostrom (eds) *Psychological Foundations of Attitudes*, pp. 147–70. San Diego, CA: Academic Press.

Grilo, C.M. and Pogue-Geile, M.F. (1991) The nature of environmental influences on weight and obesity: a behavior genetic analysis. *Psychological Bulletin*, 110: 520–37.

Grimsmo, A., Helgesen, G. and Borchgrevink, C. (1981) Short-term and long-term effects of lay groups on weight reduction. *British Medical Journal*, 283: 1093–5.

Haberman, P.W. and Baden, M.M. (1978) *Alcohol, Other Drugs and Violent Death*. New York, NY: Oxford University Press.

Haddon Jr, W. and Baker, S.P. (1981) Injury control, in D. Clark and B. MacMahon (eds) *Preventive and Community Medicine*, pp. 109–40. Boston, MA: Little, Brown.

Haddon Jr, W., Valien, P., McCarroll, J.R. and Umberger, C.J. (1961) A controlled investigation of the characteristics of adult pedestrians fatally injured by motor vehicles in Manhattan. *Journal of Chronic Diseases*, 14: 655–78.

Haddy, F.J. (1991) Roles of sodium, potassium, calcium, and natriuretic factors in hypertension. *Hypertension*, 18 (Suppl. III): III-179–III-183.

Hahn, M.E. (1966) *California-Life-Goals-Evaluation-Schedule*. Palo Alto, CA: Western Psychological Services.

Hall, S.M., Hall, R.G. and Ginsberg, D. (1990) Cigarette dependence, in A.S. Bellack, M. Hersen and A.E. Kazdin (eds) *International Handbook of Behavior Modification and Therapy*, 2nd ed., pp. 437–47. New York, NY: Plenum.

Hall, S.M., Tunstall, C.D., Vila, K.L. and Duffy, J. (1992) Weight gain and smoking cessation: cautionary findings. *American Journal of Public Health*, 82: 799–803.

Hansson, R.O. and Carpenter, B.N. (1994) *Relationships in Old Age: Coping with the Challenge of Transition*. New York, NY: Guilford Press.

Harackiewicz, J.M., Sansone, C., Blair, L.W., Epstein, J.A. and Manderlink, G. (1987) Attributional processes in behavior change and maintenance: smoking cessation and continued abstinence. *Journal of Consulting and Clinical Psychology*, 55: 372–8.

Harrison, J.A., Mullen, P.D. and Green, L.W. (1992) A meta-analysis of studies of the health belief model with adults. *Health Education Research*, 7: 107–16.

Hashim, S. and van Itallie, T. (1965) Studies in normal and obese subjects with a monitored food-dispensing device. *Annals of the New York Academy of Sciences*, 131: 654–61.

Haugvedt, C.P. and Petty, R.E. (1992) Personality and persuasion: need for cognition moderates the persistence and resistance of attitude change. *Journal of Personality and Social Psychology*, 63: 308–19.

He, Y., Lam, T.H., Li, L.S. *et al.* (1994) Passive smoking at work as a risk factor for coronary heart disease in Chinese women who have never smoked. *British Medical Journal*, 308: 380–9.

Heath, A.C. and Madden, P.A.F. (1994) Genetic influences on smoking behavior, in J.R. Turner, L.R. Cardon and J.K. Hewitt (eds) *Behavior Genetic Applications in Behavioral Medicine*, pp. 37–48. New York, NY: Plenum.

Heath, A.C. and Martin, N.G. (1993) Genetic models for the natural history of smoking: evidence for a genetic influence on smoking persistence. *Addictive Behaviors*, 18: 19–34.

Heather, N. (1995) Brief intervention strategies, in R.K. Hester and W.R. Miller (eds) *Handbook of Alcoholism Treatment Approaches*, 2nd ed., pp. 105–22. Boston, MA: Allyn and Bacon.

Heather, N., Kissoon-Singh, J. and Fenton, G. (1990) Assisted natural recovery from alcohol problems: effects of a self-help manual with and without supplementary telephone contact. *British Journal of Addiction*, 85: 1177–85.

Heather, N. and Robertson, I. (1983) *Controlled Drinking*. London: Methuen.

Heather, N., Whitton, B. and Robertson, I. (1986) Evaluation of a self-help manual for media-recruited problem drinkers: six month follow-up results. *British Journal of Clinical Psychology*, 25: 19–34.

Heatherton, T.F. and Baumeister, R.F. (1991) Binge eating as escape from self-awareness. *Psychological Bulletin*, 110: 86–108.

Heatherton, T.F., Herman, C.P. and Polivy, J. (1991) Effects of physical threat and ego threat on eating behavior. *Journal of Personality and Social Psychology*, 60: 138–43.

Heider, F. (1958) *The Psychology of Interpersonal Relations*. New York, NY: Wiley.

Helmers, K.F., Poluszny, D.M. and Krantz, D.S. (1994) Association of hostility and coronary artery disease: a review of studies, in A.W. Siegman and T.W. Smith (eds) *Anger, Hostility and the Heart*, pp. 66–96. Hillsdale, NJ: Lawrence Erlbaum.

Helzer, J.E. (1987) The epidemiology of alcoholism. *Journal of Consulting and Clinical Psychology*, 55: 284–92.

Hennekens, C.H., Willet, W., Rosner, B., Cole, D.S. and Mayrent, S.L. (1979) Effects of beer, wine, and liquor in coronary deaths. *Journal of the American Medical Association*, 242: 1973–4.

Herd, A.J. (1978) Physiological correlates of coronary-prone behavior, in T.M. Dembrowski, S.M. Weiss, J.L. Shields, S.G. Haynes and M. Feinleib (eds) *Coronary-prone Behavior*. New York, NY: Springer.

Herman, C.P. and Mack, D. (1975) Restrained and unrestrained eating. *Journal of Personality*, 43: 647–60.

Herman, C.P. and Polivy, J. (1984) A boundary model for the regulation of eating, in A.J. Stunkard and E. Stellar (eds) *Eating and its Disorders*, pp. 141–56. New York, NY: Raven Press.

Herman, C.P., Polivy, J. and Esses, V.M. (1987) The illusion of counter-regulation. *Appetite*, 9: 161–9.

Herzog, T., Abrams, D.B., Emmons, K.M., Linnan, L. and Shadel, W.G. (1999) Do processes of change predict smoking stage movements? A prospective analysis of the transtheoretical model. *Health Psychology*, 18: 369–75.

Hester, R.K. (1995) Behavioral self-control training, in R.K. Hester and W.R. Miller (eds) (1995) *Handbook of Alcoholism Treatment Approaches*, 2nd ed., pp. 148–59. Boston, MA: Allyn and Bacon.

Hester, R.K. and Miller, W.R. (eds) (1995) *Handbook of Alcoholism Treatment Approaches*, 2nd ed. Boston, MA: Allyn and Bacon.

Hibscher, J.A. and Herman, C.P. (1977) Obesity, dieting, and the expression of 'obese' characteristics. *Journal of Comparative and Physiological Psychology*, 91: 374–80.

Hiroto, D.S. (1974) Locus of control and learnt helplessness. *Journal of Experimental Psychology*, 102: 187–93.

Hiroto, D.S. and Seligman, M.E.P. (1975) Generality of learned helplessness in man. *Journal of Personality and Social Psychology*, 32: 311–27.

Hirschman, R.S. and Leventhal, H. (1989) Preventing smoking behavior in schoolchildren: an initial test of a cognitive-development program. *Journal of Applied Social Psychology*, 19: 559–83.

Holmes, T.H. and Masuda, M. (1974) Life change and illness susceptibility, in W.S. Dohrenwend and B.P. Dohrenwend (eds) *Stress for Life Events*, pp. 45–72. New York, NY: Wiley.

Holmes, T.H. and Rahe, R.H. (1967) The social readjustment rating-scale. *Journal of Psychosomatic Research*, 11: 213–18.

Holtgrave, D.R., Qualls, N.L. and Graham, J.D. (1996) Economic evaluation of HIV prevention programs. *Annual Review of Public Health*, 17: 467–88.

Horowitz, M. (1979) Psychological response to serious life events, in V. Hamilton and D.M. Warburton (eds) *Human Stress and Cognition: An Information Processing Approach*, pp. 237–65. Chichester: Wiley.

House, J.S. (1981) *Workstress and Social Support*. Reading, MA: Addison-Wesley.

House, J.S. and Kahn, R.L. (1985) Measures and concepts of social support, in S. Cohen and S.L. Syme (eds) *Social Support and Health*, pp. 83–108. Orlando, FL: Academic Press.

House, J.S., Robbins, C. and Metzner, H.L. (1982) The association of social relationships and activities with mortality: prospective evidence from the

Tecumseh Community Health Study. *American Journal of Epidemiology*, 116: 123–40.

House, J.S., Landis, K.R. and Umberson, D. (1988) Social relationships and health. *Science*, 241: 540–5.

Houston, B.K. (1994) Anger, hostility, and psychophysiological reactivity, in A.W. Siegman and T.W. Smith (eds) *Anger, Hostility, and the Heart*, pp. 97–116. Hillsdale, NJ: Lawrence Erlbaum.

Houston, B.K. and Vavak, R.C. (1991) Hostility: developmental factors, psychosocial correlates, and health behaviors. *Health Psychology*, 10: 9–17.

Hovland, C.I., Janis, I.L. and Kelley, H.H. (1959) *Communication and Persuasion: Psychological Studies of Opinion Change*. New Haven, CT: Yale University Press.

Hughes, J.R. (1986) Genetics and smoking: a brief review. *Behavior Therapy*, 17: 335–45.

Hughes, J.R. (1993) Pharmacotherapy for smoking cessation: unvalidated assumptions, anomalies, and suggestions for future research. *Journal of Consulting and Clinical Psychology*, 61: 751–60.

Hull, J., Levenson, R., Young, R. and Sher, K. (1983) The self-awareness-reducing effects of alcohol consumption. *Journal of Personality and Social Psychology*, 44: 461–73.

Hull, J., van Teuren, R. and Virnelli, S. (1987) Hardiness and health: a critique and alternative approach. *Journal of Personality and Social Psychology*, 53: 518–30.

Hull, J.G. (1981) A self-awareness model of the causes and effects of alcohol consumption. *Journal of Abnormal Psychology*, 90: 586–600.

Hull, J.G. (1987) Self-awareness model, in H.T. Blane and K.E. Leonard (eds) *Psychological Theories of Drinking and Alcoholism*, pp. 272–304. New York, NY: Guilford Press.

Hull, J.G. and Bond Jr, C.F. (1986) Social behavioral consequences of alcohol consumption and expectancy: a meta-analysis. *Psychological Bulletin*, 99: 347–60.

Hunninghake, D.B., Stein, E.A., Dujovne, C.A. *et al.* (1993) The efficacy of intensive dietary therapy alone or combined with lovastatin in outpatients with hypercholesterolemia. *New England Journal of Medicine*, 328: 1213–19.

Hunt, G.M. and Azrin, N.H. (1973) A community-reinforcement approach to alcoholism. *Behaviour, Research and Therapy*, 11: 91–104.

Hurley, J. and Horowitz, J. (eds) (1990) *Alcohol and Health*. New York, NY: Hemisphere.

Ikard, F.F. and Tomkins, S. (1973) The experience of affect as a determinant of smoking behavior: a series of validity studies. *Journal of Abnormal Psychology*, 81: 172–81.

Ikard, F.F., Green, D.E. and Horn, D.A. (1969) A scale to differentiate between types of smoking as related to management of affect. *International Journal of the Addictions*, 4: 649–59.

Imber, S., Schultz, E., Funderburk, F., Allen, R. and Flamer, R. (1976) The fate of the untreated alcoholic. *Journal of Nervous and Mental Disease*, 162: 238–47.

Ingram, R.E. and Scott, W.D. (1990) Cognitive behavior therapy, in A.S. Bellack, M. Hersen and A.E. Kazdin (eds) *International Handbook of Behavior Modification and Therapy*, 2nd ed., pp. 53–65. New York, NY: Plenum.

Irvin, J.E., Bowers, C., Dunn, M.E. and Wang, M.C. (1999) Efficacy of relapse prevention: a meta-analytic review. *Journal of Consulting and Clinical Psychology*, 67: 563–70.

Istvan, J. and Matarazzo, J.D. (1984) Tobacco, alcohol, and caffeine use: a review of their interrelationships. *Psychological Bulletin*, 95: 301–26.

Jackson, R., Scragg, R. and Beaglehole, R. (1991) Alcohol consumption and risk of coronary heart disease. *British Medical Journal*, 303: 211–16.

Jacobs Jr, D.R. (1993) Why is low blood cholesterol associated with risk of non-atherosclerotic disease death? *Annual Review of Public Health*, 14: 95–114.

Jacobs, S. (1999) *Traumatic Grief: Diagnosis, Treatment, and Prevention*. Philadelphia, PA: Brunner/Mazel.

Janis, I.L. and Mann, L. (1977) *Decision Making: A Psychological Analysis of Conflict, Choice, and Commitment*. New York, NY: Free Press.

Janis, I.L. and Terwilliger, R. (1962) An experimental study of psychological resistance to fear-arousing communication. *Journal of Abnormal and Social Psychology*, 65: 403–10.

Jansen, A., Merckelbach, H., Oosterlaan, J., Tuiten, A. and van den Hout, M.A. (1988) Nonregulation of food intake in restrained emotional and external eaters. *Journal of Psychopathology and Behavioral Assessment*, 10: 345–53.

Janssen, M., de Wit, J., Hospers, H., Kok, G. and Stroebe, W. (1998a) 'Jonge homoseksuele mannen, voorlichtingsfolders en opvattingen over risico van HIV-infectie'. Unpublished manuscript, University of Utrecht.

Janssen, M., de Wit, J., Stroebe, W. and van Griensven, F. (1998b) 'Socio-economic status and risk of HIV in young gay men'. Unpublished manuscript, University of Utrecht.

Janz, N.K. and Becker, M.H. (1984) The health belief model: a decade later. *Health Education Quarterly*, 11: 1–47.

Jeffery, R.W. (1989) Risk behaviors and health: contrasting individual and population perspectives. *American Psychologist*, 44: 1194–202.

Jeffery, R.W., Adlis, S.A. and Forster, J.L. (1991) Prevalence of dieting among working men and women: the healthy worker project. *Health Psychology*, 10: 274–81.

Jeffery, R.W., Boles, S.M., Strycker, L.A. and Glasgow, R.E. (1997) Smoking-specific weight gain concerns and smoking cessation in a working population. *Health Psychology*, 16: 487–9.

Jellinek, E.M. (1960) *The Disease Concept of Alcoholism*. Highland Park, NJ: Hillhouse.

Jepson, C. and Chaiken, S. (1990) Chronic issue-specific fear inhibits systematic processing of persuasive communications. *Journal of Social Behavior and Personality*, 5: 61–84.

Johnson, J.A. and Oksanen, E.H. (1977) Estimations of demand for alcoholic beverages in Canada from pooled time series and cross sections. *Review of Economics and Statistics*, 59: 113–18.

Johnston, J.J., Hendricks, S.A. and Fike, J.M. (1994) The effectiveness of behavioural safety belt interventions. *Accident Analysis and Prevention*, 26: 315–23.

Jonas, K. (1993) Expectancy-value models of health behaviour: an analysis by conjoint measurement. *European Journal of Social Psychology*, 23: 167–85.

Jonas, K. (1995) Der Beitrag der Einstellungsforschung zur Vorhersage präventiven und riskanten gesundheitsbezogenen Verhaltens. Habilitationsschrift (unpublished), Universität Tübingen.

Jonas, K., Stroebe, W. and Eagly, A. (1993) Adherence to an exercise program. Unpublished manuscript, University of Tübingen.

Junger, M., Stroebe, W. and van der Laan, A. (1999) Delinquency, health behavior and health. Manuscript submitted for publication.

Kalichman, S., Rompa, D., Coley, B. (1996) Experimental component analysis of a behavioral HIV–AIDS prevention intervention for inner-city women. *Journal of Consulting and Clinical Psychology*, 64: 687–93.

Kalichman, S.C. (1998) *Preventing AIDS: A Sourcebook for Behavioral Interventions*. Mahwah, NJ: Lawrence Erlbaum.

Kalichman, S.C., Nachimson, D. and Cherry, C. (1998) AIDS treatment advances and behavioral prevention setbacks: preliminary assessment of reduced perceived threat of HIV–ADS. *Health Psychology*, 17: 546–50.

Kanner, A.D., Coyne, J.C., Schaefer, C. and Lazarus, R.S. (1981) Comparison of two modes of stress measurement: daily hassles and uplifts versus major life events. *Journal of Behavioral Medicine*, 4: 1–39.

Kaplan, R.M. (1988) The value dimension in studies of health promotion, in S. Spacapan and S. Oskamp (eds) *The Social Psychology of Health*. Beverly Hills, CA: Sage.

Kaplan, R.M., Sallis, J.F. and Patterson, T.L. (1993) *Health and Human Behavior*. New York, NY: McGraw-Hill.

Karon, J.M., Rosenberg, P.J., McQuillan, G. *et al.* (1996) Prevalence of HIV infection in the United States, 1984–1992. *Journal of the American Medical Association*, 276: 1126–31.

Kashim, Y., Gallois, C. and McCamish, M. (1993) The theory of reasoned action and cooperative behavior: it takes two to use a condom. *British Journal of Social Psychology*, 32: 227–39.

Kasl, S.V. and Cobb, S. (1970) Health behavior, illness behavior, and sick role behavior. *Archives of Environmental Health*, 12: 246–66.

Keesey, R.E. (1980) The regulation of body weight: a set point analysis, in A.J. Stunkard (ed.) *Obesity*, pp. 144–65. Philadelphia, PA: Saunders.

Keesey, R.E. (1986) A set-point theory of obesity, in K.D. Brownell and J.P. Foreyt (eds) *The Physiology, Psychology, and Treatment of the Eating Disorders*, pp. 63–87. New York, NY: Basic Books.

Kelder, S.H., Perry, C.L. and Klepp, K.I. (1993) Community-wide youth exercise promotion: long-term outcomes of the Minnesota Heart Health Program and the Class of 1989 Study. *Journal of School Health*, 63: 218–23.

Kelly, J.A. and Kalichman, S.C. (1998) Reinforcement value of unsafe sex as a predictor of condom use and continued HIV/AIDS risk behavior among gay and bisexual men. *Health Psychology*, 17: 328–35.

Kelly, J.A., St Lawrence, J.S., Brasfield, T.L. and Hood, H.V. (1989) Behavioral intervention to reduce AIDS risk activities. *Journal of Consulting and Clinical Psychology*, 57: 60–7.

Kelly, J.A., St Lawrence, J., Diaz, Y. *et al.* (1991) HIV risk behavior reduction following intervention with key opinion leaders of population: an experimental analysis. *American Journal of Public Health*, 81: 168–71.

Kelly, J.A., Otto-Salaj, L.L., Sikkema, K.J., Pinkerton, S.D. and Bloom, F.R. (1998) Implications of HIV treatment advances for behavioral research on AIDS: protease inhibitors and new challenges in HIV secondary prevention. *Health Psychology*, 17: 310–19.

Kemeny, M.E., Cohen, F., Zegans, L.A. and Conant, M.A. (1989) Psychological and immunological predictors of genital herpes recurrence. *Psychosomatic Medicine*, 51: 195–208.

Kendell, R.E. and Staton, M.C. (1966) The fate of untreated alcoholics. *Quarterly Journal of Studies in Alcohol*, 27: 30–41.

Kendell, R.E., de Roumanie, M. and Ritson, E.B. (1983a) The influence of an increase in excise duty on alcohol consumption and its adverse effects. *British Medical Journal*, 287: 809–11.

Kendell, R.E., de Roumanie, M. and Ritson, E.B. (1983b) Effects of economic changes on Scottish drinking habits 1978–1982. *British Journal of Addiction*, 78: 365–79.

Kendler, K.S., Heath, A.C., Neale, M.C., Kessler, R.C. and Eaves, L.J. (1992) A population-based twin study of alcoholism in women. *Journal of the American Medical Association*, 268: 1877–82.

Kenkel, D.S. (1991) Health behavior, health knowledge, and schooling. *Journal of Political Economy*, 99: 287–305.

Kenney, W.L. (1985) Parasympathetic control of resting heart rate: relationship to aerobic power. *Medicine and Science in Sports and Exercise*, 17: 451–55.

Kent, K.M., Smith, E.R., Redwood, D.R. and Epstein, S.E. (1973) Electrical stability of acutely ischemic myocardium. Influences of heart rate and vagal stimulation. *Circulation*, 47: 291–8.

Kent, T.H. and Hart, M.N. (1987) *Introduction to Human Disease*, 2nd ed. East Norwalk, CT: Appleton-Century-Crofts.

Kessler, R.C. (1997) The effects of stressful life events on depression. *Annual Review of Psychology*, 48: 191–214.

Keys, A. (1980) *Seven Countries: A Multivariate Analysis of Death and Coronary Heart Disease*. Cambridge, MA: Harvard University Press.

Keys, A., Brozek, J., Henschel, A., Nickelson, O. and Taylor, H.L. (1950) *The Biology of Human Starvation*, Vols. 1 and 2. Minneapolis, MI: University of Minnesota Press.

Keys, A., Taylor, H.L., Blackburn, H. *et al.* (1971) Mortality and coronary heart disease among men studied for 23 years. *Archives of Internal Medicine*, 128: 201–14.

Kiecolt-Glaser, J.K. and Glaser, R. (1991) Stress and immune function in humans, in R. Ader, D.L. Felten and N. Cohen (eds) *Psychoneuroimmunology*, 2nd ed., pp. 849–67. San Diego, CA/New York, NY: Academic Press: Harcourt Brace Jovanovich.

Kiecolt-Glaser, J.K., Glaser, R., Shuttleworth, E.C. *et al.* (1987) Chronic stress and immunity in family caregivers of Alzheimers' disease victims. *Psychosomatic Medicine*, 49: 523–35.

Kiecolt-Glaser, J.K., Kennedy, S., Malkoff, S. *et al.* (1988) Marital discord and immunity in males. *Psychosomatic Medicine*, 50: 213–29.

Killen, J.D., Taylor, B.D., Hayward, C. *et al.* (1996) Weight concerns influence the development of eating disorders: a 4-year prospective study. *Journal of Consulting and Clinical Psychology*, 64: 936–40.

Killen, J.D., Robinson, T.N., Haydel, K.F. *et al.* (1997) Prospective study of risk factors for the initiation of cigarette smoking. *Journal of Consulting and Clinical Psychology*, 65: 1011–16.

Kimiecik, J. (1992) Predicting vigorous physical activity of corporate employees: comparing the theories of reasoned action and planned behavior. *Journal of Sport and Exercise Psychology*, 14: 192–206.

King, A.C., Taylor, C.B., Haskell, W.L. and DeBusk, R.F. (1989) Influence of regular aerobic exercise on psychological health: a randomized, controlled trial of healthy middle-aged adults. *Health Psychology*, 8: 305–24.

King, K.B., Reis, H.T., Porter, L.A. and Norsen, L.H. (1993) Social support and long-term recovery from coronary artery surgery: effects on patients and spouses. *Health Psychology*, 12: 56–63.

Kippax, S., Crawford, J., Davis, M., Rodden, P. and Dowsett, G. (1993) Sustaining safe sex: a longitudinal sample of homosexual men. *AIDS*, 7: 257–63.

Kippax, S., Noble, J., Prestage, G., Crawford, J.M., Campbell, D., Baxter, D. and Cooper, D. (1997) Sexual negotiation in the AIDS era: negotiated safety revisited. *AIDS*, 11: 191–7.

Kirby, D. and DiClemente, R.J. (1994) School-based interventions to prevent unprotected sex and HIV among adolescents, in R.J. DiClemente and J.L. Peterson (eds) *Preventing AIDS: Theories and Methods of Behavioural Interventions*, pp. 117–39. New York, NY: Plenum.

Kittel, F., Kornitzer, M., Dramaix, M. and Beriot, I. (1993) Health behavior in Belgian studies: who is doing best? Paper presented at the European Congress of Psychology, Tampere, Finland.

Kleinot, M.C. and Rogers, R.W. (1982) Identifying effective components of alcohol misuse prevention programs. *Journal of Studies on Alcohol*, 43: 802–11.

Klem, M.L., Wing, R.R., McGuire, M.T., Seagle, H.M. and Hill, J.O. (1998) Psychological symptoms in individuals successful at long-term maintenance of weight loss. *Health Psychology*, 17: 336–45.

Klesges, R.C. and Glasgow, R.E. (1986) Smoking modification in the worksite, in M.F. Cataldo and T.J. Coates (eds) *Health and Industry: A Behavioral Medicine Perspective*, pp. 231–54. New York, NY: Wiley.

Klesges, R.C., Benowitz, N.L. and Meyers, A.W. (1991) Behavioral and biobehavioral aspects of smoking and smoking cessation: the problem of postcessation weight gain. *Behavior Therapy*, 22: 179–99.

Klesges, R.C., Ward, K.D. and DeBon, M. (1996) Smoking cessation: a successful behavioral/pharmacologic interface. *Clinical Psychology Review*, 16: 479–96.

Klesges, R.C., Winders, S.E., Meyers, A.W. *et al.* (1997) How much weight gain occurs following smoking cessation? A comparison of weight gain using both continuous and point prevalence abstinence. *Journal of Consulting and Clinical Psychology*, 65: 286–91.

Klesges, R.C., Zbikoski, S.M., Lando, H.A. *et al.* (1998) The relationship between smoking and body weight in a population of young military personnel. *Health Psychology*, 17: 454–8.

Kobasa, S.C. (1979) Stressful life events, personality, and health: an inquiry into hardiness. *Journal of Personality and Social Psychology*, 37: 1–11.

Kobasa, S.C. and Puccetti, M.C. (1983) Personality and social resources in stress resistance. *Journal of Personality and Social Psychology*, 45: 839–50.

Kobasa, S.C., Maddi, S.R. and Courington, S. (1981) Personality and constitution as mediators in the stress–illness relationship. *Journal of Health and Social Behavior*, 22: 368–78.

Kobasa, S.C., Maddi, S.R. and Kahn, S. (1982a) Hardiness and health: a prospective study. *Journal of Personality and Social Psychology*, 42: 168–77.

Kobasa, S.C., Maddi, S.R. and Puccetti, M.C. (1982b) Personality and exercise as buffers in the stress–illness relationship. *Journal of Behavioral Medicine*, 5: 391–404.

Koopmans, H.S. (1998) Experimental studies on the control of food intake, in G.A. Bray, C. Bouchard and W.P.T. James (ed.) *Handbook of Obesity*, pp. 273–312. New York, NY: Marcel Dekker.

Kottke, T.E., Battista, R.N., DeFriese, G.H. and Brekke, M.L. (1988) Attributes of successful smoking cessation interventions in medical practice: a meta-analysis of 39 controlled trials. *Journal of the American Medical Association*, 259: 2883–9.

Kraft, P., Sutton, S.R. and Reynolds, H.M. (1999) The transtheoretical model of behavior change: are stages qualitatively different? *Psychology and Health*, 14: 433–50.

Kramsch, D.M., Aspen, A.J., Abramowitz, B.M., Kreimendahl, T. and Hood Jr, W.B. (1981) Reduction of coronary atherosclerosis by moderate conditioning exercise in monkeys on an atherogenic diet. *New England Journal of Medicine*, 303: 1483–9.

Kraus, S.J. (1995) Attitudes and the prediction of behavior: a meta-analysis of the empirical literature. *Personality and Social Psychology Bulletin*, 21: 58–75.

Kuppens, M., de Wit, J. and Stroebe, W. (1996) Angstaanjagendheid in gezondheidsvoorlichting: een dual process analyse. *Gedrag en Gezondheid*, 24: 241–8.

Kyes, K.B. (1990) The effect of a 'safer sex' film as mediated by erotophobia and gender on attitudes towards condoms. *Journal of Sex Research*, 27: 297–303.

LaCroix, A.Z., Leveille, S.G., Hecht, J.A., Grothaus, L.C. and Wagner, E.H. (1996) Does walking decrease the risk of cardiovascular disease hospitalizations and death in older adults? *Journal of the American Geriatrics Society*, 44: 113–20.

Lapidus, L., Bengtsson, C. and Lissner, L. (1990) Distribution of adipose tissue in relation to cardiovascular and total mortality as observed during 20 years in a prospective population study of women in Gothenberg, Sweden. *Diabetes Research and Clinical Practice*, 10: S185–9.

Larsson, B., Björntorp, P. and Tibblin, G. (1981) The health consequences of moderate obesity. *International Journal of Obesity*, 5: 97–116.

Larsson, B., Seidell, J., Svärdsudd, K. *et al.* (1989) Obesity, adipose tissue distribution and health in men – the study of men born in 1913. *Appetite*, 13: 37–44.

Laugesen, M. and Meads, C. (1991) Tobacco advertising restrictions, price, income and tobacco consumption in OECD countries, 1960–1986. *British Journal of Addiction*, 86: 1343–54.

Lazarus, R.S. and Folkman, S. (1984) *Stress, Appraisal, and Coping*. New York, NY: Springer.

Lazarus, R.S., DeLongis, A., Folkman, S. and Gruen, R.J. (1985) Stress and adaptational outcomes: the problem of confounded measures. *American Psychologist*, 40: 770–9.

Ledermann, S. (1956) *Alcool, alcoolisme, alcoolisation: donées scientifiques de caractère physiologique, économique et social*. Institut National D'Études Démographiques. Travaux et Documents, Cahier No. 29. Paris: Presses Universitaires de France.

Ledermann, S. (1964) *Alcool, alcoolisme, alcoolisation. Mortalité, morbidité, accidents du travail*. Institut National D'Études Démographiques. Travaux et Documents, Cahier No. 41. Paris: Presses Universitaires de France.

Leiker, M. and Hailey, B.J. (1988) A link between hostility and disease: poor health habits? *Behavioral Medicine*, 3: 129–33.

Lemers, F. and Voegtlin, W.L. (1950) An evaluation of the aversion treatment of alcoholism. *Quarterly Journal of Studies on Alcohol*, 11: 199–204.

Lepper, M.R. and Greene, D. (1978) *The Hidden Cost of Reward*. New York, NY: Wiley.

Leventhal, H. (1970) Findings and theory in the study of fear communication, in L. Berkowitz (ed.) *Advances in Experimental Social Psychology*, Vol. 5, pp. 119–86.

Leventhal, H. and Avis, N. (1976) Pleasure, addiction, and habit: factors in verbal report or factors in smoking behavior? *Journal of Abnormal Psychology*, 85: 478–88.

Leventhal, H. and Cleary, P.D. (1980) The smoking problem: a review of the research and theory in behavioral risk modification. *Psychological Bulletin*, 88: 370–405.

Lew, E.A. and Garfinkel, L. (1979) Variation in mortality by weight among 750,000 men and women. *Journal of Chronic Diseases*, 32: 563–76.

Lewit, E.M. and Coate, D. (1982) The potential for using excise taxes to reduce smoking. *Journal of Health Economics*, 1: 121–45.

Liberman, A. and Chaiken, S. (1992) Defensive processing of personally relevant health messages. *Personality and Social Psychology Bulletin*, 18: 669–79.

Lichtenstein, E. (1982) The smoking problem: a behavioral perspective. *Journal of Consulting and Clinical Psychology*, 50: 804–19.

Lichtenstein, E. and Danaher, B.G. (1975) Modification of smoking behavior: a critical analysis of theory, research, and practice, in M. Hersen, R. Eisler and P. Miller (eds) *Progress in Behavior Modification*, Vol. 3, pp. 79–132. New York, NY: Academic Press.

Locke, E.A. and Latham, G.P. (1990) *A Theory of Goal Setting and Task Performance*. Englewood Cliffs, NJ: Prentice Hall.

Longnecker, M.P. (1994) Alcoholic beverage consumption in relation to risk of breast cancer: meta-analysis and review. *Cancer Causes and Control*, 5: 73–82.

Lowe, M.R. (1993) The effects of dieting on eating behaviour: a three factor model. *Psychological Bulletin*, 114: 100–21.

Lowe, M.R., Whitlow, J.W. and Bellowoar, V. (1991) Eating regulation: the role of restraint, dieting and weight. *International Journal of Eating Disorders*, 10: 461–71.

Luepker, R.V., Murray, D.M., Jacobs, D.R. *et al.* (1994) Community education for cardiovascular disease prevention: risk factor changes in the Minnesota Heart Health Program. *American Journal of Public Health*, 84, 1383–93.

Luepker, R.V., Perry, C.L., McKinlay, S.M. *et al.* (1996) Outcomes of a field trial to improve children's dietary patterns and physical activity. *Journal of the American Medical Association*, 275: 769–76.

Luft, F.C. (1997) Salt skirmishes. *Kidney-Blood-Pressure Research*, 20: 71–3.

McCann, I.L. and Holmes, D.S. (1984) Influence of aerobics on depression. *Journal of Personality and Social Psychology*, 46: 1142–7.

McCarroll, J.R. and Haddon Jr, W. (1962) A controlled study of fatal motor vehicle crashes in New York City. *Journal of Chronic Diseases*, 15: 811–22.

McClelland, D.C., Davis, W.N., Kalin, R. and Wanner, E. (1972) *The Drinking Man*. New York, NY: Free Press.

McConnaughy, E., Prochaska, J.O. and Velicer, W.F. (1983) Stages of change in psychotherapy: measurement and sample profiles. *Psychotherapy*, 20: 368–75.

McConnaughy, E., DiClemente, C.C., Prochaska, J.O. and Velicer, W.F. (1989) Stages of change in psychotherapy: a follow-up report. *Psychotherapy*, 26: 494–503.

McCrady, S.B. and Delaney, S.I. (1995) Self-help groups, in R.K. Hester and W.R. Miller (eds) *Handbook of Alcoholism Treatment Approaches*, 2nd ed., pp. 160–75. Boston, MA: Allyn and Bacon.

McCrae, R.R. and Costa Jr, P.T. (1986) Personality, coping and coping effectiveness in an adult sample. *Journal of Personality*, 54: 385–405.

McDonald, D.G. and Hodgdon, J.A. (1991) *Psychological Effects of Aerobic Fitness Training: Research and Theory*. New York, NY: Springer.

MacDonald, T.K., Zanna, M.P. and Fong, G.T. (1995) Decision making in altered states: effects of alcohol on attitudes toward drinking and driving. *Journal of Personality and Social Psychology*, 68: 973–85.

McGinnis, J.M. and Foege, W.H. (1993) Actual causes of death in the United States. *Journal of the American Medical Association*, 270: 2207–12.

McGinnis, J.M., Shopland, D. and Brown, C. (1987) Tobacco and health: trends in smoking and smokeless tobacco consumption in the United States. *Annual Review of Public Health*, 8: 441–67.

McGue, M., Pickens, R. and Sivikis, D.S. (1992) Sex and age effects on the inheritance of alcohol problems: a twin study. *Journal of Abnormal Psychology*, 101: 3–17.

McGuire, R.J. and Vallance, M. (1964) Aversion therapy by electric shock: a simple technique. *British Medical Journal*, I: 151–3.

McGuire, W.J. (1985) Attitudes and attitude change, in G. Lindzey and E. Aronson (eds) *Handbook of Social Psychology*, 3rd ed., Vol. 2, pp. 233–346. New York, NY: Random House.

McKeown, T. (1979) *The Role of Medicine*. Oxford: Blackwell.

McKinlay, J.B. and McKinlay, S.M. (1981) Medical measures and the decline of mortality, in P. Conrad and R. Kern (eds) *The Sociology of Health and Illness*, pp. 12–30. New York, NY: St Martins.

McKinnon, W., Weisse, C.S., Reynolds, C.P., Bowles, C.A. and Baum, A. (1989) Chronic stress, leukocyte subpopulations, and humoral response to latent viruses. *Health Psychology*, 8: 389–402.

McKusick, L., Horstman, W. and Coates, T.J. (1985) AIDS and sexual behavior reported by gay men in San Francisco. *American Journal of Public Health*, 75 (15): 493–6.

Macpherson, G. (1999) *Black's Medical Dictionary*, 39th Edition. London: Black.

Maddi, S.R., Bartone, P.T. and Puccetti, M.C. (1987) Stressful events are indeed a factor in physical illness: a reply to Schroeder and Costa (1984) *Journal of Personality and Social Psychology*, 52: 833–43.

Maddi, S.R., Kobasa, S.C. and Hoover, M. (1979) An alienation test. *Journal of Humanistic Psychology*, 19: 73–6.

Maddox, G.L., Back, K.W. and Liederman, V.R. (1968) Overweight and social deviance and disability. *Journal of Health and Social Behavior*, 9: 287–98.

Maddux, J.E. and Rogers, R.W. (1983) Protection motivation and self-efficacy: a revised theory of fear appeals and attitude change. *Journal of Experimental and Social Psychology*, 19: 469–79.

Maes, S., Verhoeven, C., Kittel, F. and Scholten, H. (1998) Effects of a Dutch work-site wellness-health program: The Brabantia project. *American Journal of Public Health*, 88: 1037–41.

MAFF (Ministry of Agriculture, Fisheries and Food) (1995) *Manual of Nutrition*, 10th ed. London: The Stationery Office.

Mahoney, M.J. and Mahoney, K. (1976) *Permanent Weight Control: A Total Solution to a Dieter's Dilemma*. New York, NY: W.W. Norton.

Maisto, S.A., Lauerman, R. and Adesso, V.J. (1977) A comparison of two experimental studies of the role of cognitive factors in alcoholics' drinking. *Journal of Studies on Alcohol*, 38: 145–9.

Mandler, G. (1975) *Mind and Emotion*. New York, NY: Wiley.

Manning, W.G., Keeler, E.B., Newhouse, J.P., Sloss, E.M. and Wasserman, J. (1989) The taxes of sin: do smokers and drinkers pay their way? *Journal of the American Medical Association*, 261: 1604–9.

Manning, W.G., Blumberg, L. and Moulton, L.H. (1995) The demand for alcohol: the differential response to price. *Journal of Health Economics*, 14: 123–48.

Manstead, A.S.R., Proffitt, C. and Smart, J.L. (1983) Predicting and understanding mothers' infant-feeding intentions and behavior: testing the theory of reasoned action. *Journal of Personality and Social Psychology*, 44: 657–71.

Manuck, S.B. and Krantz, D.S. (1986) Psychophysiological reactivity in coronary heart disease and essential hypertension, in K.A. Matthews, S.M. Weiss, T. Detre, T.D. Dembrowksi, B. Falkner, S.B. Manuck and R.B. Williams Jr (eds) *Handbook of Stress, Reactivity and Cardiovascular Disease*, pp. 11–34. New York, NY: Wiley.

Marlatt, G.A. (1976) Alcohol, stress, and cognitive control, in I.S. Sarason and C.D. Spielberger (eds) *Stress and Anxiety*, Vol. 3, pp. 271–96. Washington, DC: Hemisphere.

Marlatt, G.A. (1985) Relapse prevention: theoretical rationale and overview of the model, in G.A. Marlatt and J.R. Gordon (eds) *Relapse Prevention*, pp. 3–70. New York, NY: Guilford Press.

Marlatt, G.A. and Gordon, J.R. (1980) Determinants of relapse: implications for the maintenance of behavior change, in P.O. Davidson and S.M. Davidson (eds) *Behavioral Medicine*, pp. 410–52. New York, NY: Brunner/Mazel.

Marlatt, G.A. and Rohsenow, D.J. (1980) Cognitive processes in alcohol use: expectancy and the balanced placebo design, in N.K. Mellow (ed.) *Advances in Substance Abuse*, Vol. 1, pp. 159–99. Greenwich, CT: JAI Press.

Marlatt, G.A., Demming, B. and Reid, J.B. (1973) Loss of control drinking in alcoholics: an experimental analogue. *Journal of Abnormal and Social Psychology*, 81: 233–41.

Martin, J.L. (1987) The impact of AIDS on gay male sexual behavior patterns in New York City. *American Journal of Public Health*, 77: 578–81.

Martinsen, E.W. and Morgan, W.P. (1997) Antidepressant effects of physical activity, in W.P. Morgan (ed.) *Physical Activity and Mental Health*, pp. 93–106. Philadelphia, PA: Taylor & Francis.

Martinsen, E.W., Medhus, A. and Sandvik, L. (1985) Effects of aerobic exercise on depression: a controlled study. *British Medical Journal*, 292: 109–10.

Mason, J.W. (1975) A historical view of the stress field (Part I, II). *Journal of Human Stress*, 1: 6–12, 22–36.

Matarazzo, J.D. (1984) Behavioral health: a 1990 challenge for the health sciences professions, in J.D. Matarazzo, N.E. Miller, S.M. Weiss, J.A. Herd and St M. Weiss (eds) *Behavioral Health: A Handbook of Health Enhancement and Disease Prevention*, pp. 3–40. New York, NY: Wiley.

Matthews, K.A., Glass, D.C., Rosenman, R.H. and Bortner, R.W. (1977) Competitive drive, pattern A, and coronary heart disease: a further analysis of some data from the Western Collaborative Group Study. *Journal of Chronic Disease*, 30: 489–98.

Mechanic, D. (1978) *Medical Sociology*, 2nd ed. New York, NY: Free Press.

Mechanic, D. (1979) The stability of health and illness behavior: results from a 16-year follow-up. *American Journal of Public Health*, 69: 1142–5.

Meichenbaum, P. (1977) *Cognitive Behavior Modification*. New York, NY: Plenum.

Meisel, S.R., Kutz, I., Dayan, K.I. *et al.* (1991) Effect of Iraqi missile war on incidence of acute myocardial infarction and sudden death in Israeli civilians. *Lancet*, 338: 660–1.

Meyer, A.J., Nash, J.D., McAlister, A.L., Maccoby, N. and Farquhar, J.W. (1980) Skills training in a cardiovascular health education campaign. *Journal of Consulting and Clinical Psychology*, 48: 129–42.

Meyers, A.W., Klesges, R.C., Winders, S.E. *et al.* (1997) Are weight concerns predictive of smoking cessation: a prospective analysis. *Journal of Consulting and Clinical Psychology*, 65: 448–52.

Miller, C.T. and Downey, K.T. (1999) A meta-analysis of heavyweight and self-esteem. *Personality and Social Psychology Review*, 3: 68–84.

Miller, P.M. (1972) The use of behavioral contracting in the treatment of alcoholism. *Behavior Therapy*, 3: 593–6.

Miller, S.M. (1980) Why having control reduces stress: if I can stop the roller coaster, I don't want to get off, in J. Garber and M.E.P. Selgiman (eds) *Human Helplessness: Theory and Applications*, pp. 71–95. New York, NY: Academic Press.

Miller, T.Q., Smith, T.W., Turner, C.W., Guijarro, M.L. and Hallet, A.J. (1996) A meta-analytic review of research on hostility and physical health. *Psychological Bulletin*, 119: 322–48.

Miller, W.R. and Hester, R.K. (1986) The effectiveness of alcoholism treatment: what research reveals, in W.R. Miller and N. Heather (eds) *Treating Addictive Behaviors: Processes of Change*, pp. 121–74. New York, NY: Plenum.

Miller, W.R. and Munoz, R.F. (1976) *How to Control your Drinking?* Englewood Cliffs, NJ: Prentice Hall.

Miller, W.R., Brown, J.M., Simpson, T.L. *et al.* (1995) What works? A methodological analysis of the alcohol treatment outcome literature, in R.K. Hester and W.R. Miller (eds) *Handbook of Alcoholism Treatment Approaches*, 2nd ed., pp. 12–44. Boston, MA: Allyn and Bacon.

Milstein, R.M. (1980) Responsiveness in newborn infants of overweight and normal weight parents. *Appetite*, 1: 65–74.

Monroe, S.M. (1983) Major and minor life events as predictors of psychological distress: further issues and findings. *Journal of Behavioral Medicine*, 6: 189–205.

Monti, P.M., Rohsenow, D.J., Colby, S.M. and Abrams, D.B. (1995) Coping and social skills training, in R.K. Hester and W.R. Miller (eds) *Handbook of Alcoholism Treatment Approaches*, 2nd ed., pp. 221–41. Boston, MA: Allyn and Bacon.

Mooney, A.J. (1982) Alcohol use, in R.B. Taylor (ed.) *Health Promotion: Principles and Clinical Applications*, pp. 233–58. New York, NY: Appleton-Century-Crofts.

Mooney III, A.J. and Cross, G.M. (1988) Alcoholism and substance abuse, in L.B. Taylor (ed.) *Family Medicine*, 3rd ed., pp. 690–702. New York, NY: Springer-Verlag.

Moore, M.H. and Gerstein, D.R. (eds) (1981) *Alcohol and Public Policy: Beyond the Shadow of Prohibition*. Washington, DC: National Academy Press.

Morgan, W.P. (ed.) (1997) *Physical Activity and Mental Health*. Philadelphia, PA: Taylor & Francis.

Morgenstern, J., Labouvie, B.S., McCrady, B.S., Kahler, C.W. and Frey, R.M. (1997) Affiliation with Alcoholics Anonymous after treatment: a study of its therapeutic effects and mechanism of action. *Journal of Clinical and Consulting Psychology*, 65: 768–77.

Morris, J.N., Heady, J.A., Raffle, P., Roberts, C.G. and Parks, J.W. (1953) Coronary heart disease and physical activity of work. *Lancet*, 2: 1053–7; 1111–20.

Morris, J.N., Pollard, R., Everitt, M.G. and Chave, S.P.W. (1980) Vigorous exercise in leisure-time protection against coronary heart disease. *Lancet*, 2: 1207–10.

Mulilis, J.P. and Lippa, R. (1990) Behavorial change in earthquake preparedness due to negative threat appeals: a test of protection motivation theory. *Journal of Applied Social Psychology*, 20: 619–38.

National Centers for Health Statistics (1989) *Health, United States 1988*. DHHS Publication No. (PHS) 89–1252. Washington, DC: US Government Printing Office.

National Safety Council (1986) *Accident Facts – 1986*. Chicago, IL: National Safety Council.

Neil, W.A. and Oxendine, J.M. (1979) Exercise can promote coronary collateral development without improving perfusion of ischemic myocardium. *Circulation*, 60: 1513–19.

Newcomb, M.D. (1990) What structural equation modelling can tell us about social support, in B.R. Sarason, I.G. Sarason and G.R. Pierce (eds) *Social Support: An Interactional View*, pp. 26–62. New York, NY: Wiley.

Niles, P. (1964) The relationships of susceptibility and anxiety to acceptance of fear-arousing communications. Unpublished doctoral dissertation, Yale University.

Nisbett, R.E. (1968) Taste, deprivation, and weight determinants of eating behavior. *Journal of Personality and Social Psychology*, 10: 107–16.

Nisbett, R.E. (1972) Hunger, obesity, and the ventromedial hypothalamus. *Psychological Review*, 79: 433–53.

Nolen-Hoeksema, S. and Larson, J. (1999) *Coping with Loss*. Mahwah, NJ: Lawrence Erlbaum.

Nolen-Hoeksema, S., McBride, A. and Larson, J. (1997) Rumination and psychological distress among bereaved partners. *Journal of Personality and Social Psychology*, 72, 855–62.

Novotny, T.E., Romano, R.A., Davis, R.M. and Mills, S.L. (1992) The public health practice of tobacco control: lessons learned and directions for the States in the 1990s. *Annual Review of Public Health*, 13: 287–318.

O'Leary, A.O. (1990) Stress, emotion, and human immune function. *Psychological Bulletin*, 108: 363–82.

Olson, J.M. and Zanna, M.P. (1982) *Predicting Adherence to a Program of Physical Exercise: An Empirical Study*. Toronto: Government of Ontario, Ministry of Tourism and Recreation.

Orbell, S., Hodgkins, S. and Sheeran, P. (1997) Implementation intentions and the theory of planned behavior. *Personality and Social Psychology Bulletin*, 23: 945–54.

Osmond, D.H., Page, K., Wiley, J.A. *et al.* (1994) HIV infection in homosexual and bisexual men 18 to 29 years of age: the San Francisco young gay men's health study. *American Journal of Public Health*, 84: 1933–7.

Ouelette, J.A. and Wood, W. (1998) Habit and intention in everyday life: the multiple processes by which past behavior predicts future behavior. *Psychological Bulletin*, 124: 54–74.

Paffenbarger Jr, R.S. and Hale, W.E. (1975) Work activity and coronary heart mortality. *New England Journal of Medicine*, 292: 545–50.

Paffenbarger Jr, R.S., Hyde, R.T., Wing, A.L. and Hsieh, C. (1986) Cigarette smoking and cardiovascular disease, in D.G. Zaridze and R. Peto (eds) *A Major International Hazard* (IARC Scientific Publications No. 74). Lyon: International Agency for Research on Cancer.

Paffenbarger Jr, R.S., Lee, I.M. and Leung, R. (1994) Physical activitiy and personal characteristics associated with depression and suicide in American college men. *Acta Psychiatrica Scandinavia Supplementum*, 377: 16–22.

Paffenbarger Jr, R.S., Wing, A.L. and Hyde, R.T. (1978) Chronic disease in former college students, XVI. Physical activity as an index of heart attack risk in college alumni. *American Journal of Epidemiology*, 108: 161–75.

Parker, J.D.A. and Endler, N.S. (1992) Coping with coping assessment: a critical review. *European Journal of Personality*, 6: 321–44.

Parkes, C.M. (1996) *Bereavement: Studies of Grief in Adult Life*, 3rd ed. London: Penguin.

Parkes, C.M., Benjamin, B. and Fitzgerald, R.G. (1969) Broken heart: a statistical study of increased mortality among widowers. *British Medical Journal*, 1: 740–3.

Pasternak, R.C., Grundy, S.M., Levy, D. and Thompson, P.D. (1996) Task Force 3. Spectrum of risk factors for coronary heart disease. *Journal of the American College of Cardiology*, 27: 978–90.

Pennebaker, J.W. (1989) Confession, inhibition, and disease, in L. Berkowitz (ed.) *Advances in Experimental Social Psychology*, Vol. 22, pp. 211–44. San Diego, CA: Academic Press.

Pennebaker, J. (1997) Writing about emotional experiences as a therapeutic process. *Psychological Sciences*, 8: 162–6.

Pennebaker, J.W., Kiecolt-Glaser, J.K. and Glaser, R. (1988) Disclosure of traumas and immune function: health implications for psychotherapy. *Journal of Consulting and Clinical Psychology*, 56: 239–45.

Pennebaker, J.W., Colder, M. and Sharp, L.K. (1990) Accelerating the coping process. *Journal of Personality and Social Psychology*, 58: 528–37.

Perkins, K.A. (1993) Weight gain following smoking cessation. *Journal of Consulting and Clinical Psychology*, 61: 768–77.

Perri, M.G., Martin, A.D., Leermakers, E.A., Sears, S.F. and Notelovitz, M. (1997) Effects of group- versus home-based exercise in the treatment of obesity. *Journal of Consulting and Clinical Psychology*, 65: 278–85.

Perry, C.L., William, C.L., Veblen-Mortenson, S. *et al.* (1996) Project Northland: outcomes of a community-wide alcohol use prevention program during early adolescence. *American Journal of Public Health*, 86: 956–65.

Peterson, C. and Seligman, M.E.P. (1987) Coarse explanations as a risk factor for depression: theory and evidence. *Psychological Review*, 91: 347–74.

Peterson, C., Seligman, M.E.P. and Vaillant, G.E. (1988) Pessimistic explanatory style is a risk factor for physical illness: a thirty-five-year longitudinal study. *Journal of Personality and Social Psychology*, 55: 23–7.

Peterson, C., Maier, S.F. and Seligman, M.E.P. (1993) *Learned Helplessness: A Theory for the Age of Personal Control*. New York, NY: Oxford University Press.

Petty, R. and Cacioppo, J.T. (1986) *Communication and Persuasion: Central and Peripheral Routes to Attitude Change*. New York, NY: Springer Verlag.

Petty, R., Cacioppo, J.T. and Goldman, R. (1981a) Personal involvement as a determinant of argument-based persuasion. *Journal of Personality and Social Psychology*, 41: 847–55.

Petty, R.E., Ostrom, T. and Brock, T.C. (1981b) Historical foundations of the cognitive response approach to attitudes and persuasion, in R.E. Petty, T.M. Ostrom and T.C. Brock (eds) *Cognitive responses in persuasion*, pp. 5–29. Hillsdale, NJ: Lawrence Erlbaum.

Petty, R.E., Wells, G.L. and Brock, T.C. (1976) Distraction can enhance or reduce yielding to propaganda: thought disruption versus effort justification. *Journal of Personality and Social Psychology*, 34: 874–84.

Petty, R.E., Wegener, D.T. and Fabrigar, L.R. (1997) Attitudes and attitude change. *Annual Review of Psychology*, 48: 609–47.

Pickens, R.W., Svikis, D.S., McGue, M. *et al.* (1991) Heterogeneity in the inheritance of alcoholism: a study of male and female twins. *Archives of General Psychiatry*, 48: 19–28.

Pierce, G.R., Sarason, B.R. and Sarason, I.G. (eds) (1996) *Handbook of Social Support in the Family*. New York, NY: Plenum.

Pierie, P.L., McBride, C.M., Hellerstedt, W. *et al.* (1992) Smoking cessation in women concerned about weight. *American Journal of Public Health*, 82: 1238–43.

Polich, J.M., Armor, D.J. and Braiker, H.B. (1981) *The Course of Alcoholism*. New York, NY: Wiley.

Polivy, J. and Herman, C.P. (1976) Effects of alcohol on eating behavior: influence of mood and perceived intoxication. *Journal of Abnormal Psychology*, 85: 601–6.

Polivy, J. and Herman, C.P. (1987) Diagnosis and treatment of normal eating. *Journal of Consulting and Clinical Psychology*, 28: 341–3.

Polivy, J., Heatherton, T.F. and Herman, C.P. (1988) Self-esteem, restraint and eating behaviour. *Journal of Abnormal Psychology*, 85: 338–40.

Polivy, J., Herman, P.H. and Howard, K.I. (1988) Restraint scale: assessment of dieting, in M. Hersen and A.S. Bellack (eds) *Dictionary of Behavioral Assessment Techniques*, pp. 377–80. New York, NY: Pergamon Press.

Pomerleau, O.F. and Kardia, S.L. (1999) Introduction to the featured section: genetic research on smoking. *Health Psychology*, 18: 3–6.

Pomerleau, O.F. and Pomerleau, C.S. (1989) A biobehavioral perspective on smoking, in T. Ney and A. Gale (eds) *Smoking and Behavior*, pp. 69–90. Chichester: Wiley.

Pomerleau, O.F., Pertschuk, M., Adkins, D. and Brady, J.P. (1978) A comparison of behavioral and traditional treatment for middle income problem drinkers. *Journal of Behavioral Medicine*, 1: 187–200.

Pooling Project Research Group (1978) *Relationship of Blood Pressure, Serum Cholesterol, Smoking Habit, Relative Weight and ECG-abnormality to Incidence of Major Coronary Events: Final Report of the Pooling Project*. Dallas, TX: American Heart Association Monographs, No. 60.

Powell, K.E., Thompson, P.D., Caspersen, C.J. and Kendrick, J.S. (1987) Physical activity and the incidence of coronary heart disease. *Annual Review of Public Health*, 8: 253–87.

Prochaska, J.O. and DiClemente, C.C. (1983) Stages and processes of self-change of smoking: toward an integrative model of change. *Journal of Consulting and Clinical Psychology*, 51: 390–5.

Prochaska, J.O., Velicer, W.F., DiClemente, C.C. and Fava, J.S. (1988) Measuring processes of change: applications to the cessation of smoking. *Journal of Consulting and Clinical Psychology*, 56: 520–8.

Prochaska, J.O., Velicer, W.F., Guadagnoli, E., Rossi, J.S. and DiClemente, C.C. (1991) Patterns of change: dynamic typology applied to smoking cessation. *Multivariate Behavioral Research*, 26: 83–107.

Prochaska, J.O., DiClemente, C.C. and Norcross, J.C. (1992) In search of how people change: applications to addictive behaviour. *American Psychologist*, 47: 1102–14.

Prochaska, J.O., Velicer, W.F., Rossi, J.S. *et al.* (1994) Stages of change and decisional balance for 12 problem behaviors. *Health Psychology*, 13: 39–46.

Puska, P., Nissinen, A., Tuomilehto, J. *et al.* (1985) The community-based strategy to prevent coronary heart disease: conclusions from ten years of the North Karelia Project. *Annual Review of Public Health*, Vol. 6, pp. 147–94. Palo Alto, CA: Annual Reviews Inc.

Rabkin, J.G. and Struening, E.L. (1976) Life events, stress, and illness. *Science*, 194: 1013–20.

Rahe, R.H. (1968) Life change measurement as a predictor of illness. *Proceedings of the Royal Society of Medicine*, 61: 124–6.

Rahe, R.H. and Lind, E. (1971) Psychosocial factors and sudden cardiac death. A pilot study. *Journal of Psychosomatic Research*, 15: 19–24.

Rahe, R.H. and Paasikivi, J. (1971) Psychosocial factors and myocardial infarction II. An outpatient study in Sweden. *Journal of Psychosomatic Research*, 15: 33–9.

Rahe, R.H., Romo, M., Bennett, L. and Siltanen, P. (1974) Subjects' recent life changes and myocardial infarction in Helsinki, in *Archives of Internal Medicine*, 133: 222–8.

Randall, D.M. and Wolff, J.A. (1994) The time interval in the intention–behaviour relationship: meta-analysis. *British Journal of Social Psychology*, 33: 405–18.

Ratneshwar, S. and Chaiken, S. (1991) Comprehension's role in persuasion: the case of its moderating effect on the persuasive impact of source cues. *Journal of Consumer Research*, 18: 52–62.

Remington, P.L., Forman, M.R., Gentry, E.M. *et al.* (1985) Current smoking trends in the United States: the 1981–1983 Behavioral Risk Factor surveys. *Journal of the American Medical Association*, 253: 2975–8.

Rhodewalt, F. and Zone, J.B. (1989) Appraisal of life change, depression and illness in hardy and nonhardy women. *Journal of Personality and Social Psychology*, 56: 81–8.

Richard, R. and van der Pligt, J. (1991) Factors affecting condom use among adolescents. *Journal of Community and Applied Social Psychology*, 1: 105–16.

Riddle, P.K. (1980) Attitudes, beliefs, behavioral intentions, and behaviors of men and women toward regular jogging. *Research Quarterly for Exercise and Sport*, 51: 663–74.

Riley, D.M., Sobell, L.D., Leo, G.I., Sobell, M. and Klajner, F. (1987) Behavioral treatment of alcohol: a review and a comparison of behavioral and nonbehavioral studies, in M. Wilcox (ed.) *Treatment and prevention of alcohol problems: a resource manual*, pp. 73–115. San Diego, CA: Academic Press.

Rimmele, C.T., Howard, M.O. and Hilfrink, M.L. (1995) Aversion therapies, in R.K. Hester and W.R. Miller (eds) (1995) *Handbook of Alcoholism Treatment Approaches*, 2nd ed., pp. 134–47. Boston, MA: Allyn and Bacon.

Rippetoe, P.A. and Rogers, R.W. (1987) Effects of components of protection-motivation theory on adaptive and maladaptive coping with a health threat. *Journal of Personality and Social Psychology*, 52: 596–604.

Robertson, K., Kelley, A., O'Neill, B. *et al.* (1974) A controlled study of the effect of television messages on safety belt use. *American Journal of Public Health*, 64: 1071–80.

Robertson, L.S. (1978) The seat belt use law in Ontario: effects on actual use. *Canadian Journal of Public Health*, 70: 599–603.

Robertson, L.S. (1984) Behavior and injury prevention: whose behavior?, in J.D. Matarazzo, S.M. Weiss, J.A. Herd, N.E. Miller and S.M. Weiss (eds) *Behavioral Health*, pp. 980–9. New York, NY: Wiley.

Robertson, L.S. (1986) Behavioral and environmental interventions for reducing motor vehicle trauma, in L. Breslow, J.E. Fielding and L.B. Lave (eds) *Annual Review of Public Health*, pp. 13–34. Palo Alto, CA: Annual Reviews Inc.

Robertson, L.S. (1987) Injury prevention: limits to self-protective behavior, in N.D. Weinstein (ed.) *Taking Care*, pp. 280–97. New York, NY: Cambridge University Press.

Rodin, J. (1981) Current status of the internal–external hypothesis for obesity. *American Psychologist*, 36: 361–72.

Rodin, J., Slochower, J. and Fleming, B. (1977) The effects of degree of obesity, age of onset, and energy deficit on external responsiveness. *Journal of Comparative and Physiological Psychology*, 91: 586–97.

Rogers, R.W. (1983) Cognitive and physiological processes in fear appeals and attitude change: a revised theory of protection motivation, in J.T. Cacioppo and R.E. Petty (eds) *Social Psychophysiology: A Source Book*, pp. 153–76. New York, NY: Guilford Press.

Rogers, R.W. (1985) Attitude change and information integration in fear appeals. *Psychological Reports*, 56: 179–82.

Rogers, R.W. and Mewborn, C.R. (1976) Fear appeals and attitude change: effects of anxiousness, probability of occurrence, and the efficacy of coping responses. *Journal of Personality and Social Psychology*, 34: 54–61.

Rooney, B.L. and Murray, D.M. (1996) A meta-analysis of smoking prevention programs after adjustment for errors in the unit of analysis. *Health Education Quarterly*, 23: 48–64.

Rose, J.S., Chassin, L., Presson, C.C. and Sherman, S.J. (1996) Prospective predictors of quit attempts and smoking cessation in young adults. *Health Psychology*, 15: 261–8.

Rosenberg, H. (1993) Prediction of controlled drinking by alcoholics and problem drinkers. *Psychological Bulletin*, 113: 129–39.

Rosenberg, M.J. (1960) An analysis of affective–cognitive consistency, in C.I. Hovland and M.J. Rosenberg (eds) *Attitude Organization and Change*, pp. 15–64. New Haven, CT: Yale University Press.

Rosenberg, M.J. and Hovland, C.I. (1960) Cognitive, affective, and behavioral components of attitudes, in I. Hovland and M.J. Rosenberg (eds) *Attitude Organization and Change*, pp. 1–15. New Haven, CT: Yale University Press.

Rosenman, R.H., Brand, R.J., Jenkins, C.D. *et al.* (1975) Coronary heart disease in the Western Collaborative Group Study: final follow-up experience of $8\frac{1}{2}$ years. *Journal of the American Medical Association*, 223: 872–7.

Rosenstock, I. (1974) The health belief model and preventive health behavior. *Health Education Monographs*, 2: 354–86.

Ross, C.E. and Hayes, D. (1988) Exercise and psychological well-being in the community. *American Journal of Epidemiology*, 127: 762–71.

Ross, C.E. and Mirowsky, J. (1979) A comparison of life-event weighting schemes: change, undesirability, and effect-proportional indices. *Journal of Health and Social Behavior*, 20: 166–77.

Roth, S. and Cohen, L.J. (1986). Approach, avoidance, and coping with stress. *American Psychologist*, 41: 813–19.

Rotter, J.B., Seeman, M. and Liverant, S. (1962) Internal vs. external locus of control of reinforcement: a major variable in behavior therapy, in N.F. Washburne (ed.) *Decisions, Values, and Groups*, pp. 473–516. London: Pergamon Press.

Rowe, J.W. and Kahn, R.L. (1987) Human aging: usual and successful. *Science*, 237: 143–9.

Rowe, J.W. and Kahn, R.L. (1997) Successful aging. *The Gerontologist*, 37: 433–40.

Ruberman, W., Weinblatt, E., Goldberg, J.D. and Chaudhary, B.S. (1984) Psychosocial influences on mortality after myocardial infarction. *New England Journal of Medicine*, 311: 552–9.

Ruderman, A.J. (1986) Dietary restraint: a theoretical and empirical review. *Psychological Bulletin*, 99: 247–62.

Russell, M.A.H., Wilson, C., Taylor, C. and Baker, C.D. (1979) Effect of general practitioner's advice against smoking. *British Medical Journal*, 2: 231–5.

Rzewnicki, R. and Forgays, D. (1987) Recidivism and self-cure of smoking and obesity: an attempt to replicate. *American Psychologist*, 42: 97–100.

Saffer, H. (1991) Alcohol advertising bans and alcohol abuse: an international perspective. *Journal of Health Economics*, 10: 65–79.

St Lawrence, J., Brasfield, T.L., Jefferson, K.W. *et al.* (1995a) Cognitive–behavioral intervention to reduce African American adolescents' risk for HIV infection. *Journal of Consulting and Clinical Psychology*, 63: 221–37.

St Lawrence, J., Jefferson, K.W., Alleyne, E. and Brasfield, T.L. (1995b) Comparison of education versus behavioral skill training interventions in lowering sexual HIV-risk behavior of substance-dependent adolescents. *Journal of Consulting and Clinical Psychology*, 63: 154–7.

St Lawrence, J., Eldridge, G.D., Shelby, M.C. *et al.* (1997) HIV risk reduction for incarcerated women: a comparison of interventions based on two theoretical models. *Journal of Consulting and Clinical Psychology*, 65: 504–9.

Salber, E.J., Reed, R.B., Harrison, S.V. and Green, J.H. (1963) Smoking behavior, recreational activities and attitudes towards smoking among Newton secondary school children. *Pediatrics*, 32: 911–18.

Salina, D., Jason, L.A., Hedeker, D. *et al.* (1994) A follow-up of a media-based, worksite smoking cessation program. *American Journal of Community Psychology*, 22: 257–71.

Salonen, J.T., Puska, P. and Tuomilehto, J. (1982) Physical activity and risk of myocardial infarction, cerebral stroke and death: a longitudinal study in eastern Finland. *American Journal of Epidemiology*, 115: 526–37.

Sanders, C. (1993) Risk factors in bereavement outcome, in M. Stroebe, W. Stroebe and R. Hansson (eds) *Handbook of Bereavement*, pp. 255–67. New York, NY: Cambridge University Press.

Saracco, A., Musicco, N., Nicolisi, A. *et al.* (1993) Man-to-woman sexual transmission of HIV: longitudinal study of 434 steady sexual partners of infected men. *Journal of Acquired Immune Deficiency Syndrome*, 6: 497–502.

Sarafino, E.P. (1998) *Health Psychology: Biopsychosocial Interactions*, 3rd. ed. New York, NY: Wiley.

Sarason, B.R., Shearin, E.N., Pierce, G.R. and Sarason, I.G. (1987) Interrelationships among social support measures: theoretical and practical implications. *Journal of Personality and Social Psychology*, 52: 813–32.

Sarason, B.R., Sarason, I.G. and Pierce, G.R. (1990) Traditional views of social support and their impact on assessment, in B.R. Sarason, I.G. Sarason and G.R. Pierce (eds) *Social Support: An Interactional View*, pp. 9–25. New York, NY: Wiley.

Sarason, I.G., Levine, H.M., Basham, R.B. and Sarason, B.R. (1983) Assessing social support: the social support questionnaire. *Journal of Personality*, 44: 127–39.

Scandinavian Simvastatin Survival Study Group (1994) Randomized trial of cholesterol lowering in 4444 patients with coronary heart disease: the Scandinavian Simvastatin Survival Study. *Lancet*, 344: 1384–9.

Schaalma, H., Kok, G. and Peters, L. (1993) Determinants of consistent condom use by adolescents: the impact of experience of sexual intercourse. *Health Education Research*, 8: 255–69.

Schachter, S. (1959) *The Psychology of Affiliation*. Stanford, CA: Stanford University Press.

Schachter, S. (1977) Nicotine regulation in heavy and light smokers. *Journal of Experimental Psychology: General*, 106: 5–12.

Schachter, S. (1978) Pharmacological and psychological determinants of smoking. *Annals of Internal Medicine*, 88: 104–14.

Schachter, S. (1982) Recidivism and self-cure of smoking and obesity. *American Psychologist*, 37: 436–44.

Schachter, S., Kozlowski, L.T. and Silverstein, B. (1977a) Effects of urinary pH on secret smoking. *Journal of Experimental Psychology: General*, 106: 13–19.

Schachter, S., Silverstein, B. and Perlick, D. (1977b) Psychological and pharmacological explanations of smoking under stress. *Journal of Experimental Psychology: General*, 106: 31–40.

Schaie, K.W. and Willis, S.L. (1986) Can adult intellectual decline be reversed? *Developmental Psychology*, 22: 223–32.

Scheier, M.F. and Carver, C.S. (1985) Optimism, coping, and health: assessment and implications of generalized outcome expectancies. *Health Psychology*, 4: 219–47.

Scheier, M.F. and Carver, C.S. (1987) Dispositional optimism and physical well-being: the influence of generalized outcome expectancies on health. *Journal of Personality*, 55: 169–210.

Scheier, M.F., Weintraub, J.K. and Carver, C.S. (1986) Coping with stress: divergent strategies of optimists and pessimists. *Journal of Personality and Social Psychology*, 51: 1257–64.

Scheier, M.F., Matthews, K.A., Owens, J. *et al.* (1989) Dispositional optimism and recovery from coronary artery bypass surgery: the beneficial effects on physical and psychological well-being. *Journal of Personality and Social Psychology*, 57: 1024–40.

Scheier, M.F., Carver, C.S. and Bridges, M.W. (1994) Distinguishing optimism from neuroticism (and trait anxiety, self-mastery, and self-esteem): a reevaluation of the life orientation test. *Journal of Personality and Social Psychology*, 67: 1063–78.

Schifter, D.E. and Ajzen, I. (1985) Intention, perceived control, and weight loss: an application of the theory of planned behavior. *Journal of Personality and Social Psychology*, 49: 843–51.

Schmidt, W. (1977) Cirrhosis and alcohol consumption: an epidemiological perspective, in G. Edwards and M. Grant (eds) *Alcoholism: New Knowledge and New Responses*, pp. 15–47. London: Croom Helm.

Schmidt, W. and de Lint, J. (1970) Estimating the prevalence of alcoholism from alcohol consumption and mortality data. *Quarterly Journal of Studies on Alcohol*, 31: 957–64.

Schmied, L.A. and Lawler, K.A. (1986) Hardiness, Type A behavior, and the stress–illness relationship in working women. *Journal of Personality and Social Psychology*, 51: 1218–23.

Schoenbach, V.J., Kaplan, B.H., Fredman, L. and Kleinbaum, D.G. (1986) Social ties and mortality in Evans County, Georgia. *American Journal of Epidemiology*, 123: 577–91.

Schotte, D.E., Cools, J. and McNally, R.J. (1990) Induced anxiety triggering overeating in restrained eaters. *Journal of Abnormal Psychology*, 99: 317–20.

Schroeder, D.H. and Costa Jr, P.T. (1984) Influence of life events' stress on physical illness: substantive effects on methodological floors? *Journal of Personality and Social Psychology*, 46: 853–63.

Schuler, G., Hambrecht, R., Schlierf, G. *et al.* (1992) Regular physical exercise and low-fat diet: effects on progression of coronary artery disease. *Circulation*, 86: 1–11.

Schwartz, J.L. (1987) *Smoking Cessation Methods: the United States and Canada, 1978–1985*. Division of Cancer Prevention and Control, National Cancer Institute, US Department of Health and Human Services, Public Health Service (NIH Publication No. 87-2940). Washington, DC: US Government Printing Office.

Schwarzer, R. and Fuchs, R. (1996) Self-efficacy and health behaviours, in M. Conner and P. Norman, *Predicting Health Behaviour*, pp. 163–96. Buckingham: Open University Press.

Schwarzer, R. and Leppin, A. (1989a) *Sozialer Rückhalt und Gesundheit: Eine Meta-Analyse*. Göttingen: Hogrefe.

Schwarzer, R. and Leppin, A. (1989b) Social support and health: a meta-analysis. *Psychology and Health*, 3: 1–15.

Schwarzer, R. and Leppin, A. (1992) Social support and mental health: a conceptual and empirical overview, in L. Montada, S-H. Fillipp and M. Lerner (eds) *Life Crises and Experiences of Loss in Adult Life*, pp. 435–58. Hillsdale, NJ: Lawrence Erlbaum.

Segerstrom, S.C., Taylor, S.E., Kemeny, M.E. and Fahey, J.L. (1998) Optimism is associated with mood, coping, and immune change in response to stress. *Journal of Personality and Social Psychology*, 74: 1646–55.

Seidell, J.C. and Rissanen, A.M. (1998) Time trends in world-wide prevalence of obesity, in G.A. Bray, C. Bouchard and W.P.T. James (eds) *Handbook of Obesity*, pp. 79–92. New York, NY: Marcel Dekker.

Self, C.A. and Rogers, R.W. (1990) Coping with threat to health: effects of persuasive appeals on depressed, normal and antisocial personalities. *Journal of Behavorial Medicine*, 13: 343–57.

Seligman, M.E.P. (1975) *Helplessness*. San Francisco, CA: W.H. Freeman.

Selye, H. (1976) *The Stress of Life*, 2nd ed. New York, NY: McGraw Hill.

Seydel, E., Taal, E. and Wiegman, O. (1990) Risk-appraisal, outcome and self-efficacy expectancies: cognitive factors in preventive behavior related to cancer. *Psychology and Health*, 4: 99–109.

Shaper, A.G., Wannamethee, G. and Walker, M. (1988) *Lancet*, 3: 1267–73.

Sheeran, P. and Abraham, C. (1996) The health belief model, in M. Conner and P. Norman, *Predicting Health Behaviour*, pp. 23–61. Buckingham: Open University Press.

Sheeran, P. and Orbell, S. (1999) Implementation intentions and respeated behaviors: augmenting the predictive validity of the theory of planned behavior. *European Journal of Social Psychology*, 29: 349–70.

Sheeran, P., Abraham, C. and Orbell, S. (1999) Psychosocial correlates of heterosexual condom use: a meta-analysis. *Psychological Bulletin*, 125: 90–132.

Shekelle, R.B., Hulley, S., Neaton, J. *et al.* (1985) MRFIT Research Group: the MRFIT behavior pattern study, II. Type A behavior pattern and incidence of coronary heart disease. *American Journal of Epidemiology*, 122: 559–70.

Shepherd, J., Cobbe, S.M., Ford, I. *et al.* (1995) Prevention of coronary heart disease with prevastatin in men with hypercholesterolemia. *New England Journal of Medicine*, 333: 1301–7.

Shiffman, S. (1982) Relapse following smoking cessation: a situational analysis. *Journal of Consulting and Clinical Psychology*, 50: 71–86.

Shiffman, S. (1993a) Smoking cessation treatment: any progress? *Journal of Consulting and Clinical Psychology*, 61: 718–22.

Shiffman, S. (1993b) Assessing smoking patterns and motives. *Journal of Consulting and Clinical Psychology*, 61: 732–42.

Shiffman, S., Read, L., Maltese, J., Rapkin, D. and Jarvik, M.E. (1985) Preventing relapse in ex-smokers, in G.A. Marlatt and J. Gordon (eds) *Relapse prevention: maintenance strategies in the treatment of addictive behaviors*, pp. 472–520. New York, NY: Guilford Press.

Shiffman, S., Paty, J.A., Gnys, M., Kassel, J.A. and Hickcox, M. (1996) First lapses to smoking: within-subjects analysis of real-time reports. *Journal of Consulting and Clinical Psychology*, 64: 366–79.

Shiffrin, R.M. and Schneider, W. (1977) Controlled and automatic human information processing: II. Perceptual learning, automatic attending, and general theory. *Psychological Review*, 84: 127–90.

Sibai, A.M., Armenian, H.K. and Alam, S. (1989) Wartime determinants of arteriographically confirmed coronary artery disease in Beirut. *American Journal of Epidemiology*, 130: 623–31.

Siegel, J.M. and Kuykendall, D.H. (1990) Loss, widowhood, and psychological distress among the elderly. *Journal of Consulting and Clinical Psychology*, 58: 519–24.

Siegman, A.W. (1994) From Type A to hostility and anger: reflections on the history of coronary prone behavior, in A.W. Siegman and T.W. Smith (eds) *Anger, Hostility and the Heart*, pp. 1–22. Hillsdale, NJ: Lawrence Erlbaum.

Siegman, A.W. and Smith, T.W. (eds) (1994) *Anger, Hostility and the Heart*. Hillsdale, NJ: Lawrence Erlbaum.

Sigvardsson, S., Bohman, M. and Cloninger, R. (1996) Replication of the Stockholm adoption study of alcoholism. *Archives of General Psychiatry*, 53: 681–7.

Silagy, C., Mant, D., Fowler, G. and Lodge, M. (1994) Meta-analysis on efficacy of nicotine replacement therapies in smoking cessation. *Lancet*, 343: 139–46.

Simopoulos, A.P. (1986) Obesity and body weight standards, in L. Breslow, J.E. Fielding and L.B. Lave (eds) *Annual Review of Public Health*, Vol. 7, pp. 475–92. Palo Alto, CA: Annual Reviews Inc.

Sims, E.A.H. and Horton, E.S. (1968) Endocrine and metabolic adaptation to obesity and starvation. *American Journal of Clinical Nutrition*, 21: 1455–70.

Six, B. (1996) Attitude–behavior relations: a comprehensive meta-analysis of 887 studies published between 1927 and 1993. Paper presented at the XXVI International Congress of Psychology, Montréal, Canada.

Sjöström, L. (1980) Fat cells and body weight, in A.J. Stunkard (ed.) *Obesity*. Philadelphia, PA: Saunders.

Smetana, J.G. and Adler, N.E. (1980) Fishbein's Value x Expectancy Model: an examination of some assumptions. *Personality and Social Psychology Bulletin*, 6: 89–96.

Smith, T.W. (1994) Concepts and methods in the study of anger, hostility, and health, in A.W. Siegman and T.W. Smith (eds) *Anger, Hostility and the Heart*, pp. 23–42. Hillsdale, NJ: Lawrence Erlbaum.

Smith, T.W., Pope, M.K., Rhodewalt, F. and Poulton, J.L. (1989) Optimism, neuroticism, coping, and symptom reports: an alternative interpretation of the Life Orientation Test. *Journal of Personality and Social Psychology*, 56: 640–8.

Society of Actuaries (1960) *Build and Blood Pressure Study, 1959*. Chicago, IL: Society of Actuaries.

Society of Actuaries and Association of Life Insurance Medical Directors of America (1979) *Build Study*. Chicago, IL: Society of Actuaries.

Sokol, R.J., Ager, J., Martier, S. *et al.* (1986) Significant determinants of susceptibility to alcohol teratogenicity. *Annals of the New York Academy of Sciences*, 477: 87–102.

Sonstroem, R.J. (1978) Physical estimation and attraction scales: rationale and research. *Medicine and Science in Sports*, 10: 97–102.

Sonstroem, R.J. (1988) Psychological models, in R.K. Dishman (ed.) *Exercise Adherence: Its Impact on Public Health*, pp. 125–53. Champaign, IL: Human Kinetics Books.

Sonstroem, R.J. and Kampper, K.P. (1980) Prediction of athletic participation in middle school males. *Research Quarterly for Exercise and Sport*, 51: 685–94.

Sorensen, G., Thompson, B., Glanz, K. *et al.* (1996) Work site-based cancer prevention: primary results from the Working Well Trial. *American Journal of Public Health*, 86: 939–47.

Sorensen, G., Emmons, K., Hunt, M.K. and Johnston, D. (1998) Implications of the results of community intervention trials. *Annual Review of Public Health*, 19: 379–416.

Spielberger, C.D. (1986) Psychological determinants of smoking behavior, in L.D. Tollison (ed.) *Smoking and Society*, pp. 89–132. Lexington, MA: Heath.

Spivak, K., Sanchez-Craig, M. and Davila, R. (1994) Assisting heavy drinkers to change on their own. Effects of specific and non-specific advice. *Addiction*, 89: 1135–42.

Stallones, R.A. (1983) Ischemic heart disease and lipids in blood and diet. *Annual Review of Nutrition*, 3: 155–85.

Stalonas, P.M., Johnson, W.G. and Christ, M. (1978) Behavior modification for obesity: the evaluation of exercise, contingency management and program adherence. *Journal of Consulting and Clinical Psychology*, 46: 463–9.

Stanton, A.L. and Snider, P.R. (1993) Coping with a breast cancer diagnosis: a prospective study. *Health Psychology*, 12: 16–23.

Stanton, A.L., Danoff-Burg, S., Cameron, C.L. and Ellis, A.P. (1994) Coping through emotional approach: problems of conceptualization and confounding. *Journal of Personality and Social Psychology*, 66: 350–62.

Steele, C.M. and Josephs, R.A. (1990) Alcohol myopia: its prized and dangerous effects. *American Psychologist*, 45: 921–33.

Stein, M., Keller, S.E. and Schleifer, S.J. (1985) Stress and immunomodulation: the role of depression and neuroendocrine function. *Journal of Immunology*, 135: 827s–833s.

Sternberg, B. (1985) Relapse in weight control: definitions, processes, and prevention strategies, in G.A. Marlatt and J.R. Gordon (eds) *Relapse Prevention*, pp. 521–45. New York, NY: Guilford Press.

Stokes, J.P. (1983) Predicting satisfaction with social support from social network structure. *American Journal of Community Psychology*, 11: 141–52.

Stone, A.A., Schwartz, J.E., Neale, J.M. *et al.* (1998) A comparison of coping assessed by ecological momentary assessment and retrospective recall. *Journal of Personality and Social Psychology*, 74: 1670–80.

Striegel-Moore, R. and Rodin, J. (1986) The influence of psychological variables in obesity, in K.D. Brownell and J.P. Foreyt (eds) *Handbook of Eating Disorders*, pp. 99–121. New York, NY: Basic Books.

Stroebe, M. (1992) Coping with bereavement: a review of the grief work hypothesis. *Omega*, 26: 19–42.

Stroebe, M. and Schut, H. (1999) The dual process model of coping with bereavement: rationale and description. *Death Studies*, 32: 197–224.

Stroebe, M. and Stroebe, W. (1993) Mortality of bereavement: a review, in M. Stroebe, W. Stroebe and R. Hansson (eds) *Handbook of Bereavement*, pp. 175–95. New York, NY: Cambridge University Press.

Stroebe, M., Stroebe, W. and Hansson, R. (1993) *Handbook of Bereavement*. New York, NY: Cambridge University Press.

Stroebe, W. and de Wit, J. (1996) Health-impairing behaviours, in G.R. Semin and K. Fiedler (eds) *Applied Social Psychology*, pp. 113–44. London: Sage.

Stroebe, W. and Stroebe, M. (1987) *Bereavement and Health*. New York, NY: Cambridge University Press.

Stroebe, W. and Stroebe, M. (1993) Determinants of adjustment to bereavement in younger widows and widowers, in M. Stroebe, W. Stroebe and R.O. Hansson (eds) *Handbook of Bereavement: Theory, Research, and Intervention*, pp. 208–26. New York, NY: Cambridge University Press.

Stroebe, W. and Stroebe, M. (1996) The social psychology of social support, in E.T. Higgins and A.W. Kruglanski (eds) *Social Psychology: Handbook of Basic Principles*, pp. 597–621. New York, NY: Guilford Press.

Stroebe, W., Stroebe, M. and Domittner, G. (1988) Individual and situational differences in recovery from bereavement: a risk group identified. *Journal of Social Issues*, 44: 143–58.

Stulb, S.C., McDonough, J.R., Greenberg, B.G. and Hames, C.G. (1965) The relationship of nutrient intake and exercise to serum cholesterol level in white males in Evans County, Georgia. *American Journal of Clinical Nutrition*, 16: 238–42.

Stunkard, A.J. (1984) The current status of treatment for obesity in adults, in A.J. Stunkard and E. Stellar (eds) *Eating and its Disorders*, pp. 157–74. New York, NY: Raven Press.

Stunkard, A.J. (1986) The control of obesity: social and community perspectives, in K.D. Brownell and J.P. Foreyt (eds) *Handbook of Eating Disorders*, pp. 213–28. New York, NY: Basic Books.

Stunkard, A.J. and Koch, C. (1964) The interpretation of gastric motility, I. Apparent bias in the reports of hunger by obese persons. *Archives of Genetic Psychiatry*, 11: 74–82.

Stunkard, A.J. and Sobal, J. (1995) Psychosocial consequences of obesity, in K.D. Kelley and C.G. Fairburn (eds) *Eating Disorders and Obesity*, pp. 417–21. New York, NY: Guilford Press.

Stunkard, A.J., Sorensen, T.I.A., Hanis, C. *et al.* (1986) An adoption study of human obesity. *New England Journal of Medicine*, 314: 193–8.

Suarez, E.C. and Williams Jr, R.B. (1989) Situational determinants of cardiovascular and emotional reactivity in high and low hostile men. *Psychosomatic Medicine*, 52: 558–70.

Süß, H-M. (1995) Zur Wirksamkeit der Therapie bei Alkoholabhängigen: Ergebnisse einer Meta-Analyse. *Psychologische Rundschau*, 46: 248–66.

Sutton, S. (1989) Smoking attitudes and behavior: applications of Fishbein and Ajzen's theory of reasoned action to predicting and understanding smoking decisions, in T. Ney and A. Gale (eds) *Smoking and Human Behavior*, pp. 289–312. Chichester: Wiley.

Sutton, S. (1996) Can 'stages of change' provide guidance in the treatment of addiction? A critical examination of Prochaska and DiClemente's model, in G. Edwards and C. Dare (eds) *Psychotherapy, Psychological Treatment and the Addictions*, pp. 189–205. Cambridge: Cambridge University Press.

Sutton, S., McVey, D. and Glanz, A. (1999) A comparative test of the theory of reasoned action and the theory of planned behavior in the prediction of condom use intentions in a national sample of English young people. *Health Psychology*, 18: 72–81.

Sutton, S.R. (1982) Fear-arousing communications: a critical examination of theory and research, in J.R. Eiser (ed.) *Social Psychology and Behavioral Medicine*, pp. 303–37. Chichester: Wiley.

Sutton, S.R. (1987) Social-psychological approaches to understanding addictive behaviours: attitude–behaviour and decision-making models. *British Journal of Addiction*, 82: 355–70.

Sutton, S.R. and Hallett, R. (1989) Understanding the effect of fear-arousing communications: the role of cognitive factors and amount of fear aroused. *Journal of Behavioral Medicine*, 11: 353–60.

Svetkey, L.P., Simons-Morton, D., Vollmer, W.M. *et al.* (1999) Effects of dietary patterns on blood pressure: subgroup analysis of Dietary Approaches to Stop Hypertension (DASH) randomized clinical trial. *Archives of Internal Medicine*, 159: 285–93.

Sweeney, P., Anderson, K. and Bailey, S. (1986) Attributional style in depression: a meta-analytic review. *Journal of Personality and Social Psychology*, 50: 774–91.

Tajfel, H. (1978) Social categorization, social identity and social comparison, in H. Tajfel (ed.) *Differentiation between Social Groups*. London: Academic Press.

Tanner, W.M. and Pollack, R.H. (1988) The effect of condom use and erotic instructions on attitudes towards condoms. *The Journal of Sex Research*, 25: 537–41.

Taubes, G. (1998a) As obesity rates rise, experts struggle to explain why. *Science*, 280: 1367–8.

Taubes, G. (1998b) The (political) science of salt. *Science*, 281: 898–907.

Taylor, S.E. (1995) *Health Psychology*, 3rd ed. New York, NY: McGraw-Hill.

Terborg, J.R. (1988) The organisation as a context for health promotion, in S. Spacapn and S. Oskamp (eds) *The Social Psychology of Health*, pp. 129–74. Newbury Park, CA: Sage.

Terris, M. (1967) Epidemiology of cirrhosis of the liver: national mortality data. *American Journal of Public Health*, 57: 2076–88.

Terry, D.J. and Hynes, G.J. (1998) Adjustment to a low-control situation: reexamining the role of coping responses. *Journal of Personality and Social Psychology*, 74: 1078–92.

Terry, D.J. and O'Leary, J.E. (1995) The theory of planned behaviour: the effects of perceived behavioural control and self-efficacy. *British Journal of Social Psychology*, 34: 199–220.

Theodorakis, Y. (1994) Planned behavior, attitude strength, role identity, and the prediction of exercise behavior. *The Sport Psychologist*, 8: 149–65.

Theorell, T. and Rahe, R.H. (1971) Psychosocial factors and myocardial infarction, I. An inpatient study in Sweden. *Journal of Psychosomatic Research*, 15: 25–31.

Theorell, T., Lind, E. and Floderus, B. (1975) The relationship of disturbing life changes and emotions to the early development of myocardial infarction and other serious illnesses. *International Journal of Epidemiology*, 4: 281–93.

Thompson, E.L. (1978) Smoking education programs, 1960–1976. *American Journal of Public Health*, 68: 250–7.

Thompson, J.L., Manore, M.M. and Thomas, J.R. (1996) Effects of diet and diet-plus-exercise programs on resting metabolic rate: a meta-analysis. *International Journal of Sport Nutrition*, 6: 41–61.

Thompson, P.D., Jeffery, R.W., Wing, R.R. and Wood, P.D. (1979) Unexpected degrees in plasma high density lipoprotein cholesterol with weight loss. *American Journal of Clinical Nutrition*, 32: 2016–21.

Tiffany, S.T. (1990) A cognitive model of drug urges and drug-use behavior: role of automatic and nonautomatic processes. *Psychological Review*, 97: 147–68.

Troiano, R.P., Frongillo, E.A., Sobal, J. and Levitsky, D.A. (1996) The relationship between body weight and mortality: a quantitative analysis of combined information from existing studies. *International Journal of Obesity*, 20: 63–75.

Turner, J. and Wheaton, B. (1995) Checklist measurement of stressful life events, in S. Cohen, R.C. Kessler and L. Underwood Gordon (eds) *Measuring Stress*, pp. 29–58. New York, NY: Oxford University Press.

Turpeinen, O. (1979) Effect of cholesterol-lowering diet on mortality from coronary heart disease and other causes. *Circulation*, 59: 1–7.

Uchino, B.N. and Garvey, T.S. (1997) The availability of social support reduces cardiovascular reactivity to acute psychological stress. *Journal of Behavioral Medicine*, 20: 15–27.

Uchino, B.N., Cacioppo, J.T. and Kiecolt-Glaser, J.K. (1996) The relationship between social support and physiological processes: a review with emphasis on underlying mechanisms and implication for health. *Psychological Bulletin*, 119: 488–531.

Udry, J., Clark, L., Chase, C. and Levy, M. (1972) Can mass media advertising increase contraceptive use? *Family Planning Perspectives*, 4: 37–44.

Umberson, D., Wortman, C.B. and Kessler, R.C. (1992) Widowhood and depression: explaining long-term gender differences in vulnerability. *Journal of Health and Social Behavior*, 33: 10–24.

USDHEW (US Department of Health, Education and Welfare) (1964) *Smoking and Health: A Report of the Surgeon General*. Washington, DC: US Government Printing Office.

USDHHS (US Department of Health and Human Services) (1982) *The Health Consequences of Smoking. Cancer: A Report of the Surgeon General*. Rockville, MD: Office on Smoking and Health.

USDHHS (US Department of Health and Human Services) (1984) *The Health Consequences of Smoking. Chronic Obstructive Lung Disease: A Report of the Surgeon General*. Washington, DC: US Government Printing Office.

USDHHS (US Department of Health and Human Services) (1985) *Fact Book, Fiscal Year 1985*. Bethesda, MD: National Heart, Lung, and Blood Institute.

USDHHS (US Department of Health and Human Services) (1986) *The Health Consequences of Involuntary Smoking: A Report of the Surgeon General*. Office on Smoking and Health. DHHS Publ. No. (CDC) 87-8398. Washington, DC: US Government Printing Office.

USDHHS (US Department of Health and Human Services) (1990) *The Health Benefits of Smoking Cessation: A Report of the Surgeon General*. Rockville, MD: DHHS Publication.

USDHHS (US Department of Health and Human Services) (1996a) *Clinical Practice Guidelines: Smoking Cessation*. Rockville, MD: AHCPR Publication No. 96-0692.

USDHHS (US Department of Health and Human Services) (1996b) *Physical Activity and Health: A Report of the Surgeon General*. McLean, VA: International Medical Publishing.

Vaillant, G.E. (1983) *The Natural History of Alcoholism*. Cambridge, MA: Harvard University Press.

Valleroy, L., MacKellar, D., Janssen, R. *et al.* (1996) HIV and risk behavior prevalence among young men who have sex with men sampled in six urban counties in the USA. XI International Conference on AIDS. Vancouver, July. (Abstract TuC2407)

Van den Putte, B. (1991) 20 years of the theory of reasoned action of Fishbein and Ajzen: a meta-analysis. Unpublished manuscript, University of Amsterdam.

Van der Velde, F., van der Pligt, J. and Hooykaas, C. (1994) Perceiving AIDS-related risk: accuracy as a function of differences in actual risk. *Health Psychology*, 13: 25–33.

Van Griensven, G.J.P., van den Bergh, H.S.P., Janssen, M., de Wit, J. and Keet, I.P.M. (1999) HIV prevalentie, incidentie en seksueel risicogedrag in een cohort jonge homoseksuele. Unpublished manuscript, Amsterdam: Municipal Health Service.

Velicer, W., DiClemente, C.C., Prochaska, J.O. and Brandenburg, N. (1985) Decisional balance measure for assessing and predicting smoking status. *Journal of Personality and Social Psychology*, 48: 1279–89.

Verplanken, B. and Aarts, H. (1999) Habit, attitude, planned behavior: is habit an empty construct or an interesting case of goal directed automaticity?, in W. Stroebe and M. Hewstone (eds) *European Review of Social Psychology*, Vol. 10, pp. 100–34. Chichester: Wiley.

Verplanken, B., Aarts, H., van Knippenberg, A. and Moonen, A. (1998) Habit versus planned behavior: a field experiment. *British Journal of Social Psychology*, 37: 111–28.

Vickers Jr, R.R., Conway, T.L. and Hervig, L.K. (1990) Demonstrations of replicable dimensions of health behaviors. *Preventive Medicine*, 19: 377–401.

Vinokur-Kaplan, D. (1978) To have – or not to have – another child: family planning attitudes, intentions, and behavior. *Journal of Applied Social Psychology*, 18: 710–30.

Viscusi, W.K. (1990) Do smokers underestimate risks? *Journal of Political Economy*, 98: 1253–69.

Volkmar, F.R., Stunkard, A.J., Woolston, J. and Bailey, B.A. (1981) High attrition rates in commercial weight reduction programs. *Archives of Internal Medicine*, 141: 426–8.

Wadden, T.A. (1993) The treatment of obesity: an overview, in A.J. Stunkard and T.A. Wadden (eds) *Obesity Theory and Therapy*, pp. 197–218. New York, NY: Raven Press.

Wadden, T.A. (1995) Very low-calorie diets: appraisal and recommendations, in K.D. Kelley and C.G. Fairburn, *Eating Disorders and Obesity*, pp. 484–90. New York, NY: Guilford Press.

Wadden, T.A. and Bell, S.T. (1990) Obesity, in A.S. Bellack, M. Hersen and A.E. Kazdin (eds) *International Handbook of Behavior Modification and Therapy*, 2nd ed., pp. 449–73. New York, NY: Plenum Press.

Wadden, T.A. and Stunkard, A.J. (1986) A controlled trial of very-low-calorie diet in the treatment of obesity. *Journal of Consulting and Clinical Psychology*, 54: 482–8.

Wadden, T.A., Foster, G. and Letizia, K. (1994) One-year behavioral treatment of obesity: comparison of moderate and severe caloric restriction and the effects of weight maintenance therapy. *Journal of Consulting and Clinical Psychology*, 62: 165–71.

Wagner, E.H., LaCroix, A.Z., Buchner, D.M. and Larson, E.B. (1992) Effects of physical activity on health status in older adults, I: observational studies. *Annual Review of Public Health*, 13: 451–68.

Wallace, P., Cutler, S. and Haines, A. (1988) Randomized controlled trial of general practitioner intervention in patients with excessive alcohol consumption. *British Medical Journal*, 297: 663–8.

Waller, J.A. (1987) Injury: conceptual shifts and preventive implications. *Annual Review of Public Health*, 8: 21–49.

Wallston, B.S. and Wallston, K.A. (1981) Social psychological models of health and behavior: an examination and integration, in G. Sanders and J. Suls (eds) *The Social Psychology of Health and Illness*, pp. 65–95. Hillsdale, NJ: Lawrence Erlbaum.

Walsh, D.C. and Gordon, N.P. (1986) Legal approaches to smoking deterrence, in L. Breslow, J.E. Fielding and L.B. Lave (eds) *Annual Review of Public Health*, Vol. 7, pp. 127–49. Palo Alto, CA: Annual Reviews Inc.

Warner, K.E. (1981) Cigarette smoking in the 1970's: the impact of the anti-smoking campaigns on consumption. *Science*, 211: 729–31.

Warner, K.E. (1986) Smoking and health implications of a change in the Federal Cigarette Excise Tax. *Journal of the American Medical Association*, 255: 1028–32.

Watson, D. and Pennebaker, J.W. (1989) Health complaints, stress, and distress: exploring the central role of negative effectivity. *Psychological Review*, 96: 234–54.

Watson, J.B. and Raynor, R. (1920) Conditioned emotional reactions. *Journal of Experimental Psychology*, 3: 1–14.

Weekley, C.G., Klesges, R.C. and Relya, G. (1992) Smoking as a weight-control strategy and its relationship to smoking status. *Addictive Behaviours*, 17: 259–71.

Wegner, D.M. (1994) Ironic processes of mental control, *Psychological Review*, 101: 34–52.

Weinberger, M., Hiner, S.L. and Tierney, W.M. (1987) In support of hassles as measures of stress in predicting health outcomes. *Journal of Behavioral Medicine*, 10: 19–31.

Weiner, B., Perry, R.P. and Magnusson, J. (1988) An attributional analysis of reactions to stigma. *Journal of Personality and Social Psychology*, 55: 738–48.

Weinstein, N.D. (1987) Unrealistic optimism about susceptibility to health problems: conclusions from a community-wide sample. *Journal of Behavioral Medicine*, 10: 481–500.

Weinstein, N.D. (1988) The precaution adoption process. *Health Psychology*, 7: 355–86.

Weinstein, N.D. and Sandman, P.M. (1992) A model for the precaution adoption process: evidence from home radon testing. *Health Psychology*, 11: 170–80.

Weinstein, N.D., Rothman, A.J. and Sutton, S. (1998) Stage theories of health behavior: conceptual and methodological issues. *Health Psychology*, 17: 290–99.

Welin, L., Tibblin, G., Svädsudd, K. *et al.* (1985) Prospective study of social influence on mortality. *Lancet*, 2: 915–18.

Wethington, E., Brown, G.W. and Kessler, R.C. (1995) Interview measures of stressful life events, in S. Cohen, R.C. Kessler and L. Underwood Gordon (eds) *Measuring Stress*, pp. 59–79. New York, NY: Oxford University Press.

Weyerer, S. (1992) Physical inactivity and depression in the community. *International Journal of Sports Medicine*, 13: 492–6.

WHO (World Health Organization) (1948) *Constitution of the World Health Organization*. Geneva: WHO Basic Documents.

WHO (World Health Organization) (1982) *Prevention of coronary heart disease: a report of the WHO expert committee*. Geneva: World Health Organization.

Willemsen, M.C., de Vries, H. and Genders, R. (1996) Lange-termijnresultaten van twee 'stoppen-met-roken'-bedrijfsprogramma's. *Gedrag and Gezondheid*, 24: 165–72.

Willett, W.C. and Manson, J.E. (1996) Epidemiological studies of health risks due to excess weight, in K.D. Kelley and C.G. Fairburn (eds) *Eating Disorder and Obesity*, pp. 396–405. New York, NY: Guilford Press.

Williams, D.R. and Collins, C. (1995) US socioeconomic and racial differences in health: patterns and explanations. *Annual Review of Sociology*, 21: 349–86.

Williams Jr, R.B., Haney, T.L., Lee, K.L. *et al.* (1980) Type A behavior, hostility, and coronary atherosclerosis. *Psychosomatic Medicine*, 42: 539–49.

Williams Jr, R.B., Barefoot, J.C. and Shekelle, R.B. (1985) The health consequences of hostility, in M.A. Chesney and R.H. Rosenman (eds) *Anger and Hostility in Cardiovascular and Behavioral Disorders*, pp. 173–85. New York, NY: McGraw Hill.

Williams Jr, R.B., Barefoot, J.C., Califf, R.M. *et al.* (1992) Prognostic importance of social and economic resources among medically treated patients with angiographically documented coronary artery disease. *Journal of the American Medical Association*, 267: 520–4.

Williamson, D.F. (1995) The association of weight loss with morbidity and mortality, in K.D. Brownell and C.G. Fairburn (eds) *Eating Disorders and Obesity*, pp. 411–16. New York, NY: Guilford Press.

Williamson, D.F., Serdula, M.K., Anda, R.F., Levy, A. and Byers, T. (1992) Weight loss attempts in adults: goals, duration, and rate of weight loss. *American Journal of Public Health*, 82: 1251–7.

Wilson, M. and Baker, S. (1987) Structural approach to injury control. *Journal of Social Issues*, 43: 73–86.

Wing, R.R. (1998) Behavioral approaches to the treatment of obesity, in G.A. Bray, C. Bouchard and W.P.T. James (eds) *Handbook of Obesity*, pp. 855–73. New York, NY: Marcel Dekker.

Winkelstein, W., Samuel, M., Padian, N. *et al.* (1987) The San Francisco Men's Health Study, III. Reduction in HIV transmission among gay and bisexual men, 1982–86. *American Journal of Public Health*, 76: 685–9.

Winkleby, M.A., Taylor, B., Jatulis, D. and Fortmann, S.P. (1996) The long-term effects of a cardiovascular disease prevention trial: the Stanford Five City Project. *American Journal of Public Health*, 86: 1773–9.

Wood, W. and Kallgren, C.A. (1988) Communicator attributes and persuasion: recipients' access to attitude-relevant information in memory. *Personality and Social Psychology Bulletin*, 14: 172–82.

Wood, W., Kallgren, C.A. and Preisler, R. (1985) Access to atttitude-relevant information in memory as a determinant of persuasion: the role of message attributes. *Journal of Experimental Social Psychology*, 21: 73–85.

Wooley, S.C., Wooley, O.W. and Dyrenforth, S.R. (1979) Theoretical, practical and social issues in behavioral treatments of obesity. *Journal of Applied Behavior Analysis*, 12: 3–25.

Wurtele, S.K. (1988) Increasing women's calcium intake: the role of health beliefs, intentions and health value. *Journal of Applied Social Psychology*, 18: 627–39.

Wurtele, S.K. and Maddux, J.E. (1987) Relative contributions of protection motivation theory components in predicting exercise intentions and behavior. *Health Psychology*, 6: 453–66.

Wurtele, S.K., Roberts, M.C. and Leeper, J.D. (1982) Health beliefs and intentions: predictors of return compliance in a tuberculosis detection drive. *Journal of Applied Social Psychology*, 12: 128–36.

Yanovski, S.Z. (1998) Obesity and eating disorders, in G.A. Bray, C. Bouchard and W.P.T. James (eds) *Handbook of Obesity*, pp. 115–28. New York, NY: Marcel Dekker.

Zarski, J.J. (1984) Hassles and health: a replication. *Health Psychology*, 3: 243–51.

Zierler, S. and Krieger, N. (1997) Reframing women's risk: social inequalities and HIV infection. *Annual Review of Public Health*, 18: 401–36.

AUTHOR INDEX

SUBJECT INDEX